Oxford Medical Publications

Rett Disorder and the Developing Brain

'... this is a rare but fascinating condition that is certainly of considerable interest to neurologists, developmental neuroscientists, and geneticists.'

Professor Colin Blakemore, University of Oxford.

Whilst every effort has been made to ensure that the contents of this book are as complete, accurate and up to date as possible at the date of writing, Oxford University Press is not able to give any guarantee or assurance that such is the case. Readers are urged to take appropriately qualified medical advice in all cases. The information in this book is intended to be useful to the general reader, but should not be used as a means of self-diagnosis or for the prescription of medication.

Rett Disorder and the Developing Brain

Dr Alison Kerr
Senior Lecturer in Paediatrics and Chronic Neurological Disability, Academic Centre, Department of Psychological Medicine, University of Glasgow, U.K.

And

Dr Ingegerd Witt Engerström
Senior Consultant in Paediatric Neurology and Habilitation, The Rett Centre, Frösön, Sweden

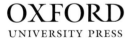

OXFORD
UNIVERSITY PRESS

Great Clarendon Street, Oxford OX2 6DP

Oxford University Press is a department of the University of Oxford.
It furthers the University's objective of excellence in research, scholarship,
and education by publishing worldwide in
Oxford New York

Athens Auckland Bangkok Bogotá Buenos Aires Calcutta
Cape Town Chennai Dar es Salaam Delhi Florence Hong Kong Istanbul
Karachi Kuala Lumpur Madrid Melbourne Mexico City Mumbai
Nairobi Paris São Paulo Singapore Taipei Tokyo Toronto Warsaw

with associated companies in
Berlin Ibadan

Oxford is a registered trade mark of Oxford University Press
in the UK and in certain other countries

Published in the United States
by Oxford University Press, Inc., New York

© Oxford University Press 2001

The moral rights of the author have been asserted

Database right Oxford University Press (maker)

First published 2001

All rights reserved. No part of this publication may be reproduced,
stored in a retrieval system, or transmitted, in any form or by any means,
without the prior permission in writing of Oxford University Press,
or as expressly permitted by law, or under terms agreed with the appropriate
reprograhics rights organization. Enquiries concerning reproduction
outside the scope of the above should be sent to the Rights Department,
Oxford University Press, at the address above.

You must not circulate this book in any other binding or cover
and you must impose this same condition on any acquirer

A catalogue record for this title is available from the British Library

Library of Congress Cataloging in Publication Data

Rett disorder and the developing brain/[edited by] Alison Kerr and Ingegerd Witt Engerström.
(Oxford medical publications)
Includes bibliographical references and index.
1. Rett syndrome. 2. Developmental neurobiology. I. Kerr, Alison, 1938–
II. Witt Engerström, Ingegerd. III. Series.
[DNLM: 1. Rett Syndrome. 2. Brain–growth & development. WL 140 R439 2000]
RJ506.R47 R475 2000   618.92´85884–dc21   00-064980
ISBN 0 19 263083 0 (Hbk.: alk. paper)

1 3 5 7 9 10 8 6 4 2

ISBN 0 19 263083 0

Typeset by Phoenix Photosetting, Chatham, Kent

Printed in Great Britain on acid free paper by
Biddles Ltd, Guildford & King's Lynn

Foreword

AN EXCITING MILESTONE

W.I. FRASER

*PROFESSOR OF DEVELOPMENTAL DISABILITIES,
UNIVERSITY OF WALES COLLEGE OF MEDICINE,
ELY HOSPITAL,
COWBRIDGE ROAD WEST,
CARDIFF CF5 5XE, UK*

I have worked in the field of Intellectual Disability since 1966, the year in which Andreas Rett first published on the condition. Rett syndrome has always engendered curiosity and excitement, but 1999 has been the most exhilarating time. I first encountered this special enthusiasm in the 1980s after the first English publication on the disorder, at a meeting at Oxford of the Forum on Mental Retardation, where there was much animated conversation among scientists deftly illustrated by their stereotyped hand movements. In 1986, that excitement mingled with helplessness when the opportunity was provided by Alison Kerr to talk to the parents and meet many of these little girls with characteristic hand movements, obvious autonomic dysregulation, able to hear and feel, and patently possessing a social awareness, their big eyes looking out on a bleak future (Kerr 1987).

Ten days before the October 1999 International Meeting at the Royal Society of Medicine, 'Rett Disorder and the Developing Brain', which brought together the authors of this book on the eve of publication, the announcement that the gene has been located renewed the exhilaration we as medical students in 1959 felt when our lecturer told us that Lejeune, Gautier and Turpin had identified the presence of an extra chromosome in Down's anomaly (Lejeune *et al.* 1959). Previous exclusion mapping using Rett families had narrowed the search to Xq28 but few anticipated that Ruthie Amir and colleagues would so rapidly identify mutations on gene MECP2 as a cause. The discovery that mutations that affect DNA methylation may lead to human disease implicates autosomal genes in the causation of other developmental disorders too. Further light has been shed on the causes of a range of developmental disorders. Over the last three decades, study of this disorder has given us insight into many aspects of child health, developmental medicine, genetics, child neurology and child psychiatry.

The study of the Rett disorder tells us so much about normal brain development. Armstrong has shown that compared with individuals with Down's syndrome, dendritic arborization in Rett shows the greatest reduction in premotor, motor and frontal cortexes, with dramatic sequelae compared with the relatively limited occipital dendritic overpruning in Down's syndrome, which leads to relatively minor limitation in visual acuity and accommodation (Woodhouse et al. 1996).

We now know that the Rett process starts at a very early stage in cortical development with very early defects in neurotransmission. Kaufmann has identified a deficiency of the microtubule-associated protein (MAP)-2 in selected cortical and subcortical neurons, a marker for the time of dendritic proliferation. Girls with Rett syndrome are small but the brain weight is decreased more than other organs. The brain weight is a reflection of this reduced branch density. Armstrong highlights a stage of dramatic and terrifying regression but this is not, strictly speaking, a progressive disorder. It is a transportation timetable gone wrong.

Dahlstrom's chapter shows how autonomic dysregulation in Rett disorder may also provide a window on the ontogeny and functioning of the autonomic nervous system.

There are lessons also from the study of the Rett disorder for understanding the development of sleep and wake cycles and how the abnormalities of sleep are modulated, particularly the circadian and ultradian rhythms. There is widespread neurotrophic deficiency affecting dopamine, acetycholine, glutamates, serotonin, substance P and nerve growth factor during the early years of life. Animal models, particularly animal studies in which MAP2 has been specifically disrupted, will enable us to model the pathways for the neurodevelopmental effects of this disorder.

The Rett disorder provides us with new insights into the prerequisites and precursors of communication. Belichenko maintains that motor speech is affected more than sensory speech. His chapter reveals an encyclopaedic knowledge of hemispheric functioning and how the resolution of modern fMRI enables us to distinguish activation in cortical areas with high accuracy. He points out how morphologically there is a small distance between cerebral representation of motor and speech areas with very high excitability of motor speech areas. His working hypothesis is that motor disturbances may significantly interfere with speech. He also believes in the existence of a 'critical period' during which language proficiency may be obtained. He reminds us that 6–12% of people with Rett do have some speech. Trevarthen and Burford point out how people with Rett, as distinct from autism, show a powerful interest in taking part in social exchanges and forming interpersonal relationships. Children with Rett do not have autism's handicap of imperviousness to other people's thoughts and feelings. They have intersubjectivity. After the 'storm' of the regression, their continuing capacities are 'all the more precious' and they do respond to 'emotional narrative and rhythms'. Children with Rett show an early interest in communication and joint attention. Twenty years ago we knew much less about how to differentiate and measure communication and stereotypies. Partly based on studies of Rett syndrome, we have developed increasingly sophisticated video analysis and event recording in real time. The Rett syndrome has been a proving ground for new methodologies and techniques.

In the study of Rett syndrome we are moving from the era of description to possibilities for intervention. Merker and Wallin discuss the potential use of music as a window on the cognitive capacities, as well as a 'potential means of enhancing the quality of life', and enjoin us to exploit the development of a musical sensibility window in the first year of life before the major deterioration occurs, particularly in focussing on rhythmic patterns, melodic content and tempo. We do not know whether later musical developments occur, such as keeping time to tunes and sensitivity to harmonization, because of their communication handicaps and instability of the autonomic nervous system, yet we are encouraged by the musical responsiveness of people with Rett disorder, providing us with powerful clues to their capacities and also giving further insights into the use of music therapy with the profoundly learning disabled.

Pharmacological interventions are the next frontier. Kaufmann points out the likely role of cholinergic deficiency in the Rett disorder. This is still uncertain, and by the time of diagnosis there is no marked choline acetyltransferase (ChAT) reduction that can justify therapeutic strategies such as those we are now using in Alzheimer's disease. Nomura suggests the possibility of turning abnormal sleep rhythms to normal after treatment with melatonin and already raised β-endorphins have led to trials of the opiate antagonist naltrexone in Rett. Sympathectomy is effective in cases of peripheral blood flow in the legs and perhaps there are hopes for better β-adrenergic agonists. Nomura, Segawa and Julu examine the evidence for early involvement of serotonin in Rett and already there are some encouraging results of intervention.

Yet even classical Rett syndrome is not homogeneous. The finding of the genetic role in the pathogenesis gives the opportunity for therapy. The window of relative normality in the first year of life may eventually allow some therapeutic interventions before the syndrome is fully clinically developed. We now have the possibility of developing a test for early diagnosis and even prenatal detection, with possibilities for intervention in the newborn state although informed genetic counselling is still some time ahead.

As an editor of a journal in the field, I await now with anticipation an explosion of knowledge about the Rett disorder. Web sites and local and regional intranets for Rett's disorder will be enriched. Space in this foreword only allows me to sample the book's richness and pay scant tribute to the many scientists who have contributed.

This book will be a valuable guide for those engaging in future research not only into the Rett disorder but also into other developmental disorders, with the intention of understanding how genetic causes lead to physical disability and behavioural disturbance and developing evidence based intervention.

This book is a milestone in bringing clarity to clinicians of many disciplines who are faced with family bewilderment and uncertainty. Parents also will value greatly the knowledge of what precisely is the cause of their daughter's disability, and will benefit from the knowledge this book contributes to advice and management.

References

Amir, R.E., Van Den Veyver, I., Wan, M., Tran, C.Q., Francke, U., and Zoghbi, H.Y. (1999). Rett's syndrome is caused by mutations in X linked MECP2 encoding methyl-CpG-binding protein. *Nature Genetics*, 23, 185–8.

Kerr, A.M. (1987). Report on the Rett Syndrome Workshop: Glasgow Scotland, 24–25 May 1986. *Journal of Mental Deficiency Research*, 31, 93–113.

Lejeune, J., Turpin, R., and Gautier, M. (1959). Le mongolisme premier exemple d'aberration autosomique humaine. *Annales de Genetique*, 1, 41.

Rett, A. (1966). Über ein cerebral-atrophisches syndrom bei Hyperammonämie. Bruder Hollinek, Vienna.

Woodhouse, J.M., Pakeman, V., Saunders, K., Parker, M., Fraser, W., Lobo, S., and Sastry, P. (1996). Visual acuity and accommodation in infants and young children with Down's syndrome. *Journal of Intellectual Disability Research*, 40, 49–55.

Preface

The Rett syndrome was doubtless observed and wondered at before Andreas Rett wrote his paper in 1966, but his was the first full clinical description and his careful observations became the foundation for the understanding of the disorder. Over 30 years later, those who first studied the disorder are reaching the end of their professional span and it is a good time to put together the evidence which has now been gathered and from it to find new directions for research.

As we go to press, mutations have been identified at Xq28 on the MECP2 gene (methyl-CpG 2) (Amir *et al.* 1999), a 'housekeeping gene' which selectively silences the expression of other genes still to be located. This important discovery powerfully supports our long-held view that the Rett syndrome represents an early developmental disorder which should be viewed in the context of early brain growth.

The disorder is an intriguing one, preferentially found in females and specifically involving the functions on which intelligence and its expression depend—learning, hand use and speech—leaving many others intact. As failure in a complex system is diagnosed through switching off individual elements and observing the selective results, so the Rett disorder explains itself by 'taking out' specific control mechanisms, effectively dismantling the early developmental process.

The authors are expert in various aspects of the development of the brain and distinguished by many years of meticulous study of the clinical, chemical, structural and physiological nature of the Rett disorder. They have been invited to share their knowledge of the normal development of the brain as well as of the problems of the disorder. The book is divided into parts according to aspects of the study—clinical, genetic and anatomical, physiological and a section on communication, with shorter papers linked to each topic.

We hope this book will be of interest to clinical and laboratory based students of human disease from neurology, genetics, neurochemistry, neuropathology, neurophysiology, brain imaging, general medicine, psychiatry and psychology, and also to educators, therapists and families of people affected by the Rett disorder who wish to understand more about its problems and to recognize the pathways to learning which remain accessible. We believe that the Rett investigation will lead to specific prevention and treatment for this devastating disease and still further to a fruitful re-examination of other developmental disorders and of the still mysterious processes by which the normal brain and mind are built.

We wish to express our thanks to the families and girls with the Rett syndrome who have provided the essential material for this research, to the Rett Associations who have given consistent encouragement, and to our professional colleagues and our co-authors who have made the joint enterprise a source of companionship and delight.

References

Amir, R.E., Van Den Veyver, I.B., Wan, M., Tran, C.Q., Francke, U., and Zoghbi, H. (1999). Rett Syndrome is caused by mutations in X-linked MECP2, encoding methyl CpG binding protein 2. *Nature Genetics*, **23**, 185–8

Rett, A. (1966). Über ein eigenartiges hirnatrophisches Syndrome bei Hyperammonämie im Kindsalter. *Wiener Medizinische Wochenschrift*, **116**, 723–6.

Alison M. Kerr
Ingegerd Witt Engerström

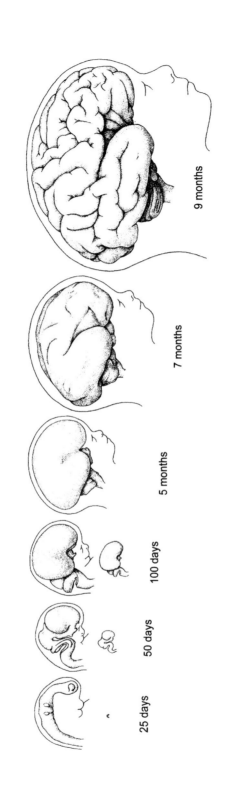

Anatomical landmarks in the developing brain	Neural plate	Neural tube	Cerebral hemispheres Hippocampus Amygdala Pons, Medulla	Superior colliculus Substantia nigra	Cortical plate Choroid plexus Globus pallidus	Cerebellum Caudate Putamen Limbic system	Corpus callosum	Thalamus Basal ganglia	Cortical gyri/sulci	Cortical lobe demarcation	Brain growth Expansion of cortical volume
Time of first appearance	17 days	26 days	5 weeks	6 weeks	7 weeks	8 weeks	9 weeks	12 weeks	6 months	6–9 months	Birth–2 years

Cellular Events	Pattern formation/ Cell proliferation	Cell migration	Neuronal / glial differentiation	Synaptogenesis	Selective cell death	Synaptic maturation and plasticity
Examples of gene products involved	SHH, Patched EGFs, FGFs, TGFs, BMPs Homeobox (Hox) transcription factors Lim1, Otx1/2, Gbx2 Pax, Nkx, Sox, Wnt families SIX3, TGIF, ZIC2/3 EMX1/2, TSC2 Delta, Notch, Numb Prospero, Inscuteable NeuroD, Noggin, Neurogenin, MASH Retinoic acid receptor Activin, En1, Cadherins	DCX Dab1, c-Abl PAFAH1B1/LIS1 XLIS NudC Filamin 1 Reelin Cdk-5, p35 PEX2/5 Neuroregulins/Erb receptors Astrotactin	Netrins/receptors Semaphorins/Neuropilin receptors Cell adhesion molecules (e.g. L1CAM, NCAM, NrCAM, TAG-1) Growth-associated proteins (e.g. GAP43, SCG10) Cytoskeletal proteins (e.g. Tau, MAP2, Tm-5, GFAP) Neurotrophins/Trks Ephrins/Eph receptors AchE, MOA, TH	Neurotrophins/Trks nNOS Presynaptic proteins (e.g. SNAREs, SNAPs, Synaptophysin, Synapsins) Postsynaptic proteins (e.g. neurotransmitter receptors, signalling proteins) Ion (e.g. sodium, potassium, calcium) channels Fasciculins Thy1	AKT Bad, Bax, Bcl-2 Caspases IAP, ICE, IL-1, JIP, JNK, c-Jun PARP IGF/receptor NGF, p75 neurotrophin receptor TNF/receptor	Glutamate receptors (e.g. NMDA, AMPA, metabotropic glutamate receptors) Acetylcholine receptors (muscarinic and nicotinic) Serotonin, dopamine receptors (e.g. 5HT1, 5HT2, D1, D2 receptors) GABA receptors Signalling proteins (e.g. G proteins, Phospholipase C-β1, Protein kinases A/C, adenylyl cyclases, CaM kinases, PSD-95, GRIP, Homer, Src, Fyn, ERK, MAPK) CREB, FMR1, Cytoskeletal proteins Neurotrophins/receptors (e.g. BDNF/TrkB)

An overview of human brain development at anatomical, cellular and molecular levels. Stages of development are illustrated in the upper panel. (Simplified from Cowan, 1979). At 25, 50 and 100 days the lower image shows the relative size of the brain at this age (approximately 80% of actual size, as for images at 5, 7 and 9 months) while an enlargement is provided in the upper image. The first appearance of brain structures is summarised in tabulated form (major source: O'Rahilly and Muller, 1994). The lower table details the sequence of cellular and intercellular events that occur in each brain area during development, with examples of genes/proteins involved in these processes listed below (abbreviated names used where possible due to space limitations). Note that many of these genes and their encoded proteins have been characterised in other species (especially rodents), and their role in human brain development is assumed by homology. Figure by A. J. Hannan.

Contents

Foreword v
Preface ix
List of Contributors xvii

1 The clinical background to the Rett disorder 1
  Alison M. Kerr and *Ingegerd Witt Engerström*

ROOTS OF DISORDER

2 Towards the genetic basis of Rett syndrome 27
  Angus Clarke, Carolyn Schanen and *Maria Anvret*
3 The neuropathology of the Rett disorder 57
  Dawna D. Armstrong and *Hannah C. Kinney*
4 Cortical development in Rett syndrome: molecular, neurochemical, and anatomical aspects 85
  Walter E. Kaufmann
5.1 The Rett syndrome: proposed mechanisms of genetic origin and inheritance 111
  Maj A. Hulten
5.2 Amino acid receptor studies in Rett Syndrome 117
  Mary E. Blue and *Michael V. Johnston*
5.3 Melatonin and Rett Syndrome disorder 121
  Sarojini S. Budden
5.4 Early abnormality in pterin levels in Rett Syndrome 125
  Souad Messahel, Anne E. Pheasant, Hardiv Pall and *Alison M. Kerr*
5.5 Neurotrophic factors in the pathogenesis of Rett Syndrome 127
  Raili Riikonen

NEURONES IN ACTION

6 The central autonomic disturbance in Rett syndrome 131
  Peter O.O. Julu
7 The role of genetic and environmental factors in brain development: development of the central monoaminergic nervous system 183
  Masaya Segawa
8 The monoamine hypothesis in Rett syndrome 205
  Yoshiko Nomura and *Masaya Segawa*
9 The central and peripheral autonomic nervous system and possible implications in Rett syndrome patients 227
  Annica Dahlström

10.1 Autonomic dysfunction and sudden death in Rett syndrome: prolonged QTc intervals and diminished heart rate variability   251
Daniel G. Glaze and *Rebecca J. Schultz*

10.2 Feeding in Rett syndrome   257
Richard Morton

10.3 Oropharyngeal dysfunction and upper gastrointestinal dysmotility, a reflection of disturbances in the autonomic nervous system in Rett syndrome   259
Kathleen J. Motil, Rebecca J. Schultz, Daniel G. Glaze and *Dawna Armstrong*

10.4 Possible link between skeletal and electrocardiographic abnormalities and autonomic dysfunction in Rett syndrome   265
Helen Leonard, Susan Fyfe and *Carolyn Ellaway*

10.5 The electroencephalogram in Rett syndrome   269
Rosemary A. Cooper

10.6 Electromagnetic stimulation of motor neurons   275
Urban M. Fietzek, F. Heinen, U. Ziemann, H. Petersen, K. Hühn, J. Schulte-Mönting, H.-J. Christen, R. Korinthenberg and *F. Hanefeld*

EXPRESSING INTELLIGENCE

11 The morphological substrate for communication   277
Pavel V. Belichenko

12 Early infant intelligence and Rett syndrome   303
Colwyn Trevarthen and *Bronwen Burford*

13 Musical responsiveness in the Rett disorder   327
Bjorn Merker and *Nils L. Wallin*

14.1 Behavioural and emotional features of Rett syndrome   339
Rebecca Mount, Richard Hastings, Tony Charman, Sheena Reilly and *Hilary Cass*

14.2 Vision in Rett syndrome: studies using evoked potentials and event-related potentials   343
Daphne L. McCulloch, Ross M. Henderson, Kathryn J. Saunders, and *R.M. Walley*

CONCLUDING CHAPTER

15 The developmental perspective in Rett disorder: where next?   349
Alison M. Kerr and *Ingegerd Witt Engerstrom*

Abbreviations and Glossary   361

Index   367

List of Contributors

Maria Anvret   Professor, Department of Clinical Genetics, Karolinska Institute, Stockholm
Dawna Armstrong   Professor, Department of Pathology, Baylor College of Medicine, 6621 Fannin Street, Houston, TX 77030, USA
Pavel Belichenko   Senior Researcher, Brain Research Institute, per obukha 5, 107120 Moscow, Russia
Mary E. Blue   Associate Professor, Department of Neurology, Johns Hopkins University School of Medicine, Kennedy Krieger Research Institute, 707 North Broadway, Baltimore, MD 21205, USA
Sarojini Budden   Director, Rett Syndrome Clinic, Associate Professor Pediatrics, Oregon Health Sciences University, Portland, Oregon, USA
Bronwen Burford   Research Fellow, Research Development Centre, Faculty of Education, Moray House Institute, University of Edinburgh, Holyrood Road, Edinburgh EH8 8AQ, UK
Anthony Charman   Behavioural Sciences, Institute of Child Health, 30 Guildford Street, London WC1N 1EH
Angus Clarke   Consultant, Department of Medical Genetics, University of Wales College of Medicine, Heath Park, Cardiff CF4 4XW, Wales, UK
Rosemary Cooper   Consultant Clinical Neurophysiologist, North Staffordshire Hospital Centre and Keele University (retired), 9 East Street, Hambledon, Hants PO7 4RX, UK
Annica Dahlström   Professor, Department of Anatomy and Cell Biology, Division of Neurobiology, Medicinare gatan 3-5, Goteborg University, Goteborg S 41390, Sweden
Ingegerd Witt Engerström   Director, Swedish Rett Centre, Frösö Strand, PO Box 601, SE83223 Frösön, Sweden
Urban M. Fietzek   Department of Neuropediatrics and Muscle Disorders, Albert-Ludwigs-University, Freiburg, Germany
William Fraser   Professor, Welsh Centre for Learning Disabilities, Clinical Studies, Meridian Court, North Road, Cardiff CF4 3BL, UK
Susan Fyfe   Department of Human Biology, School of Biomedical Sciences, Curtin University of Technology, Perth, WA 6845
Daniel G. Glaze   Associate Professor, Pediatrics and Neurology, Baylor College of

Medicine, One Baylor Plaza, Room 319C, Houston, TX 77030, USA
Anthony Hannan   Nuffield Medical Fellow, University Laboratory of Physiology, Parks Road, Oxford OX1 3PT, UK
Dr Florian Heinen   Associate Professor, Children's Hospital, Wedau Clinics, Duisburg, Zu den Rehwiesen 9, Germany
Ross Henderson   Vision Sciences, Caledonian University, Cowcaddens, Glasgow
Maj Hulten   Professor, Department of Biological Sciences, University of Warwick, Coventry CV4 7AL, UK
Michael Johnston   Professor, Departments of Neurology and Pediatrics, Johns Hopkins University School of Medicine, Kennedy Krieger Institute, 707 N. Broadway, Baltimore, MD 21205, USA
Peter Julu   Autonomic Unit, Department of Neurophysiology, Central Middlesex Hospital, Park Royal, Acton Lane, London NW10 7NS, UK
Walter E. Kaufmann   Associate Professor of Pathology, Neurology, Pediatrics and Psychiatry, Johns Hopkins University School of Medicine, Kennedy Krieger Institute, Room 522, 707 North Broadway, Baltimore, MD 21205, USA
Alison Kerr   Senior Lecturer, Honorary Consultant in Paediatrics and Learning Disability, Glasgow University Department of Psychological Medicine, Gartnavel Royal Hospital, Great Western Road, Glasgow G12 0XH, UK
Hannah C. Kinney   Associate Professor, Harvard Medical School, Department of Pathology, Boston Children's Hospital, 300 Longwood Avenue, Boston MA 02115, USA
Helen Leonard   Medical Coordinator, Australian Rett Syndrome Study, TVW Telethon Institute of Child Health Research, West Perth, Western Australia
Daphne McCulloch   Vision Sciences, Caledonian University, Cowcaddens, Glasgow, UK
Bjorn Merker   Royal University College of Music, PO Box 27711, S115 91, Stockholm
Souad Messahel   Biosciences, University of Birmingham School of Biochemistry, Edgbaston, Birmingham B15 2TT, UK
Richard Morton   Consultant Paediatrician, Ronnie MacKeith Child Development Centre, Derby City General Hospital, Derby, UK
Kathleen Motil   Blue Bird Circle Rett Centre, Baylor College of Medicine, One Baylor Plaza, Room 319C, Houston, TX 77030, USA
Rebecca Mount   Behavioural Sciences Unit, Institute of Child Health, 30 Guilford Street, London WC1N 1EH, UK
Yoshiko Nomura   Assistant Director, Segawa Institute for Paediatric Neurology, 2-8 Surugadai, Kanda, Chiyoda-ku, Tokyo, Japan
Hardiv Pall   Consultant Neurologist, Clinical Neurology, Queen Elizabeth Hospital, Birmingham 15, UK
Anne Pheasant   Biosciences, University of Birmingham School of Biochemistry, Edgbaston, Birmingham B15 2TT, UK

Raili Riikonen Professor, Department of Child Neurology, University Hospital of Kuopio, Finland

Carolyn Schanen Department of Paediatrics, UCLA School of Medicine, MDCC 398 10833, Le Conte Avenue, Los Angeles, USA

Rebecca Schultz Patient Manager, Research Coordinator, Blue Bird Circle Rett Centre, Baylor College of Medicine, One Baylor Plaza, Room 319C, Houston, TX 77030, USA

Masaya Segawa Director, Segawa Neurological Clinic for Children, 2–8 Surugadai, Kanda, Chiyoda-ku, Tokyo, Japan

Colwyn Trevarthen Emeritus Professor of Child Psychology and Psychobiology, Edinburgh University Department of Psychology, 7 George Square, Edinburgh EH8 9JZ, UK

Nils L. Wallin Via dell'Arcolaio, 31; I-50137, Florence, Italy

emails

Prof Maria Anvret <maria.anvret@arcus.se.astra.com>
Prof Dawna Armstrong <dawnaa@bcm.tmc.edu>
Prof Pavel Belichenko <pavel_belichenko@yahoo.com>
Dr Mary Blue <blue@kennedykrieger.org>
Dr Sarojini Budden <msbudden@pacifer.com>
Dr Bronwen Burford <Bronwen.Burford@ed.ac.uk>
Dr Angus Clarke <ClarkeAJ@cardiff.ac.uk>
Prof Annica Dahlström <annica.dahlstrom@anatcell.gu.se>
Dr Witt Engerström <ingegerd.witt.engerstrom@jll.se>
Dr Urban Fietzek <fietzek@KKL200.ukl.uni-freiburg.de>
Prof Fraser <fraser_bill@yahoo.com>
Dr Dan Glaze <dglaze@bcm.tmc.edu>
Dr Anthony Hannan <anthony.hannan@physiol.ox.ac.uk>
Prof Maj Hulten <ceht@dna.bio.warwick.ac.uk>
Michael Johnston <johnston@kennedykrieger.org>
Dr Peter Julu <julu@udcf.gla.ac.uk>
Prof Walter Kaufmann <wekaufma@welchlink.welch.jhu.edu>
Dr Helen Leonard <hleonard@cyllene.uwa.edu.au>
Dr Daphne McCulloch <dlmc@gcal.ac.uk>
Dr Bjorn Merker <bjorn.merker@kmh.se>
Dr Kathleen Motil <kmotil@bcm.tmc.edu>
Dr Rebecca Mount <r.mount@ich.ucl.ac.uk>
Dr Yoshiko Nomura <nomura_y@kt.rim.or.jp>
Dr Anne Pheasant (for Messahel) <a.e.pheasant@bham.ac.uk>
Prof Raili Riikonen <Raili.Riikonen@uku.fi>
Dr Carolyn Schanen <schanen@ucla.edu>
Prof Masaya Segawa <segawa@t3.rim.or.jp>
Prof Colwyn Trevarthen <C.Trevarthen@edinburgh.ac.uk>
Dr Nils L. Wallin <nils.wallin@flashnet.it>

1 The clinical background to the Rett disorder

Alison M. Kerr and Ingegerd Witt Engerström

Summary

This chapter aims to describe the clinical characteristics of the Rett syndrome and discuss briefly how they indicate the nature of underlying disorder as an introduction to the following chapters which present the evidence from laboratory investigations. Data is drawn from the authors' personal experience with the Swedish and British cohorts and a review of the scientific literature.

1.1 Introduction

Doubtless the Rett disorder has been with the human race throughout its history and we suppose that cases were hidden within such heterogeneous diagnostic categories as 'cerebral palsy' and 'autism'. Most of its features were recorded by Andreas Rett and published in German (Rett 1966). Other neurologists observed the same phenomena (Ishikawa *et al.* 1978) and Hagberg presented the first report in English (Hagberg *et al.* 1983). Early cooperation between Rett, Moser, Hagberg and Fukuyama and the family support organizations led by Mrs Kathy Hunter, founder of the International Rett Syndrome Association, encouraged the establishment of a series of international symposia attended by a wide range of clinical and laboratory based scientists and this greatly facilitated progress in research.

Early in the investigation the striking late infancy regression of the Rett syndrome led many to assume that the underlying disorder was progressive, and it has taken time for the evidence to accumulate and become widely accepted that this is indeed an essentially static early developmental problem which manifests in a predictable sequence and is accompanied by changing risks throughout life.

As so often in the history of medicine, it has been the clinical observations and surveys which have led to the laboratory discoveries. It is the informative clinical profile which indicates the neural networks which are interfered with or spared by the disorder and it is the clinical difficulties which must finally be addressed in developing intervention.

1.2 Classification

The classic Rett syndrome is defined according to an international agreement (Diagnostic Criteria Working Group 1988) developed from earlier proposals by Hagberg *et al* 1985. The purpose of this agreement was to ensure that while the diagnosis relied entirely on clinical signs researchers could select comparable groups of patients from different populations.

Adapted criteria for classic Rett syndrome
Apparently normal prenatal and perinatal period
Apparently normal psychomotor development through the first 6 months (subtle delays, see below)
Head circumference within normal centiles at birth
Deceleration of head growth between 5 months and 4 years (approx)
Reduction in acquired purposeful hand skills between 6 and 30 months (approx)
Communication dysfunction and transient social withdrawal
Appearance of severely impaired expressive and receptive language
Apparent severe psychomotor retardation
Stereotyped hand movements — wringing/squeezing/clapping/mouthing/rubbing
Gait and truncal dyspraxia appearing between 1 and 4 years

In Sweden, the symptomatic period before regression is called stage I, regression itself stage II, a following relatively unchanging 'pseudo stationary' period as stage III, and a later, non-ambulant stage as IV (Hagberg and Witt Engerström 1986, Witt Engerström 1990). The British Survey designates the period from birth to regression as 'pre-regression', the following period beginning with the first reduction in skills as 'regression' and the period which begins with the cessation of acute infancy loss of skills as 'post-regression' as it has been found unhelpful to draw a firm line between the early and later post-regression stages. Type of presentation is designated according to the predominant abnormality of muscle tone on direct examination: hypotonia (type 1), dystonia (type 2), hypertonia (type 3) and mild hypertonia ('normotonia') (type 4) (Kerr and Stephenson 1985, 1986). The Swedish and British classifications are shown together in Fig. 1.1.

Cases which fall outside the agreed definition of classic Rett syndrome in Britain are called 'atypical' and in Sweden 'variants', congenital (recognized from birth), early seizure (seizure onset before regression), forme fruste (regression after age 4), preserved speech (continuing to use phrases or sentences after

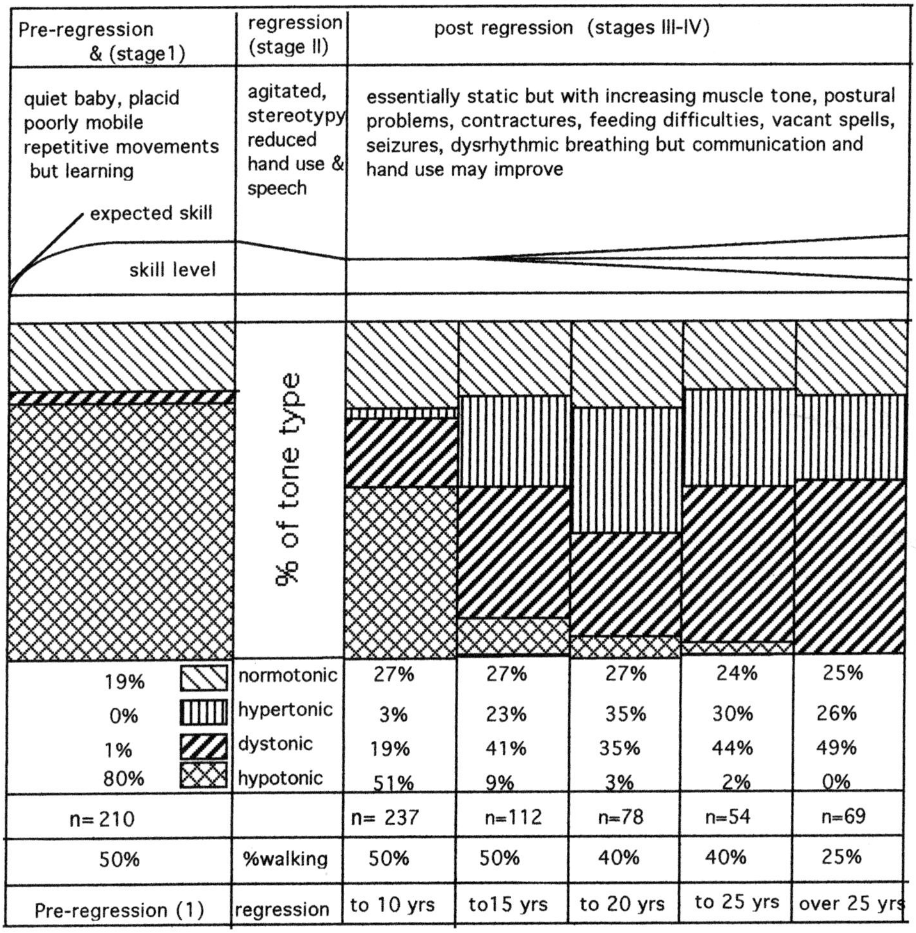
Pre-regression & (stage1)
regression (stage II)
post regression (stages III-IV)
quiet baby, placid poorly mobile repetitive movements but learning
agitated, stereotypy reduced hand use & speech
essentially static but with increasing muscle tone, postural problems, contractures, feeding difficulties, vacant spells, seizures, dysrhythmic breathing but communication and hand use may improve
expected skill
skill level
% of tone type
19% normotonic 27% 27% 27% 24% 25%
0% hypertonic 3% 23% 35% 30% 26%
1% dystonic 19% 41% 35% 44% 49%
80% hypotonic 51% 9% 3% 2% 0%
n=210 n= 237 n=112 n=78 n=54 n=69
50% %walking 50% 50% 40% 40% 25%
Pre-regression (1) regression to 10 yrs to15 yrs to 20 yrs to 25 yrs over 25 yrs

Fig. 1.1 The figure shows the changing pattern of disability throughout the life of a person with Rett Syndrome. Tone types indicate the predominant abnormality of muscle tone in the given age groups. Longditudinal data is taken from the British Rett Survey at Jan 2000 A Kerr. 'Normotonic' indicates normal or near normal tone.

regression) and male variant (Hagberg *et al.* 1985; Hagberg and Rasmussen 1986; Hagberg and Gillberg 1993; Hagberg and Skjeldal 1994).

1.3 Occurrence

Only an approximate incidence and prevalence has so far been possible for the disorder since only the full classic syndrome could be identified with certainty. Prevalence of the classic syndrome in Britain is estimated from the most completely ascertained years at not less than 1 in 10 000 females (Kerr 1992) and other estimates have ranged above and below this figure (Asthana *et al.* 1990; Kultz *et al.* 1990; Hagberg and Hagberg 1997), the highest generally where experienced clinicians have searched most assiduously. There have also been reports of high local prevalence (Zappella and Cerioli 1987; Hagberg and Hagberg 1997). In Sweden 225 cases were diagnosed and examined by May 2000. In the British Survey, 915 cases had been reported by December 1999, 689 with full data entered, of whom 7% (49/689) were considered not to have the Rett disorder although marked similarities justified keeping them under review. Of 640 considered Rett, 83% (531) were classic and 17% (109) atypical Rett. One boy with classic Rett Syndrome has been reported to the British survey with coexisting Klinefelter's syndrome (XXY) Schwartzman *et al.* 1999). There have been more reports of boys who were atypical due to frank dysmorphism and obvious early developmental problems, eight such within the UK and reports from the literature (Christen and Hanefeld 1995).

Most cases of Rett syndrome have been sporadic but 4% of British cases had a relative with Rett syndrome. It is worthy of note that classic and atypical (variant) girls and severely neurologically abnormal boys have also been reported in the same kindreds, suggesting that these people may be affected by the same clinical disorder although not showing the classic syndrome (Kerr 1992*b*). This variation within the disorder is illustrated by the illuminating case cited below with permission and advice from the family and Dr Schanen: (Schanen and Francke 1998; Amir *et al.* 1999; Wan *et al.* 1999).

A is a healthy woman in whom no Rett mutation has been found and whose X inactivation is normal. A carries the same Xq28 as her two daughters, although a mutation was not found in A and germ line mutation is thought to have occurred.

B, her daughter, has a MECP2 mutation with normal X inactivation and presents the classical Rett syndrome. She is unable to walk and has scoliosis and epilepsy.

C, another daughter of A, has the same mutation but is skewed 85.5% in favour of the normal X. She has poor fine motor skills and a mild tremor, speaks well but often parrots, reads well but solves problems very poorly. She cannot drive, ride a bicycle or light a match. Her intelligence quotient was assessed at 71 aged 8 years.

D, daughter of C, has the same mutation with normal X inactivation and classical Rett syndrome.

E, son of C by a different partner, has the same mutation and was clearly abnormal at 4 days with hypotonia, reduced head growth, seizures, repeated respiratory arrests, poorly coordinated sucking, swallowing and breathing, and extreme sensitivity to vagal stimulation such as the introduction of a naso-gastric tube. He died after such an arrest at 1 year.

Only B and D have the classical Rett syndrome, while C and E illustrate two extremes of the range of clinical expression of the same mutation, more or less masked by the pattern of X inactivation. A gonadal mutation is considered the most likely situation in A.

Several pairs of concordant monozygotic twins have been described (Perry 1991; Percy 1992; Kerr 1992*b*). Currently 12 British cases have non-twin full or half sisters with Rett (six pairs). Only once have as many as three classic affected girls been reported in one sibship and there boys have also been affected by severe neurological problems (Amir *et al.* 1999; Wan *et al.* 1999, Schanen and Francke 1998). Akesson has traced groups of Swedish cases back through nine generations, finding clusters from several small villages, suggesting that certain populations may be predisposed to the disorder. The shared ancestors of these cases have been male or female (Akesson *et al.* 1992). In Britain, of 421 families providing family information to the survey, 161 (38%) reported other conditions in siblings, parents, siblings of parents or grandparents which might relate to a genetic or neurological disorder including schizophrenia, bipolar disorder, neuromuscular disorders and autism.

1.4 Before regression

Gestation and birth of the classic Rett infant are usually uneventful (Hagberg *et al.* 1983, Kerr and Stephenson 1985; Witt Engerström 1987). The child looks normal (Fig. 1.2) and makes progress so it is easily seen why she is accepted as normal in the first months; however scrutiny of the early developmental history immediately threw doubt on this assumption (Rett 1966; Nomura *et al.* 1984; Kerr and Stephenson 1985, 1986; Kerr *et al.* 1987).

Rett indicated pre-regression problems in feeding and mobility (Rett 1966). Nomura and Segawa described the baby as 'autistic' because of disturbed sleep rhythms similar to those found in autism (Nomura and Segawa 1990, Segawa and Nomura 1990). Kerr concluded from early histories and study of videos taken by families from birth, pre-dating suspicion of disorder, that the newborn with classic Rett syndrome is already disabled in movement and cognition. This was a very quiet and placid baby, unless in pain, perceived as 'very good' but slow to learn and slow to move about, with an excess of hand patting (Kerr *et al.* 1987; Kerr 1995). Experienced parents or grandparents frequently expressed anxieties in the first days of life with regard to handling and attentiveness of the baby (Kerr *et al.* 1987; Kerr 1987; Naidu *et al.* 1995).

In a Swedish study (Witt Engerström 1987) developmental disorder could be suspected from infant screening records between 5 and 18 months (median 10) due to delay in passing gross motor milestones, unusual behaviour or weight loss. Two-thirds lay or sat with their legs in a hypotonic 'frog' position. Balancing upright was late or absent and moving about was managed by rolling or 'bottom shuffling' rather than crawling. At 1 year, 11 would not take their weight on their feet. Subtle developmental deficits could be traced from the first 6 months in 13 of 20 children. Most frequently mentioned were undue placidity, an undemanding nature suggesting poor social interaction, tremulous neck movements and reduced muscle tone. Early video recordings showed excessive bilateral hand movements.

Measures of brain growth such as occipito-frontal circumference (OFC) indicate growth within the normal range at birth and for some weeks thereafter, becoming sub-optimal during later infancy or childhood. In most, growth then resumes reaching a final head circumference near the second standard deviation, the actual size reflecting clinical severity (Stenbom *et al.* 1995, Kerr 1995, Hagberg *et al.* 2000, Percy 1992). Electroencephalographs are seldom indicated in this period and are reported normal or immature (Cooper *et al.* 1998; Chapter 10.5). Brain scans are usually reported as normal or show slight increase in the CSF space. In a Swedish study of 19 girls aged 13 to 42 months, reduced OFC growth was recorded between 5 and 22 months and brain scans showed no abnormalities (Witt Engerström 1992*a*).

In spite of these indications of the presence of the disorder long before regression in the classic Rett baby, there is also genuine developmental progress and the child frequently passes the normal developmental screening tests at 3, 6 and 9 months, sometimes even later (Witt Engerström 1987, Kerr and Stephenson 1985). While many fail to produce words some do have meaningful speech, many can feed themselves with a spoon and mug, many learn to walk, and a few climb stairs. However from the 9–12 month stage, developmental stagnation becomes increasingly obvious until regression occurs. The best levels of skill commonly reported include turning the pages of a book, sometimes with recognition of pictures, picking of fluff from the carpet, and taking and carrying a favourite toy (Kerr *et al.* 1987; Witt Engerström 1987; Leonard and Bower 1998).

In the Swedish cohort the following proportions of girls achieved the stated skills: pincer grip 11/20, walking unaided (with an immature, broad based gait) 6/20, removing socks or hat 1/20, finger feeding 7/20, single words 16/20. Only one girl achieved three-word sentences. Contact was described as weak and the child as 'not cuddly'. Babies were described as 'normal' or 'calm' in 13/20. The most advanced play involved exploratory mouthing, banging, throwing and waving of objects. Functional abilities were brushing one's own hair, holding a telephone receiver to the ear, and use of a spoon or cup. Symbolic play such as feeding a doll with a spoon or brushing the doll's hair was never recorded (Witt Engerström 1992a).

At the pre-regression stage it is therefore clear that the disorder spares some aspects of very early development while interfering selectively with the acquisition of the more sophisticated skills which should gain prominence towards the end of the first year. It is also clear that already at this early stage the clinical severity of the disorder varies considerably.

1.5 Regression (stage II)

Regression is often dramatic with reduction in skills in hand use, speech and interpersonal contact over a period of days to months. In a Swedish study onset of regression occurred at a median age of 17 months (13–25 months) and reports from the British Survey indicated a mean age of 18 months (8–40 months). It is impressive that there is no severe accompanying illness although there have been many anecdotal accounts of regression beginning after a minor event such as arrival of a new baby, a change of house, or a relatively minor respiratory or gastrointestinal disturbance.

Movement becomes poorly coordinated and girls seem unresponsive and frightened (Kerr and Stephenson 1985, 1986). As voluntary movement diminishes, involuntary movements become more obvious, twisting and patting initially mingling with normal hand use (Rett 1966; Ishikawa *et al.* 1978; Kerr *et al.* 1987, Witt Engerström 1992*a*; Nomura and Segawa 1992). Gradually frankly stereotyped involuntary movements predominate including circular hand–mouth movements, tongue movements, and tooth grinding. Transient strabismus is common during regression and this was reported in 42% of British questionnaire respondents (81/195). Hand and eye-hand coordination and trunk control tend to deteriorate with some jerky movements and dystonic postures. Sitting, shuffling, standing and walking seem more difficult but are not usually lost and some actually begin to walk alone during this period. There are spells of screaming and inappropriate night laughter, and night sleep is commonly disturbed.

Towards the end of the regression period, awake irregular breathing usually becomes noticeable with breath holding and deep breathing (Southall *et al.* 1988; Kerr *et al.* 1990; Kerr 1992*b*, 1995, Witt Engerström 1990, 1992*b*).

The electroencephalogram usually remains normal or is mildly immature until the end of regression when it becomes frankly abnormal showing paroxysms of slow waves with or without spikes in most cases. Over half have one or more seizures before the end of regression (Hagne *et al.* 1989; Glaze *et al.* 1987; Cooper *et al.* 1998; Chapter 10.5).

The regression period is very unhappy for the child whose skills become inaccessible and for her family who may lack professional support because the child still looks so 'normal' and has been making some developmental progress. In the Swedish study, regression was found to last for an average of 13 months (2–32 months), ending at a mean age of 30 months (20–51 months).

Clinical example (Swedish series no. S107, Witt Engerström 1992; Hagberg and Witt Engerström 1990a; Witt Engerström and Forslund 1992)

A daughter born to a woman with Rett syndrome (RS) has been closely followed since birth. At birth S was considered a beautiful well-grown and lively baby with normal tone and reflexes. At 6 months she gave good contact, babbled and smiled, showed hand–eye coordination and manipulated toys. She sat upright with support and turned round but would not put her feet to the ground when held to stand. No abnormal movements, reflexes or behaviours were found but she was less responsive to eye contact than to touch and did not explore her surroundings. She showed prolonged dependence on frequent feeding and sleep periods. From 6 months she followed a typical Rett course. Although she developed pincer grasp and single syllables, she did not crawl. There was a lack of reciprocal movements and persistence of an asymmetric tonic neck reflex. Held in the crawling position she displayed a general flexion of fingers, toes, knees and hips. She sat unaided, rolled and shuffled and made her first attempts to stand with support at 11 months. Her play repertoire increased very slowly showing little variey, and at 13 months she was inattentive. Her development became fragmented and her behaviour disturbed. Traces of normal skills came and went. Transient facial muscle twitches were seen with a twisting of hand and tongue. She seemed to feel sudden episodes of discomfort. After 15 months her head circumference failed to increase. At 16 months she lost single words and the control of her left hand, substituting the right hand inappropriately, as if hemiplegic, and a dystonic element was seen. She bit her left hand and put the fingers in her mouth. At times her mouth remained open and grimacing increased. However her good ability to maintain emotional contact with people was preserved. At 30 months she would still greet people with a smile and apparent interest. By this stage loss of skills had stopped. She babbled and appeared to understand words but would not look for hidden toys. Writhing tongue movements became obvious, she had difficulty with chewing and swallowing, and did not close her lips. She frequently sucked the fingers of her left hand and would unexpectedly reach out with her right hand. She did not crawl and walked only with support, preferably on tiptoe. She was basically hypotonic with lower limb dystonia. In spite of regular physiotherapy she had developed a slight scoliosis requiring later surgery. Growth of head and feet was poor. Electroencephalography showed bilateral spike-wave and poly-spike and wave activity, corresponding to eye deviations and arm movements. At 3.5 years, breath holding and tooth grinding had appeared.

1.6 Features of classic Rett syndrome after regression (stages III and IV)

From 5 years the condition is usually stable and the child becomes happier and more sociable with some capacity to learn and to display her individual personality and sensitivities. The characteristic signs of the disorder appear in a predictable sequence and we will describe these in turn, although they are not separate phenomena and difficulties in one area inevitably impact on other areas of function. The problems of the Rett disorder affect growth, movement, cognition and autonomic control and may lead to epilepsy, non-epileptic vacant spells, postural difficulties, joint deformities, nutritional and feeding problems, strange behaviours and a risk of sudden death. In spite of all these it is impressive that these people remain normal in many ways. Notwithstanding their apparently severe intellectual difficulties they look attractive and alert and they appear to see, hear, feel and enjoy experiences, continuing to relate to other people and to interact with them at an emotional level. This is quite different from the situation for an autistic person.

1.6.1 Growth

Deficient growth in the Rett disorder is reflected in early and final height and weight and in the weights of all the internal organs but disproportionately in the brain (Schultz *et al.* 1993; Armstrong 1992, 1995; Chapter 3). Stature is less than expected from about 2 years (Holm 1986) and average adult height is reduced (Thommessen *et al.* 1991). Motil and Schultz recorded an average height of 120 cm at 13, well below the normal centiles (Chapter 10.3).

The feet are commonly small, narrow and blue even in girls who walk. In the Swedish study this became apparent during regression. In a British study of girls over 10 years the fourth toe was short in 28 of 137 (20%) and in 4 of 14 adults (28%) (Kerr *et al.* 1993, 1995). Occasionally attention has been drawn to the same minor anomaly in a mother or sister. In an Australian study Glasson *et al.* reported radiographic evidence of metacarpal and metatarsal shortening (Glasson *et al.* 1998, Leonard *et al.* 1999; Chapter 10.4). This anomaly is much less common in the normal population (Ray and Haldane 1965) and we have discussed its possible significance for Rett elsewhere (Kerr *et al.* 1995, Chapter 10.4). Fractures are more common than expected in people with Rett syndrome, even in those who walk independently, and osteoporosis has been reported in several studies (Leonard *et al.* 1999; Chapter 10.4)

Although the young child with Rett syndrome looks normal, her short fourth digits are indeed a minor dysmorphism, and as she grows we have noticed that the face may develop a characteristic but not unattractive appearance with eyes rather wide set, a small chin and occasionally a broad and prominent nasal bridge. (Fig. 1.3) Thus although the early criteria for classic Rett syndrome have served a useful purpose in drawing attention to the attractive appearance of the typical affected child, it is not now strictly correct to describe her as non-dysmorphic.

The secondary sexual characteristics appear normally and menstruation does not cause exceptional problems for most people with RS. Among 52 respondents to the British Survey questions, menarche occurred at a mean age of 14 years (range 8–30, median 13 years) Women with the Rett disorder have borne children without apparent difficulty and their children appeared normal at birth, as did the parent (Witt Engerström 1992, Wan *et al.* 1999).

1.6.2 The disorder of muscle tone

Abnormal muscle tone is universal although severity varies. Before regression hypotonia is usual (Kerr and Stephenson 1985, Chapter 8). Longitudinal studies indicate that muscle tone changes over time, evolving in most people from hypotonia to hypertonia. Mild hypertonia (type 4) appears to confer the least disability in movement and in other skills (Kerr and Stephenson 1985, 1986; Fig. 1.2).

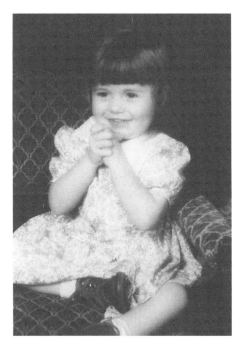

Fig. 1.2 A young child with RS.

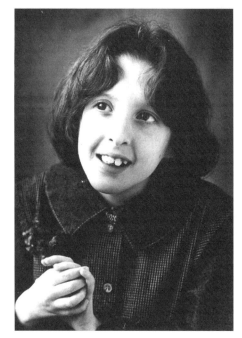

Fig. 1.3 An older girl with RS.

Muscle tone may be affected to a different degree on each side of the body. Deep tendon reflexes are increased, especially in the lower limbs, and ankle clonus is commonly present; however in our experience the Babinski response is absent (Babinski 1898; Kerr and Stephenson 1985) although it has been reported in some cases (Hagberg *et al.* 1983). Electromagnetic cortical stimulation demonstrated brisk activation of the upper motor neuron pathways, indicating an intact, although not necessarily entirely normal, upper motor neuron (Eyre *et al.* 1990, Heinen *et al.* 1996; Chapter 10.6).

With increasing muscle tone, tooth grinding moves further back in the jaw and the hand stereotypy takes on an increasingly tense and wringing character. Dystonic spasms may interrupt walking as a leg may be lifted inappropriately for several seconds at a time or the girl may bend forward at the waist, seeming puzzled yet unable to right herself. We have also seen dystonic spasms of the sterno-cleido-mastoid muscle which may be troublesome for some months and then disappear.

1.6.3 Disorder of posture and locomotion

The abnormal muscle tone in Rett is one aspect of the severely disorganized motor control affecting posture and movement. Perception seems to be involved as well as execution. Some girls who can walk seem to prefer to do so on tiptoe. It is common for a girl who is being supported to lean on the support and for a walking girl to stop and lean forward as if uncertain where she is in space. Others seem afraid to attempt to stand or walk; but righting reflexes are generally present.

In a Swedish study of 20 young girls, 12 walked by 3 years, 15 by 4 years (2 stopped at 5 and 7 years) and 5 never walked . Truncal ataxia was present in 16, shown as a jerky tremor when the individual was seated on the examiner's knee. Walking was broad based with rocking from side to side. Some turned in circles (Witt Engerström 1993).

Of 47 women with classic Rett aged 30, with continuous longitudinal records dating from before regression, 34 had walked unsupported before regression (72%). Of these 34, 22 still walked alone at 30 years (65%). Of the 12 who did not walk alone before regression, 6 learned to walk thereafter and 3 continued to do so until 30 years. This reflects not only good retention of the skill but also that the least affected women may live longer. A very few classic girls and women learn to walk up stairs and to swim with simple strokes and may do this even as adults.

Permanent contractures of the joints develop most frequently in those with the most abnormal tone, hypotonic, hypertonic or dystonic, and may occur rapidly if posture is poor (Witt Engerström 1990, Budden 1995). Particularly common are scoliosis, hip dislocation, subluxation of the knees in flexion and ankle contractures. Initially these are correctable and it is our strong impression that with suitable activity, exercises and support, deformity may often be avoided. The spinal joints being harder to control externally, scoliosis is inclined to progress and may require operative intervention (Loder *et al.* 1989; Roberts and Connor 1988; Stokland *et al.* 1992). In the British Survey 17% of classic cases have undergone scoliosis surgery, 16% in Sweden, generally during adolescence. It is of interest that this major surgery has been well tolerated in all but the most poorly nourished. By 20 years 93% of the British cohort, 85% of the Swedish, had some degree of scoliosis. Among 53 women in the 20–25 year age band, 3 (6%) were reported to have no scoliosis, 20 (38%) mild deformity, 12 (23%) moderate deformity and 13 (24%) unoperated severe scoliosis. Five (9%) had received surgical correction.

1.6.4 The disorder of voluntary movement

Voluntary movement is peculiarly disabled and we prefer to call this dyspraxia since the difficulty initiating movement seems to involve both motor and sensory mechanisms; however some spontaneous fluent and useful movement does remain after regression and this may facilitate swimming, adjustment of the sitting position even on horseback, grasping a swing appropriately, and body movement to music. Some controlled voluntary movement also remains, especially in those with relatively normal muscle tone, and new skills may develop. A few people can open a door, feed themselves with a spoon and mug and cooperate in dressing. Many continue to finger feed and to use simple switches. However the majority of people with RS have minimal hand use, and although objects of interest may be approached, studied and tapped or slapped they are not explored. Handedness is not easy to determine in view of the disabilities. Of 201 British families able to state hand preference for classic girls and women, 88 (44%) reported right preference, 54 (27%) left preference and 59 (29%) no preference. Of 84 girls and women with classic Rett in whom initial hand skills had been sufficient to allow self-feeding with spoon or mug, 31 (37%) now used the right hand, 29 (34%) the left and 24 (29%) both hands equally. Of 16 with preserved speech (both classic and atypical), 6 (38%) used the right hand, 5 (31%) the left and 5 (31%) used the hands equally.

In a Swedish study of 20 girls, 11 would reach out to grab or tap objects of interest in low stress situations. The girls used eye-pointing to achieve action and this communicative skill persisted into adulthood (Witt Engerström 1990, 1992*b*).

1.6.5 The involuntary movement disorder

Involuntary movements are universal, widespread and exacerbated by alerting (Nomura *et al.* 1984, Nomura and Segawa 1992, Kerr and Stephenson 1985, 1986, Kerr *et al.* 1987, Witt Engerström 1990). The hands are most striking with each hand developing its own sequence, slightly different from its partner although commonly meeting in the midline. The essential movement is simple — squeezing, patting or rubbing, in the hair, at the mouth, at chest level, behind the back or held out at the sides (Kerr *et al.* 1987). The tongue is usually involved in writhing movements and may flick saliva, some girls emit short cries, and tooth grinding (bruxism) is very common. There is also a general coarse tremor which increases during agitation, and dystonic posture is commonly seen.

The regularity and rate of the involuntary movements suggest an extrapyramidal disturbance at times, reminiscent of athetoid cerebral palsy or parkinsonism, disappearing during sleep and exacerbated by agitation (Kerr *et al.* 1990).

1.6.6 The seizure disorder

Epileptic seizures occur in about 75% and continue in about 50% of people (Glaze *et al.* 1987; Cooper *et al.* 1998; Hagne *et al.* 1989). There is a tendency for remission with ageing, but in a minority epilepsy is severe and difficult to control. Seizures may be generalized or partial and several types may occur in the same person. Episodes suggestive of salaam attacks have been described in young children; however true hypsarrhythmia has only rarely been reported from electroencephalographic studies (Glaze, personal communication) and we have no reports of true 'petit mal' epilepsy (3 per second spike and wave). Drugs in general use for the control of epilepsy are frequently effective and well tolerated, with the exception of Vigabatrin which has been reported to exacerbate agitated behaviour in some girls. Lamotrigine has emerged as a favoured therapy, but many are well maintained on the older anticonvulsants, sodium valproate and carbamazepine.

Although clinical epilepsy is not universal the electroencephalogram (e.e.g.) is usually very abnormal, lacking normal rhythms and poorly responsive with bursts of generalized slow high amplitude waves, sometimes with spikes, accentuated during rest and sleep (Southall *et al.* 1988, Kerr *et al.* 1987). In later years a monotonous theta rhythm is common (Verma *et al.* 1986; Cooper *et al.* 1998; Chapter 10.5).

In 20 Swedish girls, epileptic seizures were diagnosed in 11 at age 3.5 years, 13 by 5 years, and 16 by 10 years. Early e.e.g. changes generally preceded the clinical recognition of seizures and included Rolandic spikes during sleep. In 13 girls, initial focal spike activity appeared in left centro-temporal, -parietal, and -occipital leads or bilaterally. One girl was recorded before regression, seven during regression and five soon after regression. In one child there was a right occipital focus. Different epileptiform patterns appeared later, predominantly multifocal and bilaterally synchronous spike and wave discharges, suggesting a diffuse subcortical origin (Hagne *et al.* 1989). Bieber Nielsen *et al.* (1990) reported immature patterns of brain activity.

1.6.7 Autonomic disorder

Andreas Rett (1966) observed irregular breathing and it was described also by Lugaresi and colleagues (Lugaresi and Cirignotta 1982, Lugaresi *et al.* 1985; Cirignotta *et al.* 1986) who felt that it characterized the syndrome. Suggestive of autonomic dysfunction in girls with Rett are the typical agitated state with flushed face and dilated pupils, the small, narrow cold feet which become warm and pink and grow following surgical or chemical lumbar sympathectomy and the sluggish bowel function. In Britain there have been rare (personal) reports of urinary retention. Agitation is a hallmark of the syndrome as are sudden and unexplained periods of distress which may herald regression but do continue throughout life. Abnormal awake breathing has been noticed by most parents of classic girls reporting to the British Survey, hyperventilation in 78% (320/408) and breath holding in 73% (298/408). Abdominal distension with air is common and sometimes painful and it is clear that the air is forced into the stomach by poorly coordinated chest and airway activity. Among families reporting to the British Survey, 57% (103/179) reported obvious distension with air.

Episodes of abnormal breathing were noticed in 13 of the 20 Swedish girls during early post-regression (stage III) taking the form of hyperventilation and/or breath holding episodes during wakefulness. Most striking were irregular periods of intense hyperventilation interrupted by prolonged breath holding, with the air finally expelled against a more or less closed glottis and severe air swallowing. In 91 girls and women, hyperventilation was reported in 45%, breath holding in 65% and abdominal distension in 30% with no abnormalities asleep (Witt Engerström 1992*b*). Vacant spells occurred and were sometimes difficult to distinguish from the other abnormal movements.

The neuroscope (Julu 1992, Julu *et al.* 1993) has been used in accurate e.e.g. and respiratory monitoring for over 60 British girls and women and more recently for Swedish cases (Witt Engerström and Kerr 1998; Chapter 6). These techniques have demonstrated abnormal rhythms in every Rett case accompanied by low vagal tone (Julu *et al.* 1997, 1998) indicating that deficient parasympathetic restraint contributes to the autonomic imbalance in this disorder. Studies using the less direct method of heart rate variability to estimate autonomic control have also shown poor control and these together with studies of deaths in Rett syndrome suggest that this autonomic factor may be responsible for some sudden unexpected deaths (Sekul *et al.* 1994; Kerr *et al.* 1997; Chapter 6; Chapter 10.1).

Although long breath holds and forced breathing are the most obvious rhythm abnormalities and therefore most commonly reported by families, accurate 1 h recordings have shown 13 different rhythms (Julu *et al.* 1997, 1998). Each girl tends to show several different rhythms, switching between them in a manner which appears random, although on closer inspection each girl develops an individual pattern which also relates to age (Julu *et al.*, submitted; and Julu Chapter 6). The youngest girls have the greatest proportion of energetic breathing and of protracted inspiration (apneusis) whereas the oldest women have the greatest proportion of valsalva breathing (Witt Engerström and Kerr 1998). These abnormal rhythms make a major contribution to the non-epileptic vacant spells which are common at all ages (Kerr *et al.* 1990, Kerr 1992*b*, Witt Engerström 1990; Julu *et al.* 1998). The abnormal rhythms are seen only in the awake state (Lugaresi and Cirignotta 1982; Cirignotta *et al.* 1986, Southall *et al.* 1988) and there is close positive correlation between an agitated state and the breathing abnormality (Kerr *et al.* 1990).

Oxygen levels fall during and after long breath holds, particularly long central apnoeas where the inspiratory effort is delayed and we have seen loss of consciousness in such attacks. It is common for such episodes to be mistaken for epileptic seizures and ineffectively medicated as a result. The low carbon dioxide levels induced by hyperventilation may affect the behaviour of the girl through discomfort or dizziness (Southall *et al.* 1988; Chapter 6).

1.6.8 Eating and nutritional disturbance

Early feeding and weaning to soft foods is usually unremarkable but Andreas Rett (1966) and others have reported feeding difficulties from birth in some babies with poor suck and gastro-oesophageal reflux (Rett 1966, Nomura *et al.* 1990; Naidu 1997).

With the onset of regression, increasing involuntary movements and irregular breathing, various difficulties are added to the helplessness of the child and conspire to make feeding difficult. These include poor feeding posture, unhelpful movements of the jaws and tongue, inability to close the mouth firmly, lack of chewing ability and poor coordination of the palate and other oral movements. Morton *et al.* did not find swallowing to be a major difficulty in most girls (Morton *et al.* 1997) but Motil did find significant swallowing problems and gastro-oesophageal reflux (Chapter 10.2, Motil *et al.* 1994; Chapter 10.3).

A Swedish study showed disturbed oral motor function with chewing and swallowing difficulties, poor lip closure during swallowing and drooling in 10/20 at ages 3–10 years. With ageing and increasing muscle tone the tongue became more rigid, obstructing the placing and swallowing of food.

Weight is reduced in many girls even when the appetite is good and although feeding difficulties may clearly play a part in this, other constitutional factors are suspected (Rice and Haas 1988). The most agitated young girls are particularly thin and their forced breathing seems likely to demand additional calories. Increased calorie allowance has been found necessary in order to keep weight within the accepted limits for height (Rice and Haas 1988, Budden 1995). The few who have little difficulty with eating may become obese as food becomes one of the shared pleasures for the girl and her family.

Toileting is frequently abandoned by carers for a person with RS; however in our experience, girls and women are almost always capable of learning to pass a motion when habitually placed on a comfortable and secure toilet seat. A very few girls will indicate their toilet needs. Optimal physical activity, good diet and sufficient fluid help to combat constipation; however this may still remain a problem suggesting that sluggish bowel activity is part of the syndrome.

1.6.9 Sleep

Sleep is a regular problem area. Of 194 British families of girls with classic RS, 80% (156/194) reported sleep problems: 43% (84/194) had difficulties both day and night; 15% (29/194) fell asleep by day (only) and 22% (43/194) failed to sleep at night. Some of the earliest sleep laboratory studies by Nomura and Segawa indicated disrupted sleep stages (Chapter 8) and Bolthauser *et al.* (1987) reported sleep disturbance as an early sign of regression.

1.6.10 Sensory faculties

Vision and hearing are among the strengths of people with Rett disorder who appear interested in both visual and auditory stimuli; however during regression, while other internal controls seem to run into difficulties, squinting is common—reported in 81/195 classic girls in a British series (41%). However 60% of those who had squinted during regression regained control later. In detailed ophthalmic examinations of 11 Rett subjects aged 4–24 years and comparison with normal and other profoundly disabled people, Saunders *et al.* found refractive errors common but the optic fundi normal. Visual evoked potentials were demonstrated in all, indicating attention to the stimulus and function of the afferent visual pathways. The authors commented that this is unusual in such profoundly disabled people and suggested that these people might benefit from spectacle correction (Saunders *et al.* 1995; Chapter 14.2).

Auditory and somato-sensory evoked responses are present and have been reported in some studies as normal (Percy *et al.* 1985), although Pelson and Budden (1987) and Badr *et al.* (1987, 1989) found minor differences from controls in the proximal responses. It is commonly reported by families that the girls respond slowly to painful stimuli, suggesting delayed processing of this information rather than failure to receive the stimulus.

1.6.11 Speech

Babies with Rett disorder are quiet. Initially considered 'very good', this may raise suspicions in experienced carers. Most of the infants develop pre-language 'ma' and 'da' but true speech is uncommon even when regression occurs as late as 3 or 4 years; however some of the least severely affected girls and women do acquire speech and may retain it (Zappella and Cerioli 1987; Zapella 1992, 1997, Von Tetzchner 1997).

In 20 Swedish girls, the speech gained before regression was not regained. In 11 it was replaced by babbling and rare single words. Later in life, single words were unexpectedly uttered in an appropriate context when girls were highly motivated. However the girls seemed very sensitive to body language and emotional contact. Lindberg (1991) found that pictures of familiar situations appeared to be understood by most girls.

In the British Survey 71% (129 of 182) of classic girls developed words before regression and 29% (52/182) had none. One girl developed her first words only after regression. Of those 129 who had words before regression 20% (26/129) retained some of these after regression. Speech which included phrases was preserved in 4.4% of the whole group (8/182). Atypical girls are often so called due to good head growth and developmental stagnation rather than regression, although they appear to have the Rett disorder. Among 102 questionnaire responders for such girls, preserved speech in phrases and sentences was more common, 13/102 (13%). The girls with the best vocabulary may answer simple questions indicating understanding of speech. In our experience this has been at a concrete level, sufficient to indicate retention of a small vocabulary and the ability to associate objects with their labels.

1.6.12 Cognitive skills and mood

The traditional methods of psychological testing are difficult to use and perhaps inappropriate given the severe but uncertain level of executive control and irregular cognitive profile in Rett. It is clear however that within the disorder there is a wide range in mental abilities. Among the most severe there may be no sign of recognition even of a parent nor of understanding of speech, and among the least affected there may be clear recognition of both with indications of complex relationships and distinct preferences.

Lindberg (1991) studied 39 Swedish girls and women and found a neurodevelopmental level of less than 2 years regardless of age. On starting school (7 years in Sweden) all were assessed as 'severely mentally retarded'. The girls' intellectual functioning seemed to fluctuate. On some occasions they gave the impression of enjoying funny situations and jokes, and at other times they appeared quite withdrawn. Responses were delayed. Witt Engerström (1990) observed a faint reaction to pain in 9 of 20 girls. The play repertoire never matured from the functional, sensorimotor to the imaginative stage; however conditioned learning was usual.

In 18 girls Fontanesi and Haas (1988) reported relative preservation of gross motor and daily living skills at the developmental level at onset of regression, while other adaptive functions were poorer. Their results indicated that islands of motor and intellectual functions persist in RS. Lindberg (1991) emphasized the impact of 'apraxia', multiple dysfunction, and fluctuating attention on the girls' ability to achieve their potential; however she found object permanence and understanding of pictures of familiar situations. Perry et al. (1991) found social skills to be significantly correlated with age at onset of regression. Unlike Fontanesi and Haas they found mental age to decrease with increasing chronological age.

Families generally indicate that girls will 'read a situation'—for example, expecting a meal when the time and the sounds from the kitchen suggest this, fetching the coat (if able) when the family is getting ready to go out, excited when the school bus arrives, etc. Girls also seem to 'read' emotional situations, laughing when others are happy and attending to confidences; however responses are quite non-specific and even the more able classic girls who can follow a simple instruction seem unable to grasp and develop a concept. Conditioned learning seems to be universal and simple interactive games are clearly enjoyed and anticipated. Humour of the 'slap stick' variety is certainly present — dropping a plate or spilling a drink. Laughter is the usual response when someone in the family is scolded.

Memory is generally agreed to be intact at some level and ambulant girls will revisit the room where they found something agreeable. Signs of recognition are commonly seen when a favourite person appears unexpectedly.

Over-alertness or agitation are usual, especially in young post-regression girls, and sudden changes of mood occur, sometimes with screaming and tears which can switch to laughter without obvious reason. Laughter is common on waking at night. However appropriate moods also occur and sad moods do respond to gentle reassurance.

The response to music is impressive and many people show distinct preferences, often favouring a strong beat and a colourful range in pitch and timbre. Music can change the mood of the girl from sad and angry to contented, or occasionally may provoke an angry response if the 'wrong music' is offered. Most girls have favourite tunes and those which seem to satisfy them on particular occasions, and favourite tunes or videos produce highly predictable reactions. Taste in music does seem to change through life, from Teletubbies, 'Postman Pat' and the 'Singing Kettle' in early childhood to 'disco' song and dance music in adolescence. We have observed an immediate effect reducing pulse rate and blood pressure when music was introduced in the course of sessions of autonomic monitoring, strengthening the impression that music exerts a greater influence than speech (Wilson, student project (personal report); Kerr *et al.* 1987; Chapter 12, Chapter 13).

There has been much interest in the use of the computer by girls with RS. Among the girls and women with the classic syndrome we have observed such actions as switching on a radio or TV and touching a computer screen to win responses, but although we have watched girls press keys at a computer spontaneously, we have not so far observed independent selection of a sequence of meaningful letters in girls with the classic syndrome. However such skill is clearly compatible with the milder forms of the disorder (see earlier example in Section 1.3).

The evidence on cognition from clinical testing and observation in classic RS matches the results of a study by Bieber Nielsen *et al.* (1990), who found the regional blood flow in pre-frontal and temporo-parietal association regions of the telencephalon to be markedly reduced, whereas the primary sensorimotor regions were relatively spared. This suggests a distribution of brain metabolic activity comparable to that of infants of a few months of age and corresponding to the pre-reaching stage. Using single photon emission computerized tomography (SPECT) in seven girls with RS (18–48 months) Uvebrant *et al.* (1993) demonstrated hypoperfusion of the frontal lobe, especially left side, midbrain, brain stem and cerebellum.

1.7 Deaths

Deaths occur in classic Rett syndrome later than in many other profoundly intellectually disabling conditions. The annual death rate in classic Rett syndrome has been estimated at 1.4% (Sweden) and 1.2% (Britain) (Kerr *et al.* 1997). Of 31 deaths in well-documented British girls and women with the classic syndrome, 15 (48%) died in a wasted condition and these had previously been classified as 'fragile', having both very severe Rett disorder and being in poor health. These deaths mainly clustered between 15 and 20 years. Four other deaths (13%) occurred in people with severe recent epilepsy and four (13%) were due to causes apparently unrelated to Rett. However eight (26%) were completely unexpected and sudden deaths and these occurred across the age range. Poor autonomic control was considered likely to have played a significant part (Kerr *et al.* 1997).

1.8 The clinical range in Rett disorder

The wide range of clinical severity in the Rett disorder was first demonstrated by pairs of monozygotic twins who were clearly concordant for the syndrome but dissimilar in severity (Kerr 1992; Percy 1992); however it has remained difficult to reach a firm diagnosis in other cases which did not meet the criteria for the classic syndrome until the discovery of mutations on the MECP2 gene in most classic cases (Amir *et al.* 1999; Wan *et al.* 1999). The 'atypical Rett' category has therefore remained useful. It is to be expected that among these 'atypical' cases some will prove to have the Rett disorder and some to have other disorders which have affected the neural infrastructure in a similar way. Such disorders will certainly include some cases of cerebral palsy due to pre-, intra- and perinatal birth events, tuberose sclerosis with brain stem involvement, some embryonic brain stem tumours, infantile varieties of neuronal ceroid lipofuscinosis and other infantile degenerative disorders (Hagberg and Witt Engerström 1990b, Santavuouri *et al.* 1974, Santavuori 1982, 1988).

A group with atypical syndrome but Rett disorder seems likely to include some people in whom epilepsy was diagnosed before regression. Hagberg has called this the 'early seizure variant' (Hagberg and Gillberg 1993; Hagberg 1995; Hagberg and Skjeldal 1994). As seizures come under control, the signs of the classic Rett picture may appear but in others the final clinical picture remains different and the question arises whether severe early seizures have themselves damaged the brain in a similar way to the Rett disorder or altered the usual presentation. Some families with a girl with classic Rett syndrome report minor signs such as repeated blinking in the pre-regression period and these may be seen on some pre-regression videos suggesting that a minor form of epilepsy may occur before regression more often than has been recognized.

The term 'atypical Rett' presently includes people who differ from the classic picture only in degree, with developmental stagnation rather than regression and without obvious interruption of head growth. In our experience, in these people muscle tone is also less severely affected and skills are better than in classic cases and other Rett neurological signs often appear later. Hagberg has designated this as 'formes fruste' (Hagberg and Rasmussen 1986; Hagberg and Skjeldal 1994) and it is agreed that these are likely to have the Rett disorder.

Males with possible Rett disorder constitute a group of particular interest (Philippart 1990). As far as we are aware, the only males with undoubted classical Rett syndrome have also had Klinefelter's syndrome (Naidu, personal communication; Schwartzman *et al.* 1999) and the clinical characteristics of the atypical males have still to be thoroughly studied. In our experience these people are more often dysmorphic than people with classic Rett syndrome and visual defects have been found in some. The discovery of Rett mutations on the MECP2 gene will help to clarify these and the other 'atypical Rett' situations.

In future, confirmation of diagnosis is likely to depend on genetic investigation; however the clinical picture will remain of central importance. The mainly sporadic occurrence of the disorder means that in most cases the clinical signs must be recognized before the correct diagnosis can be made and early recognition will be increasingly important, mild and unusual cases presenting a particular challenge.

1.9 Conclusion

From the apparently healthy but too placid baby, through the severe but restricted regression crisis to a characteristic profile of disabilities and skills, the clinical evidence of the Rett syndrome points to a very early developmental defect and consequent failure of integration in cognitive, motor and autonomic processes. In 18 years of clinical and neuro-physiological research, observation of the many aspects of this disorder has pointed us to the brain stem as the core of the problem. This is the conductor of the growing brain, the foundation on which higher functions depend and it is here we should look for early indications of the defect in function which results from the genetic fault.

The chapters which follow present the laboratory based evidence on the disease, placing it in the context of the early growth of the brain. This evidence is essential if we are to understand, prevent and treat the condition; however the importance of the clinical picture itself cannot be overemphasized. Every detail of the girl's capacities and problems provides instruction on the neural pathways and networks which are spared and those which are impaired by the disorder. This has formed the basis for the entire investigation and so it is the attractive but profoundly disabled child who has commanded the research. It is also to this child with her problems and possibilities that the answers must finally be brought from the laboratories and it will be the quality of her life which will judge the success of that research.

Acknowledgements

A.K. has been supported by the Rett Associations in Scotland (NRSA), England (RSA UK) and the USA (IRSA) and University of Glasgow. We gladly acknowledge the assistance of the many families and girls with Rett syndrome whose presence and shared insights form the basis for the studies, and many professional colleagues and collaborators, individually referenced.

I.W.E. is supported by Östersund Hospital Foundation for Medical Research, the National Association for the Neurologically Disabled in Sweden and Marcus and Amalia Wallenberg Memorial Foundation.

References

Akesson, H.O., Hagberg, B., Wahlstrom, J., and Witt Engerström, I. (1992). Rett Syndrome a search for gene sources. *American Journal of Medical Genetics*, 42, 104–110.
Amir, R.E., Van Den Veyver, I.B., Wan, M., Tran, C.Q., Franke, U. and Zoghbi, H. (1999). Rett Syndrome is caused by mutations in X-linked MECP2, encoding methyl CpG binding protein 2. *Nature Genetics*, 23, 185–8.
Armstrong, D.D. (1992). The neuropathology of the Rett syndrome. *Brain and Development*, 14, 89–98.
Armstrong, D.D. (1995). The neuropathology of Rett Syndrome—overview 1994. *Neuropediatrics*, 26, 100–104.
Asthana, J.C., Sinha, S., Haslam, J.S., and Kingston, H.M. (1990). Survey of adolescents with severe intellectual handicap. *Archives of Disease in Childhood*, 65, 1133–6.
Babinski, J. (1898). Du phenomene des orteils et de sa valeur semiologique. *Semaine Medicale*, 18, 321–2.
Badr, G.G., Witt Engerström, I., and Hagberg, B. (1987). Brain stem and spinal cord impairment in Rett Syndrome: somatosensory and auditory evoked responses investigations. *Brain and Development*, 9, 517–22.
Bader, G.G., Witt Engerström, I. and Hagberg, B. (1989). Neurophysiological findings in the Rett Syndrome I — e.e.g. and somatosensory evoked potential studies. *Brain and Development*, 11, 102–9.
Bader, G.G., Witt Engerström, I. and Hagberg, B. (1989). Neurophysiological findings in the Rett Syndrome II — Visual and auditory brain stem middle and late evoked responses. *Brain and Development*, 11, 110–4.
Bieber Nielsen, J., Friberg, L., Lou, H., Lassen, N.A., and Sam, I.L.K. (1990) Immature pattern of brain activity in Rett syndrome. *Archives of Neurology*, 47, 982–6.
Bolthauser, E., Lange, B. and Dumermuth, G. (1987). Differential diagnosis of syndromes with abnormal respiration (tachypnea-apnea). *Brain and Development* 9, 462–5.
Budden, S.S. (1995). Management of Rett Syndrome: a ten year experience. *Neuropediatrics*, 26, 75–7.

Christen, H.-J. and Hanefeld, F. (1995). Male Rett Variant. *Neuropediatrics*, **26**, 81–2.

Cirignotta, F., Lugaresci, E., and Montagna, P. (1986). Breathing impairment in Rett Syndrome. *American Journal of Medical Genetics*, **24**, 167–73.

Cooper, R.A., Kerr, A.M., and Amos, P.M. (1998). Rett syndrome: critical examination of clinical features, serial e.e.g. and video-monitoring in understanding and management. *European Journal of Paediatric Neurology*, **2**, 127–5.

Diagnostic Criteria Working Group (1988). Diagnostic criteria for Rett syndrome. *Annals of Neurology*, **23**, 425–8.

Eyre, J.A., Kerr, A.M., Miller, S., O'Sullivan, M.C., and Ramesh, V. (1990). Neurophysiological observations on corticospinal projections to the upper limb in subjects with Rett syndrome. *Journal of Neurology, Neurosurgery and Psychiatry*, **53**, 874–9.

Fontanesi, J. and Haas, R.H. (1988). Cognitive profile of Rett syndrome. *Journal of Child Neurology*, **3** (Suppl), 20–4.

Glasson, E.J., Thomson, M.R., Leonard, S., Rousham, E., Christodoulou, J., Ellaway, C., and Leonard, H. (1998). Diagnosis of Rett Syndrome: can a radiograph help?. *Developmental Medicine and Child Neurology*, **40**, 737–42.

Glaze, D.G., Frost, J.D., Miller, H.Y., and Percy, A.K. (1987). Rett's Syndrome: correlation of electroencephalographic characteristics with clinical staging. *Archives of Neurology*, **44**, 1053–56.

Hagberg, B., Goutieres, F., Hanefeld, F., Rett, A. and Wilson, J. (1985). Rett Syndrome: criteria for inclusion and exclusion. *Brain and Development*, **7**, 372–3.

Hagberg, B. and Gillberg, C. (1993). Rett Variants — **Rettoid types**. In *Rett Syndrome — clinical and biological aspects*, Clinics in Developmental Medicine, Vol. 127 (ed. B. Hagberg, M. Anvret, M.Anvert, and J. Wahlstrom). MacKeith Cambridge University Press, Cambridge, ISBN 0 521 41283 8

Hagberg, B. and Hagberg, G. (1997). Rett Syndrome: epidemiology and geographical variability. *European Child and Adolescent Psychiatry*, **6**, 5–7.

Hagberg, B. and Rasmussen, P. (1986). Forme Fruste of Rett Syndrome — a case report. *American Journal of Medical Genetics*, **24**, 175–81.

Hagberg, B. and Skjeldal, O. (1994) Rett Variants: a suggested model for inclusion criteria. *Pediatric Neurology*, **11**, 5–11.

Hagberg, B. and Witt Engerström, I. (1986) Rett Syndrome: a suggested staging system for describing impairment profile with increasing age towards adolescence. *American Journal of Medical Genetics*, **24**, 47–59.

Hagberg, B. and Witt Engerström, I. (1990a). Swedish Rett syndrome basic data register 1960–90. In Witt Engerström, I., Rett syndrome in Sweden. Neurodevelopment—disability—pathophysiology. *Acta Paediatrica Scandinavia* (Suppl. 369), ISBN 91–628–0081–7.

Hagberg, B. and Witt Engerström, I. (1990b). Early stages Rett syndrome and infantile neuronal ceroid lipofuscinosis—a difficult differential diagnosis. *Brain and Development*, **12**, 20–2.

Hagberg, B., Aicardi, J., Dias, K., and Ramos, O. (1983). A progressive syndrome of autism, dementia, ataxia and loss of purposeful hand use in girls: Rett's syndrome—report of 35 cases. *Annals of Neurology*, **14**, 471–9.

Hagberg, B., Goutieres, F., Hanefeld, F., Rett, A., and Wilson, J. (1985). Rett syndrome—criteria for inclusion and exclusion. *Brain and Development*, **7**, 372–3.

Hagberg, G., Stenbom, Y. and Witt Engerström, I. (2000). Head growth in Rett Syndrome. *Acta Pediatrica*, **89**, 198–202.

Hagne, I., Witt Engerström, I., and Hagberg, B. (1989). EEG development in Rett syndrome. A study of 30 cases. *Electroencephalography and Clinical Neurophysiology*, **72**, 1–6.

Heinen, F. and Korinthenberg, R. (1996). Does transcranial magnetic stimulation allow early diagnosis of Rett syndrome? *Neuropediatrics*, **27**, 223–4.

Holm, V.A. (1986). Physical growth and development in patients with Rett Syndrome. *American Journal of Medical Genetics*, **24**, 119–6.

Ishikawa, A., Goto, T., Narasaki, M., Yokochi, K., Kitahra, H., and Fukuyama, Y. (1978). A new syndrome (?) of progressive psychomotor deterioration with peculiar stereotyped movement and autistic tendency: a report of three cases. *Brain and Development*, **3**, 258.

Julu, P.O.O. (1992). A linear scale for measuring vagal tone in man. *Journal of Autonomic Pharmacology*, **12**, 109–15.

Julu, P.O.O., Delamont, R.S., and Jamal, G.A. (1993). The vagal tone during non-progressing non-REM sleep in sleep deprived human subjects. *Journal of Physiology* (*London*), **459**, 146.

Julu, P.O.O., Kerr, A.M., Hansen, S., Apartopoulos, S. F., and Jamal, G.A. (1997). Functional evidence of brain stem immaturity in Rett Syndrome. *European Child and Adolescent psychiatry*, **6**, 47–54.

Julu, P.O.O., Kerr, A.M., Hansen, S., Apartopoulos, F., and Jamal, G. (1998) Cardio-respiratory instability in Rett Syndrome suggests medullary serotononergic dysfunction. In Witt Engerström I and Kerr A.M. meeting report. Workshop on Autonomic Function in Rett Syndrome. Swedish Rett Centre, Froson, Sweden, May 1998. *Brain and Development* **20**, 323–6.

Julu, P.O.O., Kerr, A.M., Hansen, S., Apartopoulos, F., Witt Engerström, I., and Engerström, L. Characterisation of the breathing and autonomic abnormality in Rett Syndrome, in preparation.

Kerr, A.M. (1987). Report on the Rett Syndrome Workshop: Glasgow, Scotland, 24–25 May 1986. *Journal of Mental Deficiency Research*, **31**, 93–113.

Kerr, A. (1992*a*). A review of the respiratory disorder in the Rett syndrome. *Brain and Development*, **14** (**Suppl**), 43–5.

Kerr, A.M. (1992*b*). Rett Syndrome British longitudinal study (1982–1990) and 1990 survey. In *Mental retardation and redical care* (ed. J.J. Roosendaal), 21–24 April **1991**, pp. 143–5. Uitgeverij Kerckbosch. Zeist ISBN 9067201219.

Kerr, A.M. (1995). Early clinical signs in the Rett Disorder. *Neuropediatrics*, **26**, 67–71.

Kerr, A.M. and Stephenson, J.P.B. (1985). Rett's Syndrome in the west of Scotland. *British Medical Journal*, **291**, 579–82.

Kerr, A.M. and Stephenson, J.B.P. (1986). A study of the natural history of Rett syndrome in 23 girls. *American Journal of Medical Genetics*, **24**, 77–83.

Kerr, A.M., Armstrong, D.D., Prescott, R.J., Doyle, D, and Kearney, D.L. (1997). Analysis of deaths in the British Rett Survey. *European Child and Adolescent Psychiatry*, **6**, 71–4.

Kerr, A.M., Mitchell, J.M., and Robertson, P. (1995). Short fourth toes in Rett Syndrome: a biological indicator. *Neuropediatics*, **26**, 72–4.

Kerr, A. M., Montague, J., and Stephenson, J.B.P. (1987). The hands, and the mind, pre- and post-regression in Rett syndrome. *Brain and Development*, **9**, 487–90.

Kerr, A.M., Robertson, P.E., and Mitchell, J. (1993). Rett Syndrome and the 4th metatarsal. *Archives of Disease in Childhood*, **68**, 433.

Kerr, A.M., Southall, D., Amos, P., Cooper, R., Samuels, M., Mitchell, J. and Stephenson, J. (1990). Correlation of electroencephalogram, respiration and movement in the Rett syndrome. *Brain and Development*, **12**, 61–8.

Kultz, J., Rohmann, E., and Hobusch, D. (1990). A study of the Rett Syndrome in the GDR. *Brain and Development*, **12**, 37–9.

Leonard, H. and Bower, C. (1998). Is the girl with Rett Syndrome normal at birth? *Developmental Medicine and Child Neurology*, **40**, 115–21.

Leonard, H., Thomson, M.M., Lasson, E., Fyfe, S., Leonard, S., Ellaway, C., Christodoulou, J., and Bower, C. (1999) Metacarpophaloangeal pattern profile and bone age in Rett Syndrome: further radiological clues to the diagnosis. *American Journal of Medical Genetics*, **83**, 88–95.

Lindberg, B. (1991). *Dealing with Rett syndrome—a practical guide for parents, teachers and psychologists*. Hogrefe & Huber, Toronto.

Loder, R.T., Lee, C.L., and Stephens Richards, B. (1989). Orthopaedic aspects of Rett Syndrome: a multicentre review. *Journal of Pediatric Orthopedics*, 9, 557–62.

Lugaresi, E. and Cirignotta, F. (1982). An unusual type of respiratory apraxia. In Henri Gastaut and the Marseilles school's contribution to the neurosciences (ed. R.J.Broughton), pp. 317–22. Elsevier, Amsterdam.

Lugaresi, E., Cirignotta, F., and Montana, P. (1985). Abnormal breathing in the Rett syndrome. *Brain and Development*, 7, 329–33.

Morton, R.E., Bonas, R., Minford, J., Kerr, A., and Ellis, R.E. (1997). Feeding ability in Rett Syndrome. *Developmental Medicine and Child Neurology*, 39, 331–5.

Motil, K.J., Schultz, R., Brown, B., Glaze, D.G., and Percy, A.K. (1994). Altered energy balance may account for growth failure in Rett Syndrome. *Journal of Child Neurology*, 9. 315–9

Naidu, S. (1997). Rett Syndrome: a disorder affecting early brain growth. *Annals of Neurology*, 42(1), 3–10.

Naidu, S., Hyman, S., Harris, E.L., Narayanan, V., Johns, D., and Castora, K. (1995). Rett syndrome studies of natural history and search for a genetic marker. *Neuropediatrics*, 26, 63–6.

Nomura, Y. and Segawa, M. (1990). Clinical features of the early stage of the Rett syndrome. *Brain and Development*, 12, 16–19.

Nomura, Y. and Segawa, M. (1992). Motor symptoms of the Rett syndrome: abnormal muscle tone, posture, locomotion and stereotyped movement. *Brain and Development*, 14(Suppl.), 21–8.

Nomura, Y., Honda, K., and Segawa, M. (1987). Pathophysiology of Rett syndrome. *Brain and Development*, 9, 506–13.

Nomura, Y., Segawa, M., and Hasegawa, M. (1984). Rett syndrome — clinical studies and pathophysiological considerations. *Brain and Development*, 6, 475–86.

Pelson, R.O. and Budden, S. (1987). Auditory brain stem response findings in Rett Syndrome. *Brain and Development*, 9, 514–16.

Percy, A.K. (1992). The Rett Syndrome: the recent advances in genetic studies in the USA. *Brain and Development*, 14(S), 104–5.

Percy, A., Zoghbi, H, and Riccardi, V. (1985). Rett Syndrome; initial experience with an emerging clinical entity. *Brain and Development*, 7, 300–4.

Percy, A. (1992). Neurochemistry of the Rett Syndrome. *Brain and Developments*, 14, (**Suppl.**): S57–S62.

Perry, A. (1991). Rett Syndrome: a comprehensive review of the literature. *American Journal on Mental Retardation*, 96, 275–90.

Philippart, M. (1990). The Rett syndrome in males. *Brain and Development*, 12, 33–6.

Ray, A. and Haldane, J. (1965).The genetics of a common Indian digital abnormality.*Proceedings of the National Academy of Sciences*, 53, 1050–53.

Rett, A. (1966). Uber ein eigenartiges hirnatrophisches Syndrome bei hyperammonamie im Kindsalter. *Wiener Medizinische Wochenschrift*, 116, 723–6.

Rice, M.A. and Haas, R.H. (1988). The nutritional aspects of Rett Syndrome. *Journal of Child Neurology*, 3, (**Suppl**), S35–42.

Roberts, A.P. and Connor, A.N. (1988). Orthopaedic aspects of Rett's Syndrome: short report. *Journal of Bone and Joint Surgery*, 70, 2079–95.

Santavuori, P. (1982). Clinical findings in 69 patients with infantile type of neuronal ceroid lipofuscinosis. In *Ceroid lipofuscinosis (Batten's disease)* (ed. D. Armstrong, N. Koppang, and J.A. Rider), pp. 23–33. Elsevier, Biomedical Press.

Santavuori, P. (1988). Neuronal ceroid-lipofuscinosis in childhood. *Brain and Development*, 10, 80–3.

Santavuori, P., Haltia, M., and Rapola, J. (1974). Infantile type of so-called neuronal ceroid-lipofuscinosis. *Developmental Medicine and Child Neurology*, 16, 644–53.

Saunders, K.J., McCulloch, D.L., and Kerr, A.M. (1995). Visual function in Rett Syndrome. *Developmental Medicine and Child Neurology*, 37, 496–504.

Schanen, C. and Francke, U. (1998). A severely affected male born into a Rett Syndrome kindred supports X-linked inheritance and allows extension of the exclusion map. *American Journal of Human Genetics*, **63**, 267–9.

Schultz, R.J., Glaze, D.G., Motil, K.J., Armstrong, D.D., Del Junco, D.J., and Percy, A.K. (1993). The pattern of growth failure in Rett syndrome. *American Journal of Disease in Childhood*, **147**, 633–7.

Schwartzman, J.S., Zatz, M., Vasquez, L.D.R., Gomez, R.R., Koiffmann, C.P., Fridman, C. and Otto, P.G. (1999). Rett Syndrome in A boy with 47, XXY karyotype. *Am. J. Hum. Genet.*, **64**, 1781–5.

Segawa, M. and Nomura, Y. (1990). The pathophysiology of the Rett syndrome from the standpoint of polysomnography. *Brain and Development*, **12**, 55–60.

Sekul, E.A., Moak, J.P., Schultz, R.J., Glaze, D.G., Dunn, J.K., and Percy, A.K. (1994). Electrocardiographic findings in Rett Syndrome: an explanation of sudden death. *Journal of Pediatrics*, **125**, 80–2.

Southall, D.P., Kerr, A.M., Tirosh, E., Amos. P., Lang. M., and Stephenson, J.B.P. (1988). Hyperventilation in the awake state potentially treatable component of Rett Syndrome. *Archives of Disease in Childhood*, **63**, 1039–48.

Stenbom, Y., Witt Engerström, I., and Hagberg, G. (1995). Gross motor disability and head growth in Rett syndrome — a preliminary report. *Neuropediatrics*, **26**, 85–6.

Stockland, E., Lidstrom J. and Hagberg, B. Scoliosis in Rett Syndrome. (1993) In *Rett Syndrome-Clinical and Biological Aspects*, Clinics in Developmental Medicine, Vol. 127 (ed B. Hagberg), pp 61–71. MacKeith. London ISBN 0 521 41283 8.

Thommessen, M., Heiberg, A., Kase, B.F., Larsen, S., and Riis, G. (1991). Feeding problems, height and weight in different groups of disabled children. *Acta Paediatrica Scandinavia*, **80**, 527–33.

Uvebrant, P., Bjure, J., Sixt, R., Witt Engerström, I., and Hagberg, B. (1993). Regional cerebral blood flow: SPECT as a tool for localisation of brain dysfunction. In *Rett syndrome—clinical and biological aspects*, Clinics in Developmental Medicine, Vol. 127 (ed. B. Hagberg), pp. 80–5. MacKeith, London.

Verma, N.P., Ramesh, L., Chheda, R.L., Nigro, M.A. and Hart, Z.H. (1986). Electroencephalographic findings in Rett syndrome. *Electroencephalography and Clinical Neurophysiology*, **64**, 394–401.

Von Tetzchner, S. (1997). Communication skills among females with Rett Syndrome. *European Child and Adolescent Psychiatry*, **6**, (Suppl. 1), 33–7.

Wan, M., Lee, S.S.J.L., Zhang, X., Houwink-Manville, I., Song, H-R., Amir, R.E., Budden, S., Naidu, S, Pereira, J.L.P., Lo, I.F.M., Zoghbi, H.Y., Schanen, N.C., and Francke, U. (1999). Rett Syndrome and beyond: recurrent spontaneous and familial MECP2 mutations at CpG hotspots. *American Journal of Human Genetics*, **65**, 1520–29.

Witt Engerström, I. (1987). Rett Syndrome: a retrospective pilot study of potential early predictive symptomatology. *Brain and Development*, **9**, 481–6.

Witt Engerström, I. (1990). Rett Syndrome in Sweden. Neurodevelopment—disability—pathophysiology. *Acta Paediatrica Scandinavica* (**Suppl.369**).

Witt Engerström, I. (1992*a*). Rett Syndrome: the late infantile regression period—a retrospective analysis of 91 cases. *Acta Paediatrica Scandinavica*, **81**, 167–72.

Witt Engerström, I. (1992b). Age related occurrence of signs and symptoms in Rett syndrome. *Brain and Development*, **14** (**Suppl**.), 11–20.

Witt Engerström, I. (1993). Evolution of clinical signs in Rett Syndrome. In *Rett Syndrome-Clinical and Biological Aspects*, Clinics in Developmental Medicine, Vol. 127 (ed B. Hagberg), pp 61–71. MacKeith. London ISBN 0 521 412838.

Witt Engerström, I. and Forslund, M. (1992). Mother and daughter with Rett Syndrome. *Developmental Medicine and Child Neurology*, **34**, 1022–23.

Witt Engerström, I. and Hagberg, B. (1990). Rett Syndrome: gross motor disability and neural impairment in adults. *Brain and Development*, **12**, 23–6.

Witt Engerström, I. and Kerr, A.M. (1998). Workshop on autonomic function in Rett Syndrome. Swedish Rett Centre, Froson, Sweden, May **1998**, *Brain and Development*, **5**, 323–6.

Woodyatt, G.C. and Ozanne, A.E. (1993). A longitudinal study of cognitive skills and communication behaviours in children with Rett Syndrome. *Journal of Intellectual Disability Research*, **37**, 419–35.

Zappella, M. (1992). The Rett girls with preserved speech. *Brain and Development*, **14**, 998–1001.

Zappella, M. (1997). The preserved speech variant of the Rett complex: a report of 8 cases. *European Child and Adolescent Psychiatry*, **6**, 23–25.

Zappella, M. and Cerioli, M. (1987). High prevalence of Rett Syndrome in a small area. *Brain and Development*, **9**, 479–80.

2 Towards the genetic basis of Rett syndrome

Angus Clarke, Carolyn Schanen, and Maria Anvret

Summary

This chapter reviews the clinical evidence that Rett Syndrome was likely to be genetic, and most probably inherited as an X-linked dominant, male-lethal disorder. We describe the molecular genetic studies that suggested the location of the Rett syndrome gene at Xq28 and the reports of mutations in the *MECP2* gene in many affected females. We discuss the implications of these findings for our understanding of the disease mechanisms that result in the typical clinical features of Rett syndrome.

2.1 Rett syndrome and inheritance

2.1.1 Sex-linked inheritance

In Andreas Rett's original description of the condition was the key observation that all affected individuals were female (Rett 1966*a,b*, 1977). Almost all definite cases of Rett syndrome (RS) described since have been female. It is this observation, together with the (almost complete) concordance of monozygotic female twins for the disorder, that has led so many investigators to conclude that RS must be genetic in origin although almost all cases are sporadic. The most convincing reports of males with RS have been of boys with mosaic or complete Klinefelter syndrome (Vorsanova *et al.* 1996; Schwartzman *et al.* 1999).

Traits that are sex-limited but not sex-linked need not be genetic in origin but will then usually manifest in a tissue affected by sexual differentiation; for example, tuberculous epididymitis would be impossible in a woman. This is an implausible explanation for the apparent sparing of males in Rett syndrome, in which the organ most seriously damaged is the brain.

Sex-linked traits have been recognized since Morgan's elucidation of the inheritance of the white-eyed trait in Drosophila melanogaster in 1911. Many such traits are recognized in Homo sapiens; the vast majority of such X-linked recessive conditions are manifest in hemizygous males whose single X chromosome carries a mutant allele at the relevant locus, whereas female carriers heterozygous for such mutant alleles—with one altered copy of the gene and one intact copy—usually have few signs. There are disorders, however, caused by mutations at X chromosome loci which manifest as readily in females as in males—X-linked dominant disorders.

What determines whether a mutation in an X chromosome gene will lead to a dominant condition or to a recessive condition? There are two principal factors influencing the degree to which an X-linked condition will manifest in a heterozygous female—the pattern of X chromosome inactivation in combination with the biology of the gene product.

A primary factor influencing the manifestation of a sex-linked disorder in a female is the process of X chromosome inactivation in the relevant tissues. Females inactivate one of their two copies of the X chromosome in each cell so that those heterozygous for X-linked mutations (having one intact copy and one altered copy of the gene) are, at the cellular level, mosaic for expression of the gene. The decision as to which X chromosome is to be inactivated is made independently and at random in different cells in the early embryo, but each cell derived from those early embryonic cells inactivates the same X as its 'parent' cell. Where the clone of cells derived from one such embryonic cell remain contiguous, as may occur in the skin, the retina and various epithelia, the tissue will consist of discrete patches of normal phenotype and other patches of mutant phenotype.

The pattern of X chromosome inactivation in the relevant tissues influences the degree to which the mutant phenotype is manifest. Most women have an approximately balanced pattern of X inactivation in most tissues, but marked skewing can occur with either the maternal or the paternal X chromosome being preferentially inactivated. This occasionally happens by chance—perhaps more frequently with female monozygotic twins because of the reduced number of cells contributing to an MZ twin at the time of X inactivation—but may also occur as a result of selection against one or the other type of cell. This can arise if one of the female's X chromosomes is involved in a reciprocal translocation with an autosome, and it leads to strong selection against those cells in which the translocated X chromosome is inactivated. Similarly, if one X chromosome carries a mutation that leads to reduced viability of cells expressing the mutant gene, then cells in the relevant tissue will preferentially utilize the intact allele. In the X-linked immunodeficiency disorders, for example, most of a female carrier's circulating B- or T-lymphocytes will have inactivated the mutant copy of the gene. Where the X chromosome carrying the disease-associated allele is preferentially active in a relevant tissue, then that female is more likely to manifest signs of the condition.

The other principal factor influencing the manifestation of a sex-linked disorder in a female is the biology of the gene product. If it has a catalytic function, as with clotting factors in the coagulation cascades (e.g. factors IX and VIII) or enzymes of intermediary metabolism (e.g. hypoxanthine–guanosine phosphoribosyl transferase), then most female carriers are likely to escape without problems so that mutations in these genes will usually act as recessive alleles. In contrast, however, if the level of enzyme activity is rate-determining for an especially critical and cell autonomous metabolic pathway (as with pyruvate dehydrogenase), then females are likely to manifest symptoms. Similarly, their status as carriers may be recognized quite readily if the gene is expressed in an epithelial tissue such as the skin, the retina or the renal tubular epithelium. For example, vitamin D-resistant, hypophosphataemic rickets is an X-linked dominant disorder that manifests in both females and males because it results from the leak of phosphate across the renal tubular epithelium. In females with normal (ie random) X inactivation, half of the epithelium leaks, leading to symptoms similar to those seen in affected males.

Certain X chromosome gene defects are frequently lethal in infancy in affected males, as with ornithine carbamoyl transferase (OCT) deficiency and Menkes disease. Female carriers of OCT deficiency only occasionally develop frank protein intolerance and carriers of Menkes disease are usually healthy.

In a few sex-linked disorders, the effects on the affected male are so severe that they are incompatible with survival of the fetus, while a female carrier of the condition is highly likely to manifest the condition in some form. The female carrier can survive because her normal tissues—those utilizing the unaffected X chromosome—rescue her from the otherwise lethal effects of the mutation. Such conditions are known as X-linked dominant, male-lethal (XDML) disorders, and they include the Goltz syndrome (of focal dermal hypoplasia), the Aicardi syndrome (if it is distinct from the Goltz syndrome) and Incontinentia Pigmenti (IP). Although the first such gene to be identified was the murine locus for 'bare patches' and 'striated', which is a 3-β-hydroxysteroid dehydrogenase involved in cholesterol metabolism (Liu *et al.* 1999), the clinically best characterized human XDML disease is Incontinentia Pigmenti (IP).

Incontinentia Pigmenti affects predominantly females and the analysis of family pedigrees reveals female-to-female transmission, an increased incidence of miscarriages and a deficit of males in the offspring of affected women (Landy and Donnai 1995). As in RS, a number of affected males have two X chromosomes, i.e. Klinefelter syndrome (Scheuerle 1998). Family linkage studies have localized the gene to Xq28, while the X chromosome breakpoints of cytogenetic rearrangements identified in a few sporadic patients with a clinical diagnosis of IP have involved the proximal short arm at Xp11. The underlying pathology in these latter cases is most likely distinct from that in familial IP, probably reflecting the partial failure of the inactivation process on the X chromosome short arm in some cells

(Hatchwell *et al.* 1996; Hatchwell 1996). Furthermore, if the gene responsible for an X-linked dominant, male-lethal Mendelian disorder is disrupted by a chromosomal translocation in a female fetus, then that fetus would be predicted to be similar to a hemizygous, male fetus and would not be expected to survive to term—so the translocations are unlikely to disrupt a locus involved in the Mendelian form of IP. In such a fetus, those cell lineages that inactivate the X chromosome involved in the translocation will often fail because of functional gene dosage problems: the X inactivation process will affect the autosomal material translocated onto the X while those X chromosome sequences translocated onto the relevant autosome will not be subject to inactivation at all.

There has been a theoretical possibility that RS could be one of the very few X-linked conditions in which females are affected and males are spared—as in one family with epilepsy and mental handicap limited to females (Ryan *et al.* 1997). This has always been most improbable, however, and we now know that it is mistaken.

It was suggested by Hagberg *et al.* (1983), Comings (1986) and Zoghbi (1988) that RS may be an XDML disorder. This has been the working hypothesis of most clinicians and researchers since 1983. We will examine this model of RS inheritance.

2.1.2 The Rett syndrome phenotype—what needs to be explained

Given that RS is most likely caused by genetic pathology, then what important phenotypic features of the disorder must be accounted for by any explanation, in addition to the mode of inheritance?

(1) High mutation rate   The largely sporadic nature of the condition and its high incidence—estimates vary, but a figure of 1 in 10000–15000 girls with the classical form of RS is a reasonable estimate—suggest that the mutation rate for the disease must be high (Kerr and Stephenson 1985; Hagberg 1985a,b; Burd *et al.* 1991; Kozinetz *et al.* 1993). The mutation rate for Duchenne muscular dystrophy (DMD) is approximately 1 in 10,000 per generation; the DMD gene is extremely large and it is thought that its size is a major reason for its high mutation rate, although a range of mutational mechanisms may contribute to this figure. In contrast, sporadic (new mutation) cases of achondroplasia occur with similar frequency to that of RS, yet a single base-pair change resulting from the deamination of a methylated cytosine in a CpG dinucleotide is responsible for the disorder in the vast majority of cases (Rousseau *et al.* 1994). What mechanisms underlie the apparently high mutation rate in RS?

(2) Apparent early normality   In considering a genetic basis for RS, the apparent normality in early infancy of girls who are later clearly affected is an important feature of the condition that needs to be explained. Although it may be

possible, in retrospect, to identify some ways in which girls with RS differ from other infants as a group (Leonard and Bower 1998), it is not usually possible to identify affected infants in the first few months. Rett syndrome pathogenesis must therefore interfere with developmental processes within the central nervous system that are operating in infancy and early childhood, and perhaps in fetal life as well.

(3) Pathological features in the central nervous system   An adequate explanation of RS pathogenesis will have to account for the pathological features evident within the central nervous system (CNS). Neuropathological studies of the brains of affected individuals report a reduction in size of the brain, partly from a reduction in the extent and complexity of the dendritic trees of neurons in layers III and V of the cortex and partly from changes in the cerebellum—a progressive loss of Purkinje cells and cerebellar white matter (Oldfors *et al.* 1990; Armstrong 1992; Chapter 3). Changes in other regions of the brain have also been described, but it is not known which are primary and which are the consequence of altered trophic influences that can reflect or be influenced by CNS function during intrauterine and post-natal development. Brain imaging studies of girls with RS have also found evidence of cortical, cerebellar, basal ganglia and midbrain atrophy; there has been uncertainty as to whether this is progressive (Murakami *et al.* 1992; Reiss *et al.* 1993) but recent results suggest that it is not.

(4) Neurochemical evidence   Changes in the levels of neurotransmitters and their metabolites have been found in the cerebrospinal fluid (CSF) of individuals affected by RS, but none have been consistent (Lekman *et al.* 1990; Percy 1992; Sekul and Percy 1992). Altered levels of homovanillic acid (Nielsen *et al.* 1992), β-endorphin (Myer *et al.* 1992), biopterin (Zoghbi *et al.* 1989) and certain gangliosides (Lekman *et al.* 1991a,b) are all likely to represent secondary changes reflecting the underlying CNS pathology. The more recent finding of reduced levels of nerve growth factor in the CSF of girls with RS is also open to more than one interpretation (Riikonen and Vanhal 1999). A trial of the opiate antagonist, naltrexone, was carried out because of reports of elevated levels of β-endorphins in the CSF; it did not prove to be helpful (Percy *et al.* 1994). Reduced levels of choline acetyltransferase activity have been found post mortem in many cortical and subcortical areas, but the significance of this is also unclear (Wenk *et al.* 1993). Changes in receptor densities for serotonin substance P and NMDA are discussed in Chapters 3, 4 and 5.2.

(5) Neurophysiological evidence   Functional disturbances of the nervous system in RS particularly affect the autonomic nervous system, and could relate to the increase in serotonin receptors found in a number of brainstem nuclei in females with RS (Armstrong *et al.* 1998). The central control of ventilation is disturbed during wakefulness, but not sleep, typically with energetic

ventilation and a difficulty in terminating inspiration (Kerr and Julu 1999). This leads to episodes of hyperventilation alternating with apnoea, resulting sometimes in hypoxemia and sometimes in a marked respiratory alkalosis (Southall *et al.* 1988; Marcus *et al.* 1994; Segawa and Nomura 1992). There is a clear potential for complex interactions in the control of ventilation between systemic CO_2 concentration and pH, localised areas of metabolic acidosis within the hindbrain, the systemic O_2 concentration and the hypoxic drive mechanisms mediated via the carotid chemoreceptors. Along with the dysfunction of other autonomic activities, these anomalies of respiration may contribute to the peripheral vasoconstriction affecting especially the feet and leading to atrophy of the skin and impaired growth. There are characteristic and evolving changes in the EEG in RS (Glaze *et al.* 1987; Hagne *et al.* 1989) as well as disturbances of cortical function identified by electrophysiological studies of motor cortex magnetic stimulation (Eyre *et al.* 1990) and of sensory evoked potentials (Bader *et al.* 1989a,b; Kimura *et al.* 1992). The ECG is also frequently abnormal, with a long QT interval perhaps contributing to the incidence of sudden, unexplained death in young women with RS (Sekul *et al.* 1994; Ellaway *et al.* 1999).

(6) Growth parameters   The genetic basis of RS need not account directly for those features of the condition that most probably arise as a secondary consequence of the disease process—such as a decline in the rate of linear growth that could occur as a result of oral-motor dysfunction, inefficient feeding behaviours, metabolic derangements or other factors (Thommessen *et al.* 1992), and the decline in the rate of growth of the head circumference that is likely to reflect the disturbance of CNS development (Schultz *et al.* 1993). It is simply not known whether the short fourth metatarsal found in 9 of 50 British cases (Kerr *et al.* 1993) and in a higher proportion of Australian cases (Leonard *et al.* 1995) is congenital or acquired. There is also a deceleration in linear growth leading to short stature by later childhood (Schultz *et al.* 1993) and there may be some other minor skeletal features (Leonard *et al.* 1999).

2.1.3 Possible familial cases of Rett syndrome

When Romeo and colleagues (1986) and Zoghbi (1988) discussed the genetics of RS, a few familial cases had been recognized: affected full sisters and half-sisters had been reported (Hagberg *et al.* 1983; Hanefeld 1985). The opportunity presented by these cases to gain an understanding of the condition was recognized. Further sister pairs have been reported since then (Haenggeli *et al.* 1990; section 2.2.4), as well as several aunt–niece pairs and one set of three affected sisters. One affected woman has transmitted RS to her daughter, who was conceived as a result of sexual abuse (Witt-Engerstrom and Forslund 1992). In addition, in at least two families with more than one female affected by classic RS, there have been males who were severely affected and died in infancy (Schanen *et al.* 1997, 1998; Schanen and Francke 1998). We will continue to discuss RS as a possible XDML disorder, even though a few affected males may survive pregnancy to be born alive, because these 'surviving' males are severely affected and either succumb in infancy or require intensive support.

In the context of an X-linked dominant, male-lethal disorder, where the great majority of cases arise as sporadic new mutations (Comings 1986), the possible mechanisms of familial recurrences are mosaicism, skewed X chromosome inactivation and the existence of unstable premutations. Either parent of two affected girls could carry a mutation causing RS in their germ cells; they would be unaffected but each daughter would have a risk of developing RS. Such families might also experience an excess of miscarriages—of the affected male conceptions—where the parent mosaic for the RS mutation is the mother, although there has been little evidence of this so far. In the usual situation of the sporadic, new mutation cases, there would be no reason to expect an increased rate of miscarriage. Skewed X inactivation could also be relevant in families with more than one affected child, because the mother of affected daughters could be an unaffected carrier of RS if the cells in the relevant tissues of her body predominantly utilized the unaffected X chromosome—i.e. if they inactivated the X chromosome on which the RS gene mutation was located. A third possible explanation would be the existence of a premutation in a parent, such as a triplet repeat expansion, which could expand when transmitted to offspring. Such unstable triplet repeat expansions are now known to underlie an increasing number of degenerative neurological disorders.

In families in which females from at least two generations have been affected—usually a niece and her maternal aunt—the intervening 'normal' female would be expected to have a pattern of X chromosome inactivation skewed very favourably, at least in the relevant cell types. The alternative explanation for such unaffected but transmitting females in two-generation RS families would be an unstable premutation.

Monozygotic twins have almost always been concordant for RS and dizygotic twins have always been discordant. It is interesting that there can be variation in the severity of the RS phenotype in monozygotic (MZ) twins, so that some twins have very similar phenotypes (Tariverdian *et al.* 1987; Tariverdian 1990) while others may show minor (Coleman *et al.* 1987) or more substantial phenotypic differences (Bruck *et al.* 1991; Kerr 1992). This is precisely what would be expected in an X-linked dominant disorder in females, with the phenotypic differences arising as a result of differences in the tissue-specific patterns of X chromosome inactivation. One pair of MZ twins has been reported as discordant for RS (Migeon *et al.* 1995); this could be accounted for by a favourable pattern of X inactivation in the relevant cells of the unaffected twin or by the post-zygotic origin of the RS mutation. It might be expected that affected MZ twins would be in some sense atypical in their manifestation of RS because of the smaller number of cells likely to contribute to each twin at the time of X inactivation (Nance 1990); this would lead to more apparent skewing of X inactivation and a tendency to both milder and more severe phenotypes.

These observations in MZ twins are important for two reasons. First, it suggests that the spectrum of RS phenotypes may be rather broader than the diagnostic criteria currently in use. The strict criteria defining a classic case of RS have been and remain thoroughly appropriate both for research and for clinical purposes—as discussed in the conclusion below—but the phenotypic spectrum resulting from mutations in the gene may well be much wider than the classic definition of RS.

Secondly, there are implications for families in which one female has classic RS and a sister or aunt has a less severe, non-classic phenotype. Some of these cases may well be affected by RD, and the findings in MZ twins encourage us to consider such families as likely representing familial cases of the RS phenotypic spectrum. There will be implications for the risk of recurrence of RD in these families. Furthermore, we must remain cautious because some families will have the misfortune of two different pathologies affecting their two daughters, so that the sister with the appearance of an atypical form of RS may in fact coincidentally have a different aetiology accounting for her condition.

2.1.4 Rett syndrome variants

The possibility that some individuals affected by RD may manifest the condition in an atypical—non-classic—manner has been reached on other grounds by some of the clinicians with most experience of the condition (Hanefeld 1985; Goutieres and Aicardi 1986; Hagberg 1993). Hagberg, in particular, has described a range of clinical phenotypes that differ from classic RS but which may represent different manifestations of the same underlying pathology. There are cases of apparently classical RS in whom the onset is earlier than 6 months and in whom seizures are very prominent. There are cases in whom there is no clear regression but whose clinical picture is otherwise classical. There are cases in whom the regression has been more gradual and of later onset than usual; some of these individuals develop a clinical picture similar to classical RS while others develop a milder condition—a 'forme fruste'—in which purposeful hand use or speech may be preserved and there may be few stereotypies (Hagberg and Gillberg 1993).

A word of caution is required here about the variant form of RS with frequent seizures from early infancy. Many causes of severe seizures at this time may disrupt the development of brain functioning at a crucial stage and thereby lead to regression—as in tuberous sclerosis (Philippart 1993) and other potential causes of West syndrome with hypsarrhythmia. We do not disagree with Hagberg's description of variant forms of RS but do seek to emphasize the difficulty of making a firm diagnosis of these variant forms.

The recognition of these phenotypes as variant forms of RS—see Chapter 1 for a systematic discussion—strengthens the view that RS may comprise a broad phenotypic spectrum and that some affected individuals may have clinical features that are not sufficiently specific for the diagnosis to be made on clinical grounds. With the arrival of molecular genetic testing for many cases of RS, our understanding of the breadth of the RS phenotypic spectrum will undoubtedly be greatly enhanced in the near future (see below).

2.1.5 Metabolic studies and mitochondria

The measurement of blood ammonia is notoriously difficult, with results being falsely elevated if the sample is not handled correctly from the moment it is drawn. The initial reports of hyperammonaemia may therefore have exaggerated this feature of RS (Rett 1977). Subsequent studies, however, have reported a transient or variable hyperammonaemia and/or an elevated urinary excretion of orotic acid in a substantial minority of affected females—especially after challenge with oral protein, intravenous alanine or oral allopurinol (Hagberg *et al.* 1983; Haas *et al.* 1986; Riederer *et al.* 1985; Bachman *et al.* 1986; Naidu *et al.* 1986). One of 12 unrelated girls with RS had increased urinary excretion of orotic acid, as did her mother and the grandmother and three of 17 other mothers of girls with RS (Thomas *et al.* 1987, 1990). Of 24 girls affected by RS in whom the studies have been reported, 12 had elevated orotic acid excretion and another two had raised ammonia levels in the blood (Clarke *et al.* 1990; Carpenter *et al.* 1990; Cameron *et al.* 1991; Pineda *et al.* 1993). Sodium valproate can lead to a similar pattern of results but these abnormalities have been found in many RS cases not taking anticonvulsant medication.

In short, the suggestion that females with RS may have a functional defect in the urea cycle is supported by far too consistent a pattern of evidence for it to be regarded as merely artefactual. Female carriers of OCT deficiency can have similar metabolic abnormalities but it would be most unlikely for the two conditions to be confused—no excess of males with OCT deficiency has been recognized in the families of females with a diagnosis of RS, and the clinical features of RS are very different from the episodic hyperammonaemia sometimes found in female carriers of OCT deficiency (Hyman and Batshaw 1986). On these grounds, it was proposed that the RS gene may be located on the X chromosome and may encode a mitochondrial protein related functionally to OCT (Thomas *et al.* 1990).

Another metabolic abnormality found in a substantial proportion of females with RS is the elevation of blood levels of lactic acid and/or pyruvic acid. Modest elevations have been found in about 50% of affected girls where evidence has been sought (Philippart and Brown 1984; Haas *et al.* 1986; Al-Mateen *et al.* 1986). Two of seven affected females with normal blood lactate and pyruvate levels had elevated levels of lactic acid in the CSF; such disturbances in intermediary metabolism can be associated with disturbances in ventilation including apnoea and hyperventilation (Matsuishi et al. 1992, 1994).

Given the location of both the urea cycle enzymes and the respiratory chain complexes within the mitochondrial compartment of the cell, the possibility that mitochondria may be involved in the pathogenesis of RS has been considered during the search for a reliable biological marker for the disorder. Structural abnormalities have been found in muscle mitochondria in RS (Ruch et al. 1989; Armstrong 1992; Eeg-Olofsson et al. 1988, 1989; Dotti et al. 1993), and functional abnormalities of the mitochondrial respiratory chain have also been recognized (Coker and Melnyk 1991; Dotti et al. 1993). In addition, a T to C transition has been found at position 10463 in the mitochondrial tRNA$_{Arg}$ in a single female affected by RS (Lewis et al. 1995), but the significance of this is uncertain.

Further evidence from three families is relevant. In each of two families, a single girl has classic RS while her full sister has had a lactic acidosis of undefined cause despite intensive investigation (cases 1, 2 and 3 in Clarke et al. 1990; Cheadle et al. 2000). In the third family, two sisters with RS have abnormalities of intermediary metabolism, with fasting hypoglycaemia and post-prandial hyperlacticacidaemia more marked in one sister than the other; one sister and the girls' mother have increased urinary excretion of orotic acid. The recognition of abnormalities in both metabolic pathways in members of the same family suggests that the underlying cause is connected—the three females in this family are now known to carry a mutation in the *MECP2* gene (Clarke et al. 1990; Cheadle et al. 2000). These findings strengthen the argument that mitochondria have an important role in the RS disease process—but this assertion must not be confused with the suggestion that the mitochondrial genome might be involved in the aetiology of RS (see below).

2.1.6 Other models of Rett syndrome inheritance

All the observations discussed so far can be accounted for by the X-linked dominant, male-lethal model of Rett syndrome aetiology. Over the course of the years since RS was defined, however, other modes of inheritance have been considered and these will be reviewed here.

The finding of structurally abnormal mitochondria in the muscle of girls with RS raised the possibility of mitochondrial inheritance of RS (Eeg-Olofsson et al. 1988). This would not account for the great dearth of males affected by RS, but another suggestion from the same group could do so. This is the proposal that RS could arise because of metabolic interference for an X-linked locus (Eeg-Olofsson et al. 1989). Metabolic interference arises from an interaction between the two different alleles in a heterozygous individual when either homozygote would be unaffected (Johnson 1980). For an X-linked locus, metabolic interference would only affect heterozygous females—the hemizygous males and both classes of homozygous females would be unaffected (so this could in principle account for male sparing).

The application of this model to RS, however, is not simple. Metabolic interference between alleles of an X chromosome locus could only occur for genes that are exempt from X inactivation or whose protein products are secreted from the cell, expressed on the cell surface or expressed in syncytial tissues such as muscle fibres. Furthermore, if inter-allelic metabolic interference were to account for RS, there would have to be a much higher incidence of familial occurrence for this usually sporadic disorder—if a woman homozygous for one allele had a male partner with the other allele at the relevant locus on the X chromosome, then *all* their daughters would have to be affected. A more complex model of allelic and non-allelic metabolic interference—involving an autosomal suppressor of the X chromosome allelic metabolic interference—has been proposed (Buhler *et al.* 1990). This has remained a formal possibility until recently, in the absence of proof for the XDML model of inheritance.

The one set of observations that seriously cast doubt on the XDML model of RS pathogenesis were the reports of common ancestry in many, apparently unrelated cases of RS. Work by genealogists in Sweden identified common districts of origin for the ancestors of about one-half of the RS classic cases studied and for about one-third of the RS 'forme fruste' cases studied (Akesson *et al.* 1991, 1992, 1995, and 1996). In some cases, the ancestry of the affected girls could be traced through their male and female antecedents to the very same homesteads. The ancestral lines linking these affected females to each other often involved 'male-to-male' transmission, and so this evidence counted against any simple idea of X-linked inheritance, including XDML with an unstable, inherited premutation. Similar findings emerged from a smaller study of RS ancestry in Northern Tuscany (Pini *et al.* 1996), where male-to-male transmission would also be required of any putative genetic factor linking the distantly related affected cousins. Both the Swedish and the Italian studies suggested an increased level of consanguinity among the grandparents but not the parents of the affected girls; it is not clear how this should have been interpreted.

Although Akesson and colleagues did carry out a similar study of the origin of cases of neurofibromatosis type I as a control measure, these genealogical studies failed to persuade most investigators that their conclusions were valid. Furthermore, the chance of two distant cousins both developing RS as a result of independent mutations becomes very substantial when the common ancestry dates back so far. In the case of seventh cousins, for example, the chance of a second new mutation causing RS, assuming a birth incidence of 1 in 12–15,000, is rather greater than the proportion of the genome likely to be held in common between the affected individuals (< 1 in 32,000). Now that the mutational basis of RS has been demonstrated in many cases, it may be possible directly to test the significance of these genealogical studies.

Another challenge to the XDML model of the genetic basis of RS came from those who argue that an extreme bias in the parental origin of mutations at the RS locus would be sufficient to account for the virtually complete restriction of RS to females (Benedetti *et al.* 1992; Thomas 1996). While considerable differences in rates of mutation at many loci are known between males and females, with new point mutations occurring more frequently in spermatozoa and new deletion mutations at some loci occurring more frequently in oocytes, there is no precedent for a mutational mechanism that will occur exclusively at spermatogenesis. The recent molecular insights into the genetic basis of RS will allow these hypotheses to be tested.

2.2 Genetic investigations in Rett syndrome

2.2.1 Cytogenetic studies of Rett syndrome

Children with RS usually have cytogenetic investigations as a standard part of their diagnostic assessment, and it was long hoped that such studies might identify an important clue as to the underlying genetic basis of RS. Unfortunately, that did not happen. A few children were identified who broadly satisfied the diagnostic criteria for RS but who had a cytogenetic anomaly not involving the X chromosome—such as a deletion of 18q, a duplication of 6p (Wahlstrom and Anvret 1986; Gordon *et al.* 1993) or a deletion of 3p (Wahlstrom *et al.* 1999). It is unclear to what extent the symptoms in these individuals are caused by their various cytogenetic anomalies or whether they may have RS in addition to other problems. No association between RS and any autosomal site has been found on more than one occasion. A somewhat increased frequency of chromosome breaks has been reported in lymphocyte cultures from a series of 15 affected females (Telvi *et al.* 1994) but this observation has not been confirmed by others.

In relation to the X chromosome, increased expression of the common fragile site at Xp22 was found in one small series of females affected by RS (Gillberg *et al.* 1984), but this was not confirmed by further studies (Archidiacono *et al.* 1985; Romeo *et al.* 1986; Wahlstrom and Anvret 1986; Martinho *et al.* 1990; Telvi *et al.* 1994). A deletion of distal Xp was reported in a single affected girl (Wahlstrom and Anvret 1986), but the RS phenotype was not found in other females carrying terminal deletions of distal Xp. Two females with a phenotype resembling RS have also been described with X autosome translocations and these warrant further comment. Zoghbi and colleagues reported a girl with apparently typical RS who had a *de novo* translocation involving the X chromosome and chromosome 3 (Zoghbi *et al.* 1990*a*). The X breakpoint is located at Xp21.3 (Ellison *et al.* 1992)—not at Xp22 as had originally been reported. The other translocation case involved chromosome 22 and Xp11.22, although the girl's history is not entirely typical of

RS. She had an early onset of seizures and her mother and sister also had the same chromosomal translocation but did not have definite clinical features of RS (Journel *et al.* 1990).

Females with X chromosome translocations disrupting important X chromosome disease loci often suffer from the relevant sex-linked disease as if they were affected, hemizygous males (see above). This casts doubt upon the relevance of any such translocation cases to our understanding of a male-lethal disorder such as RS. Females being investigated for suspected Rett syndrome, however, should continue to have chromosomal analyses performed because an unusual finding, such as a chromosomal translocation, could help to account for the clinical disorder and might modify the risk of recurrence of similar problems in another child; it might also be of value for research into the basis of RS.

2.2.2 Uniparental disomy for the X chromosome

Uniparental disomy (UPD) for a number of chromosomes and chromosomal segments is known to cause at least some cases of a diverse range of developmental disorders including Angelman and Prader–Willi syndromes, Beckwith–Wiedemann syndrome and the Silver–Russell syndrome. The suggestion that RS might be caused by uniparental disomy for the X chromosome has been made by several authors. The lack of similar phenotypic features in either Klinefelter syndrome or Turner syndrome—in both of which disorders, the affected individual may have his or her X chromosome(s) derived from just one parent—made it implausible for UPD of the X chromosome to lead to such a disorder, but studies to exclude this possibility as a frequent event in RS were considered worthwhile (Rivkin *et al.* 1992; Benedetti *et al.* 1992; Webb *et al.* 1993; Migeon *et al.* 1995).

2.2.3 X chromosome inactivation

Given that RS occurs only in females, it is not unreasonable to consider what biological and genetic processes occur only in the human female. One of these female-specific processes is X chromosome inactivation, and it is therefore entirely reasonable to examine this process in RS (Riccardi 1986).

Cytogenetic studies of X chromosome inactivation suggested that the sequence in which X chromosome bands are replicated differs in RS from the usual sequence of replication (Martinho *et al.* 1990; Kormann-Bortolotto *et al.* 1992). Further work, however, failed to confirm this—no evidence of an altered pattern of X chromosome replication exists in RS (Kormann-Bortolotto and Webb 1995).

Molecular genetic studies of X inactivation in RS have generally employed the variable number of tandem repeats (VNTR) marker M27-Beta (DXS255) which indicates the parental origin of each allele as well as its methylation status; other markers have also been employed in some studies. Evidence of marked skewing of X inactivation in individuals affected by classic, sporadic RS or in the healthy, potentially 'carrier' relatives of familial cases could be taken to support the X-linked dominant, male-lethal model of RS. Two reports have indicated no significant excess of skewing among affected girls or their close relatives (Webb *et al.* 1993; Anvret and Wahlstrom 1994).

Other reports have indicated a higher rate of skewed X inactivation in the lymphocytes of affected females (Zoghbi *et al.* 1990*b*; Camus *et al.* 1996) and also skewing in the lymphocytes of the mother of two half-sisters with RS (Zoghbi *et al.* 1990*b*) but not in the unaffected mother and grandmother of the niece in a family from Sweden in which the niece and her aunt both have RS (Anvret and Wahlstrom 1994). In contrast, Schanen found skewing of X inactivation in the obligate gene carrier in an RS aunt–niece family but not in the probably mosaic mothers in two families with two affected half-sisters (Schanen *et al.* 1997). In studies where skewing has been apparent, it has more often favoured inactivation of the paternal X chromosome (Camus *et al.* 1996; Krepischi *et al.* 1998). The few samples of brain or liver examined from affected females have shown no evidence of skewed X inactivation (Zoghbi *et al.* 1990b; Anvret *et al.* 1993).

The absence of UPD or of markedly skewed patterns of X inactivation in females with RS was interpreted by one group as evidence that the genetic factor 'causing' RS could not be located on the X chromosome (Migeon *et al.* 1995). The XDML model of RS, however, does not predict UPD as a cause of RS nor does it require skewing of X inactivation in lymphocytes, liver or even the brain as a whole organ, although skewing in some cell types within the brain would be compatible with it.

2.2.4 Molecular genetic studies

Until very recently, the only feasible approach to molecular genetic studies of RS has been the use of genetic markers—variant forms found along the length of all chromosomes—to identify regions of the X chromosome that are shared by the affected individuals within a family. More recently, it has become possible to seek out plausible candidate genes and examine their DNA sequence in affected females.

The use of genetic linkage studies to exclude those regions of the X chromosome that are not shared by the affected members of a family was proposed by Romeo and colleagues (1986) and Zoghbi (1988). The first linkage analysis in a family with RS tracked a set of 11 X chromosome markers through a two-generation family in which both an aunt and a niece were affected (Anvret *et al.* 1990). Few conclusions could be drawn from that study in isolation, and different loci on the X could be regarded as 'excluded' if different assumptions were made about the possible parental origin of the mutation and its penetrance in females.

Archidiacono and colleagues then reported their studies on material from two Swedish affected half-sisters, their unaffected mother and her healthy son (Archidiacono *et al.* 1991). They excluded the areas around four of the 34 X chromosome markers used in the analysis. The same family was studied by Ellison and colleagues along with another RS family with affected maternal half-sisters (Ellison *et al.* 1992). Multipoint linkage analysis suggested that the length of chromosome from the Duchenne muscular dystrophy locus at Xp21 across the centromere to Xq21 or q22 was unlikely to contain the RS locus. The same laboratory team cloned the region of the X breakpoint from the X;3 translocation case of RS and concluded that it was unlikely to contain the RS gene—this area was effectively excluded as the RS locus in the two families with affected half-sisters (Ellison *et al.* 1993).

Curtis and colleagues examined 24 markers in four families—in two affected sisters, in the Swedish half-sisters and two families (one Swedish, one British) with an affected aunt and niece (Curtis *et al.* 1993). Beuten and colleagues reported studies of three families with affected sisters (Beuten *et al.* 1993). These reports suggested that the RS locus was unlikely to be located at the X chromosome centromere or on proximal Xp or proximal Xq. Further linkage analyses on European families demonstrated concordance between affected sisters for markers in Xq28 and Xp23 but did not adequately exclude the rest of the X chromosome long arm (Thomas *et al.* 1995). The region of exclusion was extended by Schanen *et al.* (1997) in their studies of an aunt–niece family and of the families reported by Ellison *et al.* (1992). Schanen and Francke (1998) extended the region of exclusion still further when a severely affected male was born into the aunt–niece kindred used for their earlier studies (Schanen *et al.* 1998).

Three further recent reports, including two that examine the pattern of X chromosome segregation in a Brazilian family with three sisters affected by RS, all indicated that the RS locus was effectively excluded from most of the X chromosome in as large a pool of families as could realistically be gathered (Sirianni *et al.* 1998; Xiang *et al.* 1998; Webb *et al.* 1998). The most probable location of the RS locus was indicated as being Xq28, although there was residual uncertainty about the sites of 'exclusion' of RS from the X chromosome so that the confidence with which RS had been excluded from much of the X chromosome was open to debate. Furthermore, there was some overlap of the families included in these studies so that their results were not entirely independent.

2.2.5 Candidate genes in Xq28

Given the paucity of families with multiple affected females, it was clearly going to be difficult to define the RS gene locus very much more precisely by further linkage analyses within Xq28. The focus of research therefore had to change to a systematic search in silico of Xq28 gene sequences that could plausibly relate to RS gene candidates, using bioinformatic approaches to examine the sequences stored in publicly accessible genome databases. Because the confidence with which RS had been excluded from other areas of the X was not absolute, however, it was not appropriate to completely exclude from consideration all sequences except those in Xq28.

Laboratory research was then required to search for potentially disease-causing mutations in these candidate genes. This phase of research lasted for rather more than 2 years and mutations in six potential RS candidate genes were excluded to a reasonable degree of confidence: *M6b* (Narayanen *et al.* 1998), glutamate dehydrogenase-2 and Rab GDP-dissociation inhibitor I (Wan and Francke 1998), gastrin-releasing peptide receptor (Heidary *et al.* 1998), glycine receptor α2 subunit (Cummings *et al.* 1998) and holocytochrome c-type synthetase (van den Veyver *et al.* 1998). Other groups searched for mutations in other X chromosome loci such as the γ-aminobutyric acid receptor components at Xq28.

During this phase of research, criteria for the most plausible candidate loci were discussed. There are so many genes expressed in the brain that this mere fact—expression in the brain or even selective expression in the brain—was clearly not going to be very helpful in selecting loci for mutation searches. Apart from their location at Xq28, or other X chromosome regions of interest, genes were regarded as potentially interesting candidates if they were involved in one or more of the following biological processes:

(1) neurotransmitter function (synthesis, release, reception);
(2) neurodevelopment—such as members of the neurotrophin gene family, the neurotrophin receptors and structural proteins implicated in axon guidance and related functions, including peptides and neurotransmitters with a neurotrophic role in early development;
(3) synapse plasticity, especially the reinforcement of synapses through 'molecular learning';
(4) nuclear encoding of mitochondrial proteins involved as enzymes in intermediary metabolism or having a structural or a protein import role in the mitochondrion. A parallel here could be with the hyperornithinaemia–hyperammonaemia–homocitrullinuria (HHH) syndrome, where the various metabolic anomalies are caused by a common underlying defect—mutations in the mitochondrial ornithine transporter gene *ORNT1* (Camacho *et al.* 1999).

2.2.6 The methyl-CpG-binding protein 2

At this point, the 'educated guessing' process outlined above came to a halt because two collaborating research groups announced their finding of mutations in one of the two copies of the methyl-CpG-binding protein 2 (MeCP2) gene in seven girls

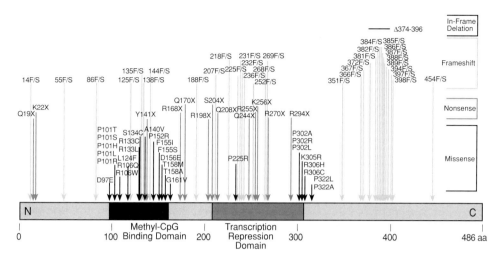

Fig. 2.1 Disease-causing mutations in MeCP2. Amino acid positions of disease-causing mutations in *MECP2* are indicated along a schematic of the protein. The two known functional domains, the methyl-CpG binding domain and the transcription repression domain, are indicated. Mutations resulting a change of amino acid (missense) are indicated as black lines, mutations causing the introduction of a stop codon (nonsense) are indicated as dark grey lines, and mutations resulting in a change of frame (frameshift) are indicated as light grey lines. One in-frame deletion is also indicated. Both nonsense and frameshift mutations result in the truncation of the MeCP2 protein and are thus truncating mutations. Mutations have been taken from the following references: Amir, R. E., *et al*. (2000). *Ann Neurol* **47**, 670–9; *et al*. (1999). *Nat Genet* **23**, 185–8; Bienvenu, T., *et al*. (2000). *Hum Mol Genet* **9**, 1377–84; Cheadle, J. P., *et al*. (2000). *Hum Mol Genet* **9**, 1119–1129; Clayton-Smith, J., *et al*. (2000). *Lancet* **356**, 830–2; De Bona, C., *et al* (2000). *Eur J Hum Genet* **8**, 325–30; Hampson, K., *et al*. (2000). *J Med Genet* **37**, 610–2; Hupple, P., *et al*. (2000). *Hum Mol Genet* **9**, 1369–75; Kim, S. J., and Cook, E. H., Jr. (2000). *Hum Mutat* (Online) **15**, 382–3; Meloni, I., *et al*. (2000). *Am J Hum Genet* **67**, 982–985; Obata, K., *et al*. (2000). *J Med Genet* **37**, 608–10; Orrico, A., *et al*. (2000). *FEBS Lett* **481**, 285–288; Vacca, M., *et al*. (2000) *J Mol Med*, In press; Wan, M., *et al*. (1999). *Am J Hum Genet* **65**, 1520–1529; Xiang, F., *et al*. (2000). *J Med Genet* **37**, 250–5. http://expage.com/page/rettmecp2 Figure by B Hendrich, Edinburgh

affected by RS out of at least 23 who had been studied (Amir *et al.* 1999). The protein is known by the symbol MeCP2 and the gene encoding it is known by the symbol *MECP2*.

First, it is necessary to explain a few terms relating to the methylation of deoxyribonucleic acid (DNA). When a cytosine residue is followed by a guanine residue along the length of DNA, read in the 5′–3′ direction, this is termed a CpG dinucleotide; the complementary bases on the other strand will also be CpG when it is read from 5′ to 3′. The cytosine residues in these CpG dinucleotides are frequently—more often than not—methylated. Such methylated CpG groups are the binding sites of the widely distributed DNA-binding protein, MeCP2. These CpG dinucleotides are interesting for a number of reasons, including their high mutation rate and their non-random distribution in the genome. CpG dinucleotides are clustered at the 5′ end of many 'housekeeping'—widely expressed—genes, and in these 'CpG islands' they are usually exempt from methylation. In contrast, CpGs at other sites—in the 5′ region of tissue-specific genes and in constitutive heterochromatin—are more usually methylated.

It is interesting that, of the seven independent mutations identified in the paper of Amir *et al.*, four probably occurred by the deamination of a methyl-CpG group. A second paper from the same research teams (Wan *et al.* 1999) discussed a wider range of mutations in *MECP2* and the pattern of recurrent mutations in the gene at specific methylated CpG sites. The reasons why only some methylated CpGs are mutational hot-spots remain unclear, and other types of recurrent mutation are also found in the gene (Cheadle *et al.* 2000).

It must be appreciated that DNA does not exist in physical isolation within the cell nucleus but is intimately associated with a wide range of structural proteins, enzymes and transcription factors. The structural proteins include the histones, around which the DNA double helix is wrapped to form nucleosomes. Other proteins help the chromatin to maintain its higher level three-dimensional structure. Other structural proteins found in chromatin and enzymes that modify the histone proteins can make the DNA more or less accessible to transcription.

MeCP2 was identified in 1992 by scientists interested in the role of DNA methylation, as a protein that specifically bound to methylated CpG dinucleotides (Lewis *et al.* 1992) See Fig. 2.1. It is an abundant protein and its distribution along rodent chromosomes was shown to parallel the distribution of methylated CpGs. It includes a methyl-CpG binding domain and a transcription repression domain (Meehan *et al.* 1992; Nan *et al.* 1993,1997), and the transcription repression domain itself incorporates the nuclear localization signal (Nan *et al.* 1996). The gene is unusual in that it has a long, well-conserved 3′ untranslated region incorporating some blocks of striking sequence conservation and therefore perhaps of particular functional (regulatory) importance (Coy *et al.* 1999). We know that MeCP2 is required for embryonic development in the mouse and that male chimaeric embryos, mosaic for intact and non-functional MeCP2, were structurally abnormal if the proportion of cells without MeCP2 was at least 80% (Tate *et al.* 1996).

MeCP2 can repress transcription even in the presence of histone H1, which it can displace from chromatin to access methyl-CpG sites (Nan *et al.* 1997) and to bind stably to the nucleosomal core, for which activity the carboxy-terminal segment of the protein must be intact (Chandler *et al.* 1999).

When MeCP2 is bound to methyl-CpGs, it is associated with the transcriptional repressor Sin3 and with histone deacetylase (Jones *et al.* 1998). The acetylation of histone proteins is generally associated with the activation of transcription from their associated genes (Ng and Bird 1999), although this is not invariably true (De Rubertis *et al.* 1996), and the inhibition of histone deacetylase relieves the repression of transcription achieved by the binding of MeCP2 to methylated DNA (Jones *et al.* 1998). This understanding of the inhibition of gene transcription by MeCP2—its being achieved through the functional association of MeCP2 with

Sin3 and with histone deacetylases—has been confirmed by studies of methylation and transcription at the fragile X site, FRAXA, in the *FMR1* gene locus. Expansion of the CGG triplet repeat at this locus is associated with methylation of several CpG groups; this is associated with deacetylation of the histone proteins at the FRAXA site (Coffee *et al.* 1999).

It can thus be appreciated that one likely effect of mutations in *MECP2* will be to impair the binding of MeCP2 to methylated CpG sites; this in turn will lead to increased transcriptional 'noise'—non-specifically increased transcription from a large number of genes, some widely expressed 'housekeeping' genes but also the more tissue-specific genes, and perhaps especially those genes which are subject to imprinting (although that remains to be seen).

Most of the *MECP2* mutations identified so far in females with RS are predicted to either disrupt the synthesis of the MeCP2 protein (nonsense mutations that terminate translation of the protein) or to cause substitutions of one amino acid for another in one of the two major functional domains (the methylated CpG binding domain, amino acids 79–162, and the transcription repression domain, amino acids 207–305). In general, mutations predicted to result in the termination of protein translation are associated with a somewhat more severe RS phenotype than the missense (amino acid substitution) mutations, and mutations predicted to terminate protein translation earlier (nearer the amino-terminus of the MeCP2 protein) are associated with a somewhat more severe phenotype than those that allow a larger portion of the protein to be synthesized (Cheadle *et al.* 2000). It must also be remembered that the nuclear localisation signal (amino acids 255–271) is incorporated within the transcription repression domain and the carboxyl-terminus includes a nucleosome-binding domain consisting of the 63 C-terminal amino acids, so mutations disrupting these sites may have specific additional consequences.

2.2.7 Speculation

How then do mutations in *MECP2* lead to the Rett syndrome? There are two possible approaches to understanding this. First, there is the conventional, linear approach. This will entail measuring the effect of *MECP2* gene mutations on the expression of downstream, 'regulated' genes in the hope of finding a specific causal mechanism. Everything we know about MeCP2, however, suggests that it will not have a major role in the regulation of transcription from specific loci. It is more likely that there is a general effect on the derepression of transcription from multiple loci, giving generally increased levels of protein synthesis. Some loci may be affected more than others—imprinted loci especially, perhaps—but we would expect the number of affected loci to be very large indeed, too many to permit the tracing of a simple linear causal chain. This derepression of transcription caused by mutations in *MECP2*—the increased transcriptional noise postulated by Nan *et al.* (1997)—may be tolerated relatively well in some tissues, especially where the metabolic demands on individual cells are modest or where many cells carry out effectively the same set of functions, but may not be tolerated well in other tissues.

The second approach to understanding the pathogenesis of Rett syndrome, therefore, is to speculate that it could arise where cells are metabolically very active and where the function of single cells cannot be substituted by their neighbours—as in the developing brain, once the early neuronal plasticity and substitutability have been lost. Such cells, or at least their more delicate functions such as the formation or maintenance of synapses, may be more vulnerable than others to disturbances in metabolism. If such a cell is lost in fetal life, its functions may be taken over by its neighbours—but such plasticity is progressively less likely to occur as the infant matures into a child. If the same cell were to degenerate or become functionally impaired in infancy, its tasks would not be taken over so readily by its neighbours.

The tissue specificity of the features of Rett syndrome would result in large part, on this model, from the lack of substitutability by one neuron for the functions of another. In addition, post-mitotic cells may be more at risk because they are not reassembling their chromatin during cycles of cell division. Occasional involvement of other tissues will depend upon the individual's pattern of X inactivation; metabolic anomalies, for example, might arise if the pattern of X inactivation deviated substantially from 50:50 towards a majority of the cells in the liver, or other relevant tissue, inactivating the intact *MECP2* gene. Similarly, the timing of the onset of symptoms in Rett syndrome would result from either the greater vulnerability of neurons to metabolic disarray in infancy as compared to fetal life or the loss of neuronal plasticity at this time, or both.

The characteristic clinical features of the Rett syndrome could therefore be the result of processes that are only apparent at the level of whole organ, or even whole organism, development and function; they could not be predicted from even a 'complete' understanding of the molecular biology of individual neurons.

This model would satisfactorily account for many features of Rett syndrome but will be difficult to confirm experimentally. Like Rett syndrome itself, it may remain a model of exclusion—to be accepted only after specific hypotheses of linear causality have been found to be inadequate. It is also possible that some mutations cause Rett syndrome through mechanisms compatible with our model while others, perhaps including particular missense mutations, may lead to specific 'toxic' consequences or dominant negative effects on gene transcription. A similar type of explanation for the pattern of tissue involvement in a group of diseases has been proposed in relation to diseases caused by mutations in the mitochondrial genome (Clarke 1990).

2.2.8 Unanswered questions

Future work in RS research will need to seek evidence of disturbed expression of 'downstream' genes as a consequence of the *MECP2* mutations, and thereby to challenge the model of RS pathogenesis outlined above. In addition, there are some specific questions that can be addressed through a combination of clinical and laboratory work.

(1) How wide is the phenotypic spectrum of *MECP2* mutations in females?
(2) How commonly do *MECP2* mutations account for mild, non-progressive intellectual disability, autism or other developmental disorders in females?
(3) How wide is the phenotypic spectrum of *MECP2* mutations in males?
(4) How often do *MECP2* mutations account for otherwise unexplained encephalopathies in male infants?
(5) How often is RS associated with *MECP2* mutations outside the coding region—in the promoter or the untranslated regions?
(6) How do mutations in *MECP2* lead to the usual Rett phenotype?
(7) Does RS display genetic heterogeneity—are there other gene loci in which mutations can give rise to the Rett phenotype?

Answers to some of these questions can already be formulated, but further work is required before we can have any confidence that we 'understand' Rett syndrome. In the meantime, we must be very careful in our use of words if we are to avoid confusing ourselves and others. We must remember that a female with the clinical 'Rett syndrome' has this as a useful clinical diagnosis whether or not she also has a *MECP2* mutation. Similarly, someone with a *MECP2* mutation may be entirely normal clinically—perfectly healthy, with no signs of a clinical disorder until investigated—or may have a mild intellectual impairment, or the classic form of Rett syndrome, or (if male) a lethal encephalopathy. 'Rett syndrome' refers to a clinical diagnosis and *MECP2* refers to the result of a laboratory investigation; the two terms must be used with care and precision because they are not equivalent. Future research will be needed to clarify the relationship between these entities.

References

Akesson, H.O., Hagberg, B., Wahlstrom, J., and Witt Engerström, I. (1991). Common origins in Rett's syndrome. *Lancet*, **337**, 184.

Akesson, H.O., Hagberg, B., Wahlstrom, J., and Witt Engerstrom, I. (1992). Rett syndrome: a search for gene sources. *Am. J. Med. Genet.*, **42**, 104–8.

Akesson, H.O., Wahlstrom, J., Witt Engerstrom, I., and Hagberg, B. (1995). Rett syndrome: potential gene sources—phenotypical variability. *Clin. Genet.*, **48**, 169–72.

Akesson, H.O., Hagberg, B., and Wahlstrom, J. (1996). Rett syndrome, classical and atypical: genealogical support for common origin. *J. Med. Genet.*, **33**, 764–6.

Al-Mateen, M., Philippart, M., and Shields, W.D. (1986). Rett syndrome—a commonly overlooked progressive encephalopathy in girls. *Am. J. Dis. Child.,* **140,** 761–5.

Amir, R.E., van den Veyver, I.B,, Wan, M., Tran, C.Q., Francke. U,, and Zoghbi, H.Y. (1999). Rett syndrome is caused by mutations in X-linked MECP2, encoding methyl-CpG-binding protein. *Nature Genetics,* **23,** 185–8.

Anvret, M., Wahlstrom, J., Skogsberg, P., and Hagberg, B. (1990). Segregation analysis of the X-chromosome in a family with Rett syndrome in two generations. *Am. J. Med. Genet.,* **37,** 31–5.

Anvret, M., Wahlstrom, J., and Akesson, H.-O. (1993). Genetic considerations and clues from molecular genetics. In *Syndrome—clinical and biological aspects*(ed. B. Hagberg), ch. 10, pp.99–107. Cambridge University Press for the MacKeith Press, Cambridge.

Anvret, M., and Wahlstrom, J. (1994). Rett syndrome: random X chromosome inactivation. *Clin. Genet.,* **45,** 274–5.

Archidiacono, N., Rett, A., Rocchi, M., Rolando, S., Lugaresi, E., and Romeo, G. (1985). Rett syndrome and fragile site in Xp22. *Lancet,* **ii,** 1242–3.

Archidiacono, N., Lerone, M., Rocchi, M., Anvret, M., Ozcelik, T., Francke, U., and Romeo, G. (1991). Rett syndrome: exclusion mapping following the hypothesis of germinal mosaicism for new X-linked mutations. *Hum. Genet.,* **86,** 604–6.

Armstrong, D.D. (1992). The neuropathology of the Rett syndrome. *Brain Dev.,* **14 (Suppl):** S89–S98.

Armstrong, D.D., Panigrahy, A., Sleeper, L.A., and Kinney, H.C. (1998). Preliminary studies demonstrating increased [3H]lysergic acid diethylamide ([3H]LSD) binding to serotonin receptors in selected nuclei of the brain stem in Rett syndrome. Abstract of presentation in Meeting Report by Witt Engerström I. and Kerr A.: Workshop on Autonomic function in Rett syndrome. Swedish Rett Center, Froson, Sweden, May 1998. *Brain Dev.* **20,** 323–6.

Bachmann, C., Colombo, J.P., Gugler, E., Killian, W., Rett, A., and da Silva, V. (1986). Biotin and Rett syndrome. *Am. J. Med. Genet.,* **24,** 323–30.

Bader, G.G., Witt Engerström, I., and Hagberg, B. (1989a). Neurophysiological findings in the Rett syndrome, I: EMG, conduction velocity, EEG and somatosensory-evoked potential studies. *Brain Dev.,* **11,** 102–9.

Bader, G.G., Witt Engerström, I., and Hagberg, B. (1989b). Neurophysiological findings in the Rett syndrome, II: visual and auditory brainstem, middle and late evoked responses. *Brain Dev.,* **11,** 110–4.

Benedetti, L., Munnich, A., Melki, J., Tardieu, M., and Turleau, C. (1992). Parental origin of the X chromosomes in Rett syndrome. *Am J Med Genet.,* **44,** 121–2.

Beuten, J., van Roy, B., Vits, L., Hanefeld, F., Begeer, J.H., de Muynck, L., and Willems, P.J. (1993). Molecular analysis of the X chromosome in 24 patients with Rett syndrome. *International Rett Syndrome Congress,* Antwerp, Belgium, October 1993.

Bolthauser, E., Niederwieser, A., and Kierat, L. (1986). Pterins in patients with Rett syndrome. *Am. J. Med. Genet.,* **24,** 317–21.

Bruck, I., Philippart, M., Giraldi, D., and Antoniuk, S. (1991). Difference in early development of presumed monozygotic twins with Rett syndrome. *Am J Med Genet.,* **39,** 415–7.

Buhler, E.M., Malik, H.J., and Alkan, M. (1990). Another model for the inheritance of Rett syndrome. *Am. J. Med. Genet.,* **36,** 126–31.

Burd, L., Martsolf, J.T., and Randall, T. (1990). A prevalence study of Rett syndrome in an institutionalised population. *Am. J. Med. Genet.,* **36,**33–36

Burd, L., Vesley, B., Martsolf, J.T., and Kerbeshian, J. (1991). Prevalence study of Rett syndrome in North Dakota children. *Am. J. Med. Genet.,* **38,** 565–8.

Camacho, J.A., Obie, C., Biery, B., Goodman, B.K., Hu, C.-A., Almashanu, S., Steel, G., Casey, R., Lambert, M., Mitchell, G.A., and Valle, D. (1999). Hyperornithinaemia-hyperammonaemia-homocitrullinuria syndrome is caused by mutations in a gene encoding a mitochondrial ornithine transporter. *Nature Genetics.,* **22,** 151–8.

Cameron, D., Losty, H., and Wallace, S. (1991). The Rett syndrome and ornithylcarbamoyl transferase deficiency. *Brain Dev.,* **13,** 138.

Camus, P., Abbadi, N., Perrier, M.-C., Chery, M., and Gilgenkrantz, S. (1996). X chromosome inactivation in 30 girls with Rett syndrome: analysis using the probe M27Beta. *Hum Genet.,* **97,** 247–50.

Carpenter, K.H., Bonham, J.R., and Clarke, A. (1990). Rett's syndrome and ornithine carbamoyltransferase deficiency. *J. Inher. Metab. Dis.,* **13,** 308–10.

Chandler, S.P., Guschin, D., Landsberger, N., and Wolffe, A.P. (1999). The methyl-CpG binding transcriptional repressor MeCP2 stably associates with nucleosomal DNA. *Biochemistry.,* **38,** 7008–18.

Cheadle, J.P., Gill, H., Fleming, N., Maynard, J., Kerr, A., Leonard, H., Krawczak, M., Cooper, D.N., Lynch, S., Thomas, N.S.T., Hughes, H.E., Hulten, M., Ravine, D., Sampson, J.R., and Clarke, A.J. (2000). Long-read sequence analysis of the MECP2 gene in Rett syndrome patients: correlation of disease severity with mutation type and location. *Hum. Molec. Genet.,* **9,** 7: 1119–29.

Clarke, A. (1990). Mitochondrial genome: defects, disease and evolution. *J. Med. Genet.,* **27,** 451–6

Clarke, A. (1996). Rett syndrome. *J. Med. Genet.* **33,** 693–9.

Clarke, A., Gardner-Medwin, D., Richardson, J. *et al.* (1990). Abnormalities of carbohydrate metabolism and of OCT gene function in the Rett syndrome. *Brain Dev.,* **12,** 119–24.

Coffee, B., Zhang, F., Warren, S.T., and Reines, D. (1999). Acetylated histones are associated with FMR1 in normal but not fragile X-syndrome cells. *Nature Genetics.,* **22,** 98–101.

Coker, S.B., and Melnyk, A.R. (1991). Rett syndrome and mitochondrial enzyme deficiencies. *J. Child Neurology.,* **6,** 164–6.

Coleman, M., Naidu, S., Murphy, M., Pines, M., and Bias, W. (1987). A set of monozygotic twins with Rett syndrome. *Brain Dev.,* **9,** 475–8.

Comings, D.E. (1986). The genetics of Rett syndrome: the consequence of a disorder where every case is a new mutation. *Am. J. Med. Genet.,* **24,** 383–8.

Coy, J.F., sedlacek, Z., Bachner, D., Delius, H., and Poustka, A. (1999). A complex pattern of evolutionary conservation and alternative polyadenylation within the long 3'-untranslated region of the methyl-CpG-binding protein 2 gene (MeCP2) suggests a regulatory role in gene expression. *Hum. Mol. Gene.,* **8,** 1253–62.

Cummings, C.J., Dahle, E.J.R., and Zoghbi, H.Y. (1998). Analysis of the genomic structure of the human glycine receptor alpha2 subunit gene and exclusion of this gene as a candidate for Rett syndrome. *Am. J. Med. Genet.,* **78,** 176–8.

Curtis, A.R.J., Headland, S., Lindsay, S., Thomas, N.S.T., Boye, E., Kamakari, S., Roustan, P., Anvret, M., Wahlstrom, J., McCarthy, G., Clarke, A., and Bhattacharya, S. (1993). X chromosome linkage studies in familial Rett syndrome. *Hum. Genet.,* **90,** 551–5.

De Rubertis, F., Kadosh, D., Henchoz, S., Pauli, D., Reuter, G., Struhl, K., Spierer, P. (1996). The histone deacetylase RPD3 counteracts genomic silencing in Drosophila and yeast. *Nature.,* **384,** 589–91.

Dotti, M.T., Manneschi, L., Malandrini, A., De Stefano, N., Caznerale, F., and Federico, A. (1993). Mitochondrial dysfunction in Rett syndrome. An ultrastructural and biochemical study. *Brain Dev.,* **15,** 103–6.

Eeg-Olofsson, O., Al-Zuhair, A.G.H., Teebi, A.S., and Al-Essa, M.M.N. (1988). Abnormal mitochondria in Rett syndrome. *Brain Dev.,* **10,** 260–2.

Eeg-Olofsson, O., Al-Zuhair, A.G.H., Teebi, A.S., and Al-Essa, M.M.N. (1989). Rett syndrome: genetic clues based on mitochondrial changes in muscle. *Am. J. Med. Genet.,* **32,** 142–4.

Ellaway, C.J., Sholler, G., Leonard, H., and Christodoulou, J. (1999). Prolonged QT interval in Rett syndrome. *Arch. Dis. Child.,* **80,** 470–2.

Ellison, K.A., Fill, C.P., Terwilliger, J., DeGennaro, L.J., Martin-Gallardo, A., Anvret, M., Percy, A.K., Ott, J., and Zoghbi, H. (1992). Examination of X chromosome markers in Rett syndrome:

exclusion mapping with a novel variation on multilocus linkage analysis. *Am. J. Hum. Genet.,* **50**, 278–7.

Ellison, K.A., Roth, E.J., McCabe, E.R.B., Chinault, A.C., and Zoghbi, H.Y. (1993). Isolation of a yeast artificial chromosome contig spanning the X chromosomal translocation breakpoint in a patient with Rett syndrome. *Am. J. Med. Genet.,* **47**, 1124–34.

Eyre, J.A., Kerr, A.M., Miller, S., O'Sullivan, M.C., and Ramesh, V. (1990). Neurophysiological observations on corticospinal projections to the upper limb in subjects with Rett syndrome. *J. Neurol. Neurosurg. Psychiatr.,* **53**, 874–9.

Gillberg, C., Wahlstrom, J., and Hagberg, B. (1984). Infantile autism and Rett's syndrome: common chromosomal denominator. *Lancet,* **ii**, 1094–95.

Glaze, D.G., Frost, J.D., Zoghbi, H.Y., and Percy, A.K. (1987). Rett's syndrome: correlation of electroencephalographic characteristics with clinical staging. *Arch Neurol.,* **44**, 1053–56.

Gordon, K., Siu, V.M., Sergovich, F., and Jung, J. (1993). 18q- Mosaicism associated with Rett syndrome phenotype. *Am. J. Med. Genet.,* **46**,142–4.

Goutieres, F., and Aicardi, J. (1986). Atypical forms of Rett syndrome. *Am. J. Med. Genet.,* **24**, 183–194.

Haas, R.H., Rice, M.A., Trauner, D.A., and Merritt, T.A. (1986). Therapeutic effects of a ketogenic diet in Rett syndrome. *Am. J. Med. Genet.,* **24**, 225–46.

Haenggeli, C.-A., Moura-Serra, J., and DeLozier-Blanchet, C.D. (1990). Two sisters with Rett syndrome. *J. Autism Dev. Disord.,* **20**, 129–138.

Hagberg, B. (1985). Rett's syndrome: prevalence and impact on progressive severe mental retardation in girls. *Acta. Paediatr. Scand.,* **74**, 405–8.

Hagberg, B. (1985). Rett syndrome: Swedish approach to analysis of prevalence and cause. *Brain Dev.,* **7**, 277–80.

Hagberg, B. (1993). Clinical criteria, stages and natural history. In *Rett syndrome—clinical and biological aspects,* Clinics in Developmental Medicine, No. 127(ed. B. Hagberg, M.Anuret and J. Wahlstrom), ch. 2, pp.4–20. MacKeith Press/Cambridge University Press.

Hagberg, B., Aicardi, J., Dias, K. and Ramos, O. (1983). A progressive syndrome of autism, dementia, ataxia and loss of purposeful hand use in girls: Rett's syndrome: report of 35 cases. *Ann. Neurol.,* **14**, 471–9.

Hagberg, B., and Witt-Engerstrom, I. (1986). Rett syndrome: a suggested staging system for describing impairment profile with increasing age towards adolescence. *Am. J. Med. Genet.,* **24**, 47–59.

Hagberg, B., and Gillberg, C. (1993). Rett variants—Rettoid phenotypes. In *Rett Syndrome—clinical and biological aspects,* Clinics in Developmental Medicine, No. 127. (ed. B. Hagberg, M. Anuret, and J.wahlstrom), ch.5, pp. 40–60. MacKeith Press/Cambridge University Press.

Hagne, I., Witt-Engerstrom, I., and Hagberg, B. (1989). EEG development in Rett syndrome. A study of 30 cases. *Electroencephalogr. Neurophysiol,* **72**, 1–6.

Hanefeld, F. (1985). The clinical pattern of the Rett syndrome. *Brain Dev.,* **7**, 320–5.

Hatchwell, E. (1996). Hypomelanosis of Ito and X;autosome translocations: a unifying hypothesis. *J. Med. Genet.,* **33**, 177–83.

Hatchwell, E., Robinson, D., Crolla, J.A., and Cockwell, A.E. (1996). X inactivation analysis in a female with hypomelanosis of Ito associated with a balanced X;17 translocation: evidence for functional disomy of Xp. *J. Med. Genet.,* **33**, 216–20.

Heidary, G., Hampton, L.L., Schanen, N.C., Rivkin, M.J., Darras, B.T., Battey, J., and Francke, U. (1998). Exclusion of the gastrin-releasing peptide receptor (GRPR) locus as a candidate gene for Rett syndrome. *Am. J. Med. Genet.,* **78**, 173–5.

Hyman, S.L., and Batshaw, M.L. (1986). A case of ornithine transcarbamylase deficiency with Rett syndrome manifestations. *Am. J. Med. Genet.,* **24**, 339–343.

Jellinger, K., and Seitelberger, F. (1986). Neuropathology of Rett syndrome. *Am. J. Med. Genet.,* **24,** 259–88.

Johnson, W.G. (1980). Metabolic interference and the + and—heterozygote. A hypothetical form of simple inheritance which is neither dominant nor recessive. *Am. J. Hum. Genet.,* **32,** 374–86.

Jones, P.L., Veenstra, G.J.C., Wade, P.A., Vermaark, D., Kass, S.U., Landsberger, N., Strouboulis, J., and Wolffe, A.P. (1998). Methylated DNA and MeCP2 recruit histone deacetylase to repress transcription. *Nature Genetics,* **19,** 187–91.

Journel, H., Melki, J., and Turleau, C. et al. (1990). Rett phenotype with X/autosome translocation: possible mapping to the short arm of chromosome X. *Am. J. Med. Genet.,* **35,** 142–7.

Kerr, A. (1992). Rett syndrome: British longitudinal study (1982–1990) and 1990 survey, In *Mental retardation and medical care,* (ed. J.J. Roosendaal), Conference Proceedings, April 1991. Uitgeverij Kerckbosch, Zeist.

Kerr, A.M., and Stephenson, J.B.P. (1985). Rett's syndrome in the west of Scotland. *BMJ,* **291,** 579–82.

Kerr, A., Robertson, P., and Mitchell, J. (1993). Rett syndrome and the 4th metatarsal. *Arch. Dis. Child.,* **68,**433–4.

Kerr, A., and Julu, P.O.O. (1999). Recent insights into hyperventilation from the study of Rett syndrome. *Arch. Dis. Child.,* **80,** 384–7.

Kimura, K., Nomura, Y., and Segawa, M. (1992). Middle and short latency somatosensory evoked potentials (SEPm,SEPs) in the Rett syndrome: chronological changes of cortical and subcortical involvements. *Brain Dev.,* **14 (Suppl)**, S37–42.

Kormann-Bortolotto, M.H., Woods, C.G., Green, S.H., and Webb, T. (1992). X-inactivation in girls with Rett syndrome. *Clin. Genet.,* **42,** 296–301.

Kormann-Bortolotto, M.H., and Webb, T. (1995). Alterations in replication timing of X-chromosome bands in Rett syndrome. *J. Intellectual Disability Research,* **39,** 91–6.

Kozinetz, C.A., Skender, M.L., MacNaughton, M., Almes, M.J., Schultz, R.J., Percy, A.K., and Glaze, D.G. (1993). Epidemiology of Rett syndrome: a population-based registry. *Pediatrics,* **91,**445–50.

Krepischi, A.C.V., Kok, F., and Otto, P.G. (1998). X chromosome-inactivation patterns in patients with Rett syndrome. *Hum. Genet.,* **102,** 319–21.

Landy, S.J., and Donnai, D. (1995). Incontinentia pigmenti (Bloch–Sulzberger syndrome). In *Congenital malformation syndromes* (ed. D. Donnai, and R.M. Winter,)ch. 52, pp. 399–411. Chapman and Hall, London:

Lekman, A., Witt-Engerstrom, I., Holmberg, B., Percy, A., Svennerholm, L., and Hagberg, B. (1990). CSF and urine biogenic amine metabolites in Rett syndrome. *Clin. Genet.,* **37,** 173–8.

Lekman, A., Hagberg, B., and Svennerholm, L. (1991a). Membrane cerebral lipids in Rett syndrome. *Pediatr. Neurol.,* **7,** 186–90.

Lekman, A., Hagberg, B., and Svennerholm, L. (1991b). Altered cerebellar ganglioside pattern in Rett syndrome. *Neurochem. Internat.,* **19,** 505–9.

Leonard, H., Thomson, M., Bower, C., Fyfe, S., and Constantinou, J. (1995). Skeletal abnormalities in Rett syndrome: increasing evidence for dysmorphological defects. *Am. J. Med. Genet.,* **58,** 282–5.

Leonard, H., and Bower, C. (1998). Is the girl with Rett syndrome normal at birth? *Dev. Med and Child Neurol.,* **40,** 115–21.

Leonard, H., Thomson, M., Glasson, E., Fyfe, S., Leonard, S., Ellaway, C., Christodoulou, J., and Bower, C. (1999). Metacarpophalangeal pattern profile and bone age in Rett syndrome: further radiological clues to the diagnosis. *Am. J. Med. Genet.,* **83,** 88–95.

Lewis, J.D., Meehan, R.R., Henzel, W.J., Maurer-Fogy, I., Jeppesen, P., Klein, F., and Bird, A. (1992). Purification, sequence and cellular localization of a novel chromosomal protein that binds to methylated DNA. *Cell* **69,** 905–14.

Lewis, D.W., Burgess, C.E., Naidu, S., and Castora, F.J. (1995). Single-strand conformational polymorphism analysis of mtDNA in Rett syndrome. *Ann. Neurol.,* **38,** 532 (abstract 115 from 24th Annual Meeting of Child Neurology Society, Baltimore, Maryland; October 1995).

Lin, M-.Y., Wang, P-.J., Lin, L-.H., Shen, Y-.Z. (1991). The Rett and Rett-like syndromes: a broad concept. *Brain Dev.,* **13,** 228–31.

Liu, X.Y., Dangel, A.W., Kelley, R.I., Zhao, W., Denny, P., Botcherby, M., Cattanach, B., Peters, J., Hunsicker, P.B., Mallon, A-.M, Strivens, M.A., Bate, R., Miller, W., Rhodes, M., Brown, S.D.M., and Herman, G.E. (1999). The gene mutated in bare patches and striated mice encodes a novel 3beta-hydroxysteroid dehydrogenase. *Nature Genetics.,* **22,** 182–7.

Marcus, C.L., Carroll, J.L., McColley, S.A., Loughlin, G.M., Curtis, S., Pyzik, P., and Naidu, S. (1994). Polysomnographic characteristics of patients with Rett syndrome. *J. Pediatr.,* **125,** 218–24.

Martinho, P.S., Otto, P.G., Kok, F., Diament, A., Marques-Dias, M.J., and Gonzalez, C.H. (1990). In search of a genetic basis for the Rett syndrome. *Hum. Genet.,* **86,** 131–4.

Matsuishi, T., Urabe, F., Komori, H., Yamashita, Y., Naito, E., Kuroda, Y., Horikawa, M., and Ohtaki, E. (1992). The Rett syndrome and CSF lactic acid patterns. *Brain Dev.,* **14,** 68–70.

Matsuishi, T., Urabe, F., Percy, A.K., Komori, H., Yamashita, Y., Schultz, R.S., Ohtani, Y., Kuriya, N., and Kato, H. (1994). Abnormal carbohydrate metabolism in cerebrospinal fluid in Rett syndrome. *J. Child Neurol.,* **9,** 26–30.

Meehan, R.R., Lewis, J.D., and Bird, A.P. (1992). Characterisation of MeCP2, a vertebrate DNA binding protein that binds specifically to DNA that contains methylated CpGs. *Cell,* **58,** 499–507.

Migeon, B.R., Dunn, M.A., Thomas, G., Schmeckpeper, B.J., and Naidu, S. (1995). Studies of X inactivation and isodisomy in twins provide further evidence that the X chromosome is not involved in Rett syndrome. *Am. J. Hum. Genet.,* **56,** 647–53.

Murakami, J.W., Courchesne, E., Haas, R.H., Press, G.A., and Yeung-Courchesne, R. (1992). Cerebellar and cerebral abnormalities in Rett syndrome: a quantitative MR analysis. *Am. J. Radiol.,* **159,** 177–83.

Myer, E.C., Tripathi, H.M., Brase, D.A., and Dewey, W.L. (1992). Elevated CSF beta-endorphin immunoreactivity in Rett's syndrome: report of 158 cases and comparison with leukemic children. *Neurology,* **42,** 357–60.

Naidu, S., Murphy, M., Moser, H.W., and Rett, A. (1986). Rett syndrome—natural history in 70 cases. *Am. J. Med. Genet.,* **24,** 61–72.

Nan, X., Meehan, R.R., and Bird, A. (1993). Dissection of the methyl-CpG binding domain from the chromosomal protein MeCP2. *Nuc. Acids Res.,* **21,** 4886–92.

Nan, X., Tate, P., Li, E., and Bird, A. (1996). DNA methylation specifies chromosomal lcalization of MeCP2. *Mol. Cell Biol.,* **16,** 414–21.

Nan, X., Campoy, F.J., and Bird, A. (1997). MeCP2 is a transcriptional repressor with abundant binding sites in genomic chromatin. *Cell,* **88,** 471–81.

Nance, W.E. 1990 Invited Editorial: Do Twin Lyons Have Larger Spots? *Am. J. Hum. Genet.,* **46,** 646–48.

Narayanen, V., Olinsky, S., Dahle, E., Naidu, S., and Zoghbi, H.Y. (1998). Mutation analysis of the M6b gene in patients with Rett syndrome. *Am. J. Med. Genet.,* **78,** 165–8.

Ng, H-.H., and Bird, A. (1999). DNA methylation and chromatin modification. *Curr. Opin. Gene. Dev.,* **9,** 158–63.

Nielsen, J.B., Bertelsen, A., and Lou, H.C. (1992). Low CSF HVA levels in the Rett syndrome: a reflection of restricted synapse formation. *Brain Dev.,* **14 (Suppl),** S63–5.

Oldfors, A., Hagberg, B.A., Nordgren, Y.H., Sourander, P., and Witt-Engerstrom, I. (1988). Rett syndrome: spinal cord neuropathology. *Pediatric Neurology,* **4,** 172–4.

Oldfors, A., Sourander, P., Armstrong, D.L., Percy, A.K., Witt-Engerstrom, I., and Hagberg, B.A. (1990). Rett syndrome: cerebellar pathology. *Pediatric Neurology,* **6,** 310–4.

Percy, A.K. (1992). Neurochemistry of the Rett syndrome. *Brain Dev.,* **14 (Suppl),** S57–62.

Percy, A.K., Zoghbi, H.Y., Lewis, K.R., and Jankovic, J. (1988). Rett syndrome: qualitative and quantitative differentiation from autism. *J. Child Neurology*, **3**, 65–7.

Percy, A.K., Glaze, D.G., Schultz, R.J., Zoghbi, H.Y., Williamson, D., Frost, J.D., Jankovic, J.J., del Junco, D., Skender, M., Waring, S., and Myer, E.C. (1994). Rett syndrome: controlled study of an oral opiate antagonist, naltrexone. *Ann. Neurol.*, **35**, 464–70.

Pereira, J.L.P., and Pilotto, R.F. (1992). A new set of sisters with Rett syndrome. In *2nd International Workshop and Symposium on Rett Syndrome*, Orlando, Florida, October 1992.

Philippart, M. (1986). Clinical recognition of Rett syndrome. *Am. J. Med. Genet.*, **24**, 111–8.

Philippart, M., and Brown, W.J. (1984). Dystonia and lactic acidosis: new features of Rett's syndrome. *Ann. Neurol.*, **16**, 387.

Philippart, M. (1993). Rett syndrome associated with tuberous sclerosis in a male and in a female: evidence for arrested motor and mental development. *Am. J. Med. Genet. (Neuropsychiatric Genetics)* **48**, 229–30.

Pineda, M., Vilaseca, M.A., Vernet, A., Campistol, J., Mas, A., and Fabrega, C. (1993). The allopurinol test in patients with Rett syndrome. *J. Inher. Metab. Dis.*, **16**, 577–80.

Pini, G., Milan, M., and Zappella, M. (1996). Rett syndrome in Northern Tuscany (Italy): family tree studies. *Clin Genet.*, **50**, 486–90.

Reiss, A.L., Faruque, F., Naidu, S., Abrams, M., Beaty, T., Bryan, R.N., and Moser, H. (1993). Neuroanatomy of Rett syndrome: a volumetric imaging study. *Ann. Neurol.*, **34**, 227–34.

Rett, A. (1966a). *Ueber ein cerebral-atrophisches Syndrom bei Hyperammonamie*. Bruder Hollinek, Vienna.

Rett, A. (1966b). Uber ein eigenartiges hirnatrophisches Syndrom in Kindesalter. *Wien Med Wochenschr.*, **116**, 723–38.

Rett, A. (1977). Cerebral atrophy associated with hyperammonaemia. Ch 16 in Vinken PJ and Bruyn GW in association with Klawans HL (eds) *Metabolic and deficiency diseases of the nervous system III. Handbook of Clinical Neurology*, Vol. 26 (ed. P.J. Vinken and G.W. Bruyn). Elsevier/North Holland Biomedical Press.

Rett Syndrome Diagnostic Criteria Working Group (1988). Diagnostic criteria for Rett syndrome. *Ann Neurol* **23**, 425–8.

Riccardi, V.M. (1986). The Rett syndrome: genetics and the future. *Am. J. Med. Genet.*, **24**, 389–402.

Riederer, P., Brucke, T., Sofic, E., Kienzl, E., Schnecker, K., Schay, V., Kruzik, P., Killian, W., and Rett, A. (1985). Neurochemical aspects of the Rett syndrome. *Brain Dev.*, **7**, 351–60.

Riikonen, R., and Vanhala, R. (1999). Levels of cerebrospinal fluid nerve-growth factor differ in infantile autism and Rett syndrome. *Dev. Med. and Child Neurol.*, **41**, 148–52.

Rivkin, M.J., Zhen, Ye, Mannheim, G.B., and Darras, B.T. (1992). A search for X chromosome uniparental disomy and DNA rearrangements in the Rett syndrome. *Brain Dev.*, **14**, 273–5.

Romeo, G., Archidiacono, N., Ferlini, A., and Rocchi, M. (1986). Rett syndrome: lack of association with fragile site Xp22 and strategy for genetic mapping of X-linked new mutations. *Am. J. Med. Genet.*, **24**, 355–9.

Rousseau, F., Bonaventure, J., Legeai-Mallet, L., Pelet, A., Rozet, J.-M., Maroteaux, P., Le Merver, M., and Munnich, A. (1994). Mutations in the gene encoding fibroblast growth factor receptor-3 in achondroplasia. *Nature* **371**, 252–4.

Ruch, A., Kurczynski, T.W., and Velasco, M.E. (1989). Mitochondrial alterations in Rett syndrome. *Pediatr. Neurol.*, **5**, 320–3.

Ryan, S.G., Chance, P.F., Zou, C-.H., Spinner, N.B., Golden, J.A., and Smietana, S. (1997). Epilepsy and mental retardation limited to females: an X-linked dominant disorder with male sparing. *Nature Genetics*, **17**, 92–5.

Sansom, D., Krishnan, V.H.R., Corbett, J., and Kerr, A. (1993). Emotional and behavioural aspects of Rett syndrome. *Dev. Med. Child Neurol.*, **35**, 340–5.

Schanen, N.C., Dahle, E.J.R., Capozzoli, F., Holm, V.A., Zoghbi, H.Y., and Francke, U. (1997). A New Rett syndrome family consistent with X-linked inheritance expands the X chromosome exclusion map. *Am. J. Hum. Genet.,* **61** 634–41.

Schanen, N.C., and Francke, U. (1998). A severely affected male born into a Rett syndrome kindred supports X-linked inheritance and allows extension of the exclusion map. *Am. J. Hum. Genet.,* **63,** 267–9.

Schanen, N.C., Kurczynski, T.W., Brunelle, D., Woodcock, M.W., Dure, L.S. IV, and Percy, A.K. (1998). Neonatal encephalopathy in two boys in families with recurrent Rett syndrome. *J. Child Neurol.,* **13,** 229–31.

Scheuerle, A.E. (1998). Male cases of incontinentia pigmenti: case report and review. *Am. J. Med. Genet.,* **77,** 201–18.

Schultz, R.J., Glaze, D.G., Motil, K.J., Armstrong, D.D., del Junco, D.J., Hubbard, C.R., and Percy, A.K. (1993). The pattern of growth failure in Rett syndrome. *Am. J. Dis. Child.,* 147:633–7.

Schwartzman, J.S., Zatz, M., Vasquez, L.D.R., Gomes, R.R., Koiffmann, C.P., Fridman, C., and Otto, P.G. (1999). Rett syndrome in a boy with a 47,XXY karyotype. *Am. J. Hum. Genet.,* **64**: 1781–5.

Segawa, M., and Nomura, Y. (1992). Polysomnography in the Rett syndrome. *Brain Dev.,* **14 (Suppl),** S46–54.

Sekul, E.A., and Percy, A.K. (1992). Rett Syndrome: Clinical features, genetic considerations, and the search for a biological marker. *Ch 7, pp 173–200, In Current neurology, Vol. 12,* Mosby-Year Book.

Sekul, E.A., Moak, J.P., Schultz, R.J., Glaze, D.G., **Dunn, K.,** and Percy, A.K. (1994). Electrocardiographic findings in Rett syndrome: **an explanation for sudden death?** *J. Pediatr.,* **125**: 80–2.

Sirianni, N., Naidu, S., Pereira, J., Pillotto, R.F., and **Hoffman, E.P. (1998).** Rett syndrome: confirmation of X-linked dominant inheritance and localization of the gene to Xq28. *Am. J. Hum. Genet.,* **63,** 1552–8.

Southall, D.P., Kerr, A.M., Tirosh, E., Amos, P., Lang, M.H., and Stephenson, J.B.P. (1988). Hyperventilation in the awake state: potentially treatable component of Rett syndrome. *Arch. Dis. Childhood,* **63,** 1039–48.

Tariverdian, G., Kantner, G., and Vogel, F. (1987). A monozygoytic twin pair with Rett syndrome. *Hum. Genet.,* **75,** 88–90.

Tariverdian, G. (1990). Follow-up of monozygotic twins concordant for the Rett syndrome. *Brain Dev.,* **12,** 125–7.

Tate, P., Skarnes, W., and Bird, A. (1996). The methyl-CpG binding protein MeCP2 is essential for embryonic development in the mouse. *Nature Genetics,* **12,** 205–8.

Telvi, L., Leboyer, M., Chiron, C., Feingold, J., and Ponsot, G. (1994). Is Rett syndrome a chromosome breakage syndrome? *Am. J. Med. Genet.,* **51**: 602–5.

Thomas, G.H. (1996). High male:female ratio of germ-line mutations: an alternative explanation for postulated gestational lethality in males in X-linked dominant disorders. *Am. J. Hum. Genet.,* **58,** 1364–8.

Thomas, S., Hjelm, M., Oberholzer, V., Brett, E.M., and Wilson, J. (1987). Rett's syndrome and ornithine carbamoyltransferase deficiency. *Lancet,* **ii,** 1330–1.

Thomas, S., Oberholzer, V., Wilson, J., and Hjelm, M. (1990). The urea cycle in Rett syndrome. *Brain Dev.,* **12**: 93–6.

Thomas, N.S.T., Davies, K., Williams, N., Price, W., Owen, M., Pereira, J., Kerr, A., Anvret, M., Hanefeld, F., and Clarke, A. (1995). Molecular genetic studies in familial Rett syndrome (Poster Abstract 183). *Psychiatric Genetics,* **5 (Suppl. 1),** August 1995, S88–9.

Thommessen, M., Kase, B.F., and Heiberg, A. (1992). Growth and nutrition in 10 girls with Rett syndrome. *Acta. Pediatr.,* **81,** 686–90.

van den Veyver, I.B., Subramanian, S., and Zoghbi, H.Y. (1998). Genomic structure of a human holocytochrome c-type synthetase gene in Xp22.3 and mutation analysis in patients with Rett syndrome. *Am. J. Med. Genet.,* **78,** 179–81.

Vorsanova, S.G., Demidova, I.A., Ulas, V. Yu, Soloviev, I.V., Kazantzeva, L.Z., and Yurov, Yu B. (1996). Cytogenetic and molecular-cytogenetic investigation of Rett syndrome: analysis of 31 cases. *Neuroreport* **8,** 187–9.

Wahlström, J., and Anvret, M. (1986). Chromosome findings in the Rett syndrome and a test of a two-step mutation theory. *Am. J. Med. Genet.,* **24,** 361–8.

Wahlström, J., Uller, A., Johannesson, T., Holmquist, D., Darnfors, C., Vujic, M., Tonnby, B., Hagberg, B., Martinsson, T. (1999). Congenital variant of Rett syndrome in a girl with terminal deletion of chromosome 3p. *J. Med. Genet.,* **36,** 343–5.

Wan, M., and Francke, U. (1998). Evaluation of two X chromosomal candidate genes for Rett syndrome: glutamate dehydrogenase-2 (GLUD2) and Rab GDP-dissociation inhibitor (GDII). *Am. J. Med. Genet.,* **78,** 169–72.

Wan, M., Lee, S.S.J., Zhang, X., Houwink-Manville, I., Song, H-.R., Amir, R.E., Budden, S., Naidu, S., Pereira, J.L.P., Lo, I.F.M., Zoghbi, H., Schanen, N.C., and Francke, U. (1999). Rett syndrome and beyond: recurrent spontaneous and familial MECP2 mutations at CpG hotspots. *Am. J. Hum. Genet.,* **65,** 1520–9.

Webb, T., Watkiss, E., Woods, C.G. (1993). Neither uniparental disomy nor skewed X inactivation explains Rett syndrome. *Clin. Genet.,* **44:** 236–40.

Webb, T., Clarke, A., Hanefeld, F., Pereira, J-.L., Rosenbloom, L., and Woods, C.G. (1998). Linkage analysis in Rett syndrome families suggests that there may be a critical region at Xq28. *J. Med. Genet.,* **35,** 997–1003.

Wenk, G.L., O'Leary, M., Nemeroff, C.B., Bissette, G., Moser, H., and Naidu, S. (1993). Neurochemical alterations in Rett syndrome. *Dev. Brain Res.,* **74,** 67–72.

Witt-Engerstrom, I. (1987). Rett syndrome: a retrospective pilot study on potential early predictive symptomatology. *Brain Dev.,* **9,** 481–6.

Witt-Engerstrom, I. (1990). Rett syndrome in Sweden: neurodevelopment, disability, pathophysiology. Thesis, University of Goteborg.

Witt-Engerstrom, I. (1992). Rett syndrome: the late infantile regression period—a retrospective analysis of 91 cases. *Acta. Paediatr.,* **81,** 167–72.

Witt-Engerstrom, I., and Gillberg, C. (1987). Autism and Rett syndrome. A preliminary epidemiologic study of diagnostic overlap. *J. Autism. Dev. Dis.,* **17,** 149–50.

Witt-Engerstrom, I., and Forslund, M. (1992). Mother and daughter with Rett syndrome. *Dev. Med. Child Neurol.,* **34,** 1022–5.

Xiang, F., Zhang, Z., Clarke, A., Pereira, J., Naidu, S., Budden, S., Delozier-Blanchet, C.D., Hansmann, I., Edstrom, L., and Anvret, M. (1998). Chromosome mapping of Rett syndrome: a liklely candidate region on the telomere of Xq. *J. Med. Genet.,* **35,** 297–300.

Zapella, M. (1992). The Rett girls with preserved speech. *Brain Dev.,* **14,** 98–101.

Zoghbi, H. (1988). Genetic aspects of Rett syndrome. J. Child Neurol., **3** (**Suppl.**), S76–8.

Zoghbi, H.Y., Milstien, S., Butler, I.J., Smith, EO'.B., Kaufman, S., Glaze, D.G., and Percy, A.K. (1989). Cerebrospinal fluid biogenic amines and biopterin in Rett syndrome. *Ann. Neurol.,* **25,** 921–4.

Zoghbi, H.Y., Ledbetter, D.H., Schultz, R. *et al.* (1990a). A de novo X;3 translocation in Rett syndrome. *Am. J. Med. Genet.,* **35,** 148–51.

Zoghbi, H.Y., Percy, A.K., Schultz, R.J., Fill, C. (1990b). Patterns of X chromosome inactivation in the Rett syndrome. *Brain Dev.,* **12,** 131–5.

3 The neuropathology of the Rett disorder

Dawna D. Armstrong and Hannah C. Kinney

Summary

Many of the clinical, functional, anatomic and chemical features of Rett syndrome suggest that normal growth and maturation of the nervous system have been interrupted before or during infancy. Parts of the nervous system are not affected equally and there are preserved lacunae of function, anatomy and chemistry which contribute to the difficulty in defining the pathoetiology of the disorder. However, the identification of the deficiencies may lead to treatments, and to further investigations that will elucidate the pathogenesis of this maldevelopment. Although the deficits of the higher cortical functions in Rett syndrome seem most obvious and severe, the problems within the brainstem may be primary, and should be the focus of our research efforts.

3.1 Introduction

Rett syndrome is a disorder which affects between 1/10000–1/23,000 infant girls throughout the world (Hagberg *et al.* 1983; Burd *et al.* 1990; Kozinetz *et al.* 1993). It is associated with profound intellectual and motor disability and is diagnosed in typical cases by a unique phenotype (Chapter 1).The disorder is sporadic but rarely occurs in families and there is one example of vertical transmission from mother to daughter (Chapters 1, 2.) The infants 'seem' almost normal at birth (Chapter 1; Kerr 1995) and develop slowly, but into the second year of life the disorder becomes apparent, and the classic phenotype unfolds. A period of extreme agitation, suggesting an encephalopathy, heralds the appearance of the severe deficits: loss of hand use, loss of speech, sometimes loss of the ability to walk, growth delay, hand stereotypies, breathing irregularities, feeding problems and other subtle symptoms of autonomic dysfunction (Hagberg *et al.* 1983). There are frequently seizures, scoliosis, and Parkinsonian symptoms (FitzGerald *et al.* 1990).

The girls are small but mature sexually and, although there is an increased incidence of sudden death (Sekul et al. 1994), they may survive for decades.

This unusual disorder appears to be primarily a disease of the nervous system exhibiting functional impairment of the cerebral cortex, basal ganglia, limbic system, cerebellum, brainstem, spinal cord, skeletal muscles, pain sensation and autonomic nervous system. There are no obvious alterations in the morphology of any of these systems but special techniques have disclosed structural and chemoarchitectural defects which help to explain the functional deficits. There is, as yet, no consistent biochemical alteration that is pathognomonic of Rett syndrome, but the long awaited Rett gene, MECP2, has finally been identified (Amir et al. 1999). A definite diagnosis may now be made in some cases, and our understanding of the biology and the pathogenesis of this enigmatic disease process will be forthcoming.

In Rett syndrome, in spite of a predictable sequence of clinical symptoms that suggests a progressive pathology we have not identified any recognized process which characterizes degenerations associated with progressive brain disorders. That is, there is no continuing deterioration in serial clinical examinations (Kerr and Stephenson 1986), no progressive alteration in the magnetic resonance imaging (MRI) (Reiss et al. 1993), no evidence of progressive deterioration in the electroencephalogram (EEG) (Glaze et al. 1987) nor brain atrophy as defined by brain weight (Armstrong et al. 1999). Also, in the central nervous system there is no recognizable malformation, degeneration or inflammatory process, nor any consistent evidence of a cellular disorder involving cytoskeleton, lysosomes or myelin. The alterations, as described below, appear rather to be a deficiency of the dendritic and synaptic apparatus of selected neurons, their neurotransmitters and possibly some cellular proteins. The cause of these deficiencies is not understood.

Rett syndrome was initially described as being a progressive syndrome of autism, dementia, ataxia and loss of purposeful hand use in girls (Hagberg et al.1983). Since 1983 these features have been carefully re-evaluated. Rett syndrome can now be differentiated from autism (Percy et al. 1988). There is doubt about the progressive nature of the disorder and about whether 'dementia' is an appropriate interpretation of the mental handicap. Because of the absence of a recognizable disease process, and because of various functional, physical, anatomic and chemical features, it has been hypothesized that Rett syndrome could be a disorder of development. This chapter presents some of the observations pertaining to physical, functional, anatomic and chemical features of Rett syndrome which would support this hypothesis.

3.2 The physical aspects of Rett syndrome

3.2.1 The Rett girl is small

The Rett child is not dysmorphic; however, she is small for her age (Thommessen *et al.* 1992; Schultz *et al.* 1993) and appears to have a pervasive growth disorder. The etiology for this is being investigated. No consistent definition of a hormonal abnormality has been found (Holm 1986; Cooke *et al.* 1995). There is a difficulty with food intake, because of the lack of hand use and because of oropharyngeal and gastroesophageal incoordination (Morton *et al.* 1997; Motil *et al.* 1999). The increased energy expenditure associated with the continuous activity in the Rett child, such as the hand wringing, does not contribute to growth failure (Motil *et al.* 1998).

The pattern of growth failure is characterized by a deceleration of the growth of the head circumference, with deviation from the 50th percentile beginning in some infants at 3 months. Weight may begin to deviate at 4 months and height at 16 months (Schultz *et al.* 1993). The hands and feet are small (Schultz *et al.*1998). The hand length is proportionate to the height of the child whereas foot length is less than expected for height, suggesting that additional factors, such as decreased blood flow in the foot, may be influencing the foot size.

The pattern of decelerated head growth rate after birth appears to be unique for Rett syndrome, separating it from other disorders with microencephaly and some chromosomal disorders (Cronk 1978). The head does not appear to be disproportionately microcephalic because of the small size of the Rett girl. Head circumference has been correlated with the degree of motor handicap (Stenbom *et al.* 1995) and this measurement may be useful in recognizing forms of Rett syndrome with preserved speech and some hand use (Zappella 1992; Hagberg 1995).

3.2.2 The Rett brain is especially small

Data pertaining to brain size has been obtained through imaging studies and autopsy examinations. MRI studies have defined a reduced brain volume. There are however conflicting reports about whether the loss of brain volume is progressive. Murakami *et al.* (1992) reported global hypoplasia of the brain and a progressive atrophy of the cerebellum with age. Casanova *et al.* (1991) reported reduced area of the whole brain hemispheres and of the caudate nuclei. Reiss *et al.* (1993) reported that cerebral volume is reduced and that there is no decrease in brain volume over time. His more recent study, examining more cases (Subramaniam *et al.* 1997; Chapter 4), confirms this and observes that the white matter is more affected than the cortex.

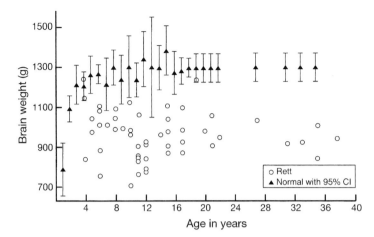

Fig. 3.1 The brain weight of 51 Rett girls and women at autopsy is designated as an open circle. The normal weight for each age is designated as a closed triangle. Note that, in this sample, there is no obvious decline in the weight of the Rett brain with increasing age.

The brain weight is reduced in Rett syndrome. In Fig. 3.1 the brain weights of 51 Rett girls and women, gathered from published reports (Jellinger and Seitelberger 1986; Riederer et al. 1986; Cornford et al. 1994; Bauman et al. 1995) and from the autopsy reports collected by the Rett Tissue Consortium, are compared with the published normal brain weights for girls and women. The mean Rett brain weight is 993 grams. In this sample there is no consistent decline in brain weight with age, an observation supporting the hypothesis that Rett syndrome is not the result of a progressive degenerative process.

Because there is a generalized growth arrest in the Rett girl, the weights of all organs were compared with established normal weights for girls and women. In Rett syndrome the heart, liver, spleen, kidneys, and adrenal glands all weigh less than the control values for age, but their weight is appropriate for height. The brain, however, is significantly reduced in weight for both age and height (Armstrong et al. 1999). This suggests that the brain in Rett syndrome is particularly vulnerable to the influences affecting growth in Rett syndrome.

3.3 The functional aspects of Rett Syndrome

3.3.1 Behaviour

The functional deficits of the Rett girl have been carefully recorded by clinicians around the world (Rett 1977; Hagberg et al. 1983; Nomura et al. 1984; Kerr and Stephenson, 1986; Aicardi, 1988; Witt Engerström 1991). Some abnormalities, disguised as 'good behaviour', are present at birth (Kerr 1995). This observation is extremely important as we attempt to understand the pathogenesis of the Rett disorder in relation to brain development. By the end of the first, year gross motor delays become apparent and hand stereotypies may be present. Non-specific abnormalities of tone, balance, coordination, feeding and involuntary movements are observed near the end of infancy. Then there follows a dramatic and terrifying period of regression, when acquired skills, particularly hand use and speech, are lost. This critical period is difficult to explain on the basis of arrested normal brain development. Some functions are conserved but the motor functions essential to independent survival, hand use and speech, cannot be maintained, or fail to develop. The absence of these skills makes the utility of formal neuropsychological testing questionable. However, such testing has defined the overall function of the Rett girl to be at a pre-intentional level consistent with a profound intellectual disability (Woodyatt and Ozanne 1992). Individual observations have suggested a range of developmental levels. Hand function in the classic Rett child is considered to be at the 4 month level. She can grasp and bring her hands to the midline (Nomura and Segawa 1990). Visual assessment (using a Teller procedure) defines a resolution acuity similar to unaffected 12–24 month infants (von Tetzchner *et al.* 1996).

3.3.2 Neurophysiology

Neurophysiological studies in Rett syndrome identify defective central processing of auditory stimuli (Strach *et al.* 1994), and defective sleep and respiratory patterns (Nomura *et al.* 1984; Piazza *et al.* 1990; Glaze *et al.* 1987; Kerr, 1992). Some studies suggest that the function of the brain is at an infantile level. Brainstem frequency-following responses in Rett syndrome are the same as those observed in control infants (Galbraith *et al.* 1996). EEG studies in 82 Rett girls (2–30 years, Glaze *et al.* 1987) demonstrate that the EEG pattern is appropriate for age at 5–18 months when signs of Rett syndrome are beginning to appear. Thereafter the EEG is abnormal exhibiting slowing, a loss of the occipital dominant rhythm, a loss of the non-rapid eye movement (NREM) sleep characteristics, and the presence of focal sharp wave discharges during sleep. In most of the girls in the post-regression period, the EEG is diffusely slow with poorly defined sleep patterns. But, in some girls in the later stages, there is a reappearance of the more normal occipital dominant rhythm and the NREM sleep characteristics.

Photon emission computed tomography reveals a global decrease in cerebral blood flow in Rett syndrome. There is a marked reduction in the prefrontal and temporoparietal association regions with relative sparing of the primary sensory-motor areas. The distribution of brain blood flow is considered to be similar to that associated with the metabolic activity of normal infants a few months of age (Nielsen *et al.* 1990).

Rett girls demonstrate episodic and profound irregularities of body homeostasis which include abnormalities of breathing pattern, blood pressure, arousal, nociception, eating and metabolism. Details of the autonomic dysfunction in Rett syndrome are presented in Chapters 1, 6 and 8, and in Nomura *et al.* (1984) and Kerr (1992). Haas *et al.* (1995), Glaze *et al.* (1987), Motil *et al.* (1999) have studied these significant autonomic abnormalities using continuous neurophysiological and metabolic recordings. Some of the alterations in autonomic function, e.g. the alterations in heart rate variability (Johnsrude *et al.* 1995) and the cardiorespiratory instability (Julu *et al.* 1997; Witt Engerström and Kerr 1998; and Julu Chapter 2), have been interpreted to reflect an immaturity of autonomic nervous control.

3.3.3 Neuroendocrinology

The functional abnormalities in Rett syndrome present a confusing picture, with deficits in some areas and preservation of others. For example, in spite of the abnormalities listed above, the maturation and functioning of the neuroendocrine system is apparently normal. The girls pass through menarche, develop secondary sexual characteristics and one pregnancy has been recorded (Witt Engerström and Forslund 1992).

3.4 The neuroanatomy Rett syndrome

Investigation of the neuroanatomy of Rett syndrome has been challenging and it is incomplete. The informative studies have required specialized histological and neurochemical techniques. The examinations that have been done were chosen on the basis of leads from other disciplines. Most of the anatomic studies have been performed on the cerebral cortex because the deficits of cortical function in Rett syndrome are immediately apparent. There are still regions to be examined in detail: the basal ganglia and thalamus, the amygdala and the brainstem. The studies presented here summarize the anatomic studies that add support to the hypothesis that Rett syndrome is a disorder of development.

3.4.1 The Rett brain is small

The Rett brain is decreased in size, with the average weight being similar to a 12 month infant (Fig. 3.1). However, the gross appearance of the cerebral cortex, myelin, ventricular system, basal ganglia, cerebellum and brainstem resembles that of a mature brain. In the first extensive report on the neuropathology of Rett syndrome, Jellinger and Seitelberger (1986) described the decreased size of the brain and, using quantitative techniques, made the astute observation that the neurons of the pars compacta of the substantia nigra contained less melanin than age matched control brains. All subsequent anatomic studies of the Rett brain have concentrated on the further definition and understanding of these two initial observations.

3.4.2 The Rett brain has decreases in volume and in neuronal dendritic arborization in specific cortical regions

The first volumetric MRI studies of 11 girls with RS (4–20 years) revealed that there is a general decrease in the amount of cortical grey matter, but that the volumes of the frontal lobe, caudate nucleus and midbrain are especially decreased (Reiss *et al.* 1993). However, in a subsequent study with more patients, the midbrain volume was found to be similar in Rett syndrome to that from age matched controls (Subramaniam *et al.* 1997; Chapter 4).

The brain volume is determined by neuronal and glial cell number, cell size, extent of dendritic arborization, amount of myelin, volume of the ventricles, and the number and size of blood vessels. In the Rett brain there is no apparent alteration in the ventricular size or in myelination. Bauman *et al.* (1995) have observed that individual neuronal size is reduced and that the packing density (the number of neurons per $0.1\,mm^3$ area) is increased in the hippocampus and entorhinal cortex. This observation implies that there may be a reduction in dendritic arborization. We have verified this in selected neuronal population in several specific brain regions (Armstrong *et al.*1995). In 16 Rett brains, ages 2.9–35 years, the premotor frontal (area 6), motor (area 4), inferior temporal (area 20), hippocampus (areas 34, 28), and visual cortex (area 17) were studied using a rapid Golgi technique. Pyramidal neurons of layers III and V were examined except in the hippocampus. Drawings of the dendritic branches, basilar and apical, were submitted to the Sholl analysis, which revealed a paucity of dendrite numbers and a simplified branching pattern. These alterations were not obvious without analysis. The pyramidal neurons in frontal, motor and inferior temporal regions had significantly less dendritic branching than those of the non-Rett brains. Within these cortical regions, basal and apical dendrites were affected differently; basal dendrites of layers III and V in the frontal and motor cortex were decreased. Basal dendrites of layer IV of the subiculum and apical dendrites of layer V of the motor cortex were significantly decreased in their dendritic arborization. Since our first report we have analysed additional cases and find that the subicular region approaches significant alteration whereas the basilar dendrites of the inferior temporal gyrus are now significantly reduced (Fig. 3.2). These observations suggest that synaptic input into the cortex at these sites would be less than normal, an idea supported by Belichenko and Dahlstrom's (1995) observations in the Rett frontal cortex (using confocal laser scanning microscopy) of a regional 'loss' of dendritic spines. The Golgi studies have identified a deficiency of dendrites in frontal, motor and temporal cortex, brain regions associated with many of the functions which are deficient in Rett syndrome. Such regional

64 | Rett disorder and the developing brain

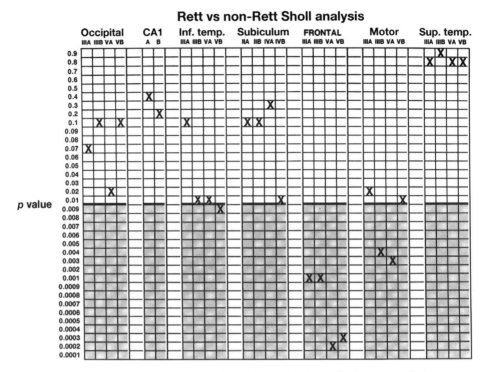

Fig. 3.2 The significance of the decrease in dendritic arborizations in Rett brains compared with non-Rett brains is depicted graphically. Seveb cortical regions are analysed and the apical and basilar dendrites of pyramidal neurons in the third and fifth, or second and fourth, layers are compared. Note that the Rett brains show highly significant decreases in dendritic branching in the frontal and motor cortex, and notable involvement also of the temporal cortex.

selectivity raises the possibility that the 'factor' responsible for Rett syndrome has its greatest effect in these specific cortical regions.

3.4.3 The dendritic branching deficits in Rett syndrome are not seen in trisomy-21, another disorder with psychomotor delay

Reduced dendritic arborization is not pathognomonic of a particular disease process and could reflect either a lack of dendrite formation or atrophy. In Rett syndrome, as stated above, there is no convincing evidence, such as gliosis, that the dendrites are degenerating, or becoming atrophic, so that a lack of formation is a plausible explanation of the small dendrites. Malformed and reduced dendrites have also been recorded in various other forms of mental retardation, so that this observation in Rett syndrome is not unexpected (Huttenlocher 1974; Marin-Padilla 1976; Takashima *et al.* 1981; Bauman and Kemper 1982; Jagadha and Becker 1989). In these previous studies of the brain in mental retardation only one or two brain regions were examined. To determine whether the selective alterations observed in the Rett brain were unique to Rett syndrome, a similar study was undertaken of the same six brain regions in Down's syndrome (Armstrong *et al.* 1998). Six trisomy-21 brains (0.6–11 years) were evaluated. In Rett syndrome the dendritic arborization in the basal dendrites of layers III and V of the frontal cortex, layer IV of the subiculum and layer V of the motor cortex and the apical dendrites of layer III of the frontal cortex were significantly smaller than those of trisomy-21. This observation adds supports to our hypothesis that there is a selective 'malformation' of specific neurons in Rett syndrome.

3.4.4 The Rett brain shows regional deficiencies of neuronal proteins

There are several ongoing studies attempting to characterize specific neuronal cell populations in Rett syndrome. Belichenko (Witt Engerström and Kerr 1998; Chapter 11) has evaluated the speech areas 4, 45, 22, and 40 in Rett brains and identified in them a 'normal pattern of asymmetry' in which the pyramidal neurons in cortical layers III are larger in the left speech area than in the right speech area. However, he also observed that the numbers of interneurons, as identified with antibodies to parvalbumin, are reduced in the Rett brain. In the Rett speech areas too he has found less synaptophysin immunoreactivity suggesting that there is a decrease in the numbers of synaptic sites within the speech areas.

Kauffman (Kaufmann *et al.* 1995; Chapter 4) has evaluated the neocortex of three Rett brains (8, 12, and 18 years) for the presence of specific neuronal markers, and demonstrated that pyramidal neurons as defined with anti-neurofilament (monoclonal SMI-32 Sternberger), anti calbindin-D-28K (monoclonal CL-300 Sigma), and anti neuropeptide Y (polyclonal Inkstar) were normal except for their reduced size and ramification. In ten Rett brains (ages 5–34) he found decreased expression of cyclooxygenase (an enzyme which is normally-present in dendritic spines) in the deeper layers of the motor and frontal cortex (Kaufmann *et al.*1997). In the three cases (8–18 years) he has defined an abnormality of a microtubulin associated protein (MAP2, monoclonal SMI-52 Sternberger) (Kaufmann *et al.*1995) which exhibits reduced staining in the deepest layers of the cortex, and an absence of MAP2 staining in the subplate neurons. The prefrontal cortex was more involved than the premotor and orbitofrontal cortex, and he suggests that the earliest migrating neurons of the cortex and the subplate neurons are defective in this major protein. MAP2 is regulated by several neurotransmitter systems, which may be abnormal in Rett syndrome. Kaufmann's observations support the concept of specific neuronal anomalies or deficiencies in Rett syndrome.

3.4.5 Some unanswered questions about the histopathology of Rett syndrome

(a) *Are there reduced numbers of neurons in the Rett brain?*
The decreased brain weight and volume of the Rett brain has been partially explained by the decrease in dendritic arborization (Armstrong *et al*.1995) which could account for the observed increase in packing density in selected brain regions (Baumann *et al*.1995) In addition, as described above, there may be an absence of specific populations of neurons in Rett syndrome (Witt Engerström and Kerr 1998; Kaufmann *et al.* 1995). However, quantitative studies of neurons in Rett syndrome are incomplete. Actual neuronal counts of brain regions in Rett syndrome have been reported in only a few regions.

Jellinger and Seitelberger (1986) evaluated the nucleus basalis of Meynert and the nucleus raphe dorsalis and found no difference in neuronal number or density in two Rett brains compared with age matched controls. Bauman (Bauman and Kemper 1995) has found increased the packing density (the neuronal nucleoli/0.1 mm^3) and decreased cell size in the hippocampus, subiculum and entorhinal cortex of three Rett brains compared with age matched controls. Kitt reported a 30% reduction of neurons in the substantia nigra with decreased melanin in the pars compacta in one 21 year old Rett brain compared to an age matched control. Jellinger and Seitelberger (1986) examined the substantia nigra for pigmented cells in two Rett brains and observed that about 30% of the neurons in the zona compacta contained little or no melanin whereas only 7% of the neurons in controls had no melanin. The total number of neurons was not significantly reduced.

(b) *Is there neuronal degeneration in Rett syndrome?*
The original report of Rett syndrome, using light microscopy but no quantitative evaluations, reported that there was 'mild to very mild spotty loss of neurons with occasional astrogliosis but no definite increase in GFAP reactivity' (Jellinger and Seitelberger 1986). These observations and others must be considered (Armstrong 1997). Belichenko in four brains, reports a loss of pyramidal neurons in layers II and III compared with layers V and VII, with more loss in frontal and temporal cortex than in visual cortex. Kitt (Kitt and Wilcox 1995), using the TUNEL method and an age matched control, reported apoptosis in the substantia nigra of one case (age 21 years). They also observed ubiquitin positive intraneuronal inclusions, suggesting that this represented neurodegeneration. Wenk and Hauss-Wegrzyniak (1999) studied three Rett brains with the TUNEL technique and found positive cells in the basal forebrain of a 4 and 21 year old, but none in a 35 year old. Cornford *et al.* (1994) found evidence of increased lipofuscin in the cortex and basal ganglia in one case of Rett syndrome (age 15 years), and suggestive evidence of neuronal degeneration in the basal ganglia. Jellinger and Seitelberger (1986) observed axons with a reactive or degenerative change in the

caudate nucleus, and Belichenko (Armstrong 1997) reported that there was degeneration in the hand region of the pallidus. Oldfors *et al*. (1990) studied the cerebellum in five brains (ages 7–30 years) and observed gliosis and some foliar atrophy in the older brains. He studied two spinal cords (20 and 30 years) and reported gliosis, loss of dorsal root ganglia and motor neurons and degenerating axons. Jellinger *et al*. (1990) studied the peripheral nerves in four Rett girls (9–19 years) and muscle in two of them. He found no evidence of motor neuron degeneration in any case but only of a late onset denervation related to distal axonopathy of unknown etiology.

There is lack of agreement about some other observations which suggest degeneration. Belichenko *et al*. (1994) report normal lipofuscin in Rett brains compared with controls, but Jellinger and Seitelberger (1986) and Cornford *et al*. (1994) have observed increased lipofuscin. Belichenko *et al*. (1997) report a 20–40% decrease in synaptophysin in four Rett cases whereas Cornford found normal synaptophysin in frontal cortex, basal ganglia and substantia nigra in a 15 year old Rett brain. Some of these differences may be explained on the basis of age and brain sites studied. In all of the reports there does not seem to be a unanimous conviction that degeneration occurs in Rett syndrome. However, on the other hand, there is agreement, using evidence from several techniques, confocal microscopy, immunocytochemistry, quantitation and Golgi studies (Belichenko *et al*. 1994; Kaufmann *et al*. 1995; Baumann *et al*. 1995; Armstrong *et al*. 1995), that the projection neurons of selected cortical regions are small or have decreased branches. As yet there is no morphologic study that proves this to be the result of hypoplasia or of atrophy. But, as outlined above, there are several observations from other disciplines to support a hypothesis of 'underdevelopment'.

(c) *Is there delayed maturation or dysmaturation in the Rett brain?*
The average weight of the Rett brain for girls and women is comparable to that of a 12 month infant. But the brain has features of an older brain; the myelination appears to be complete, the external granular cell layer of the cerebellum has migrated appropriately; the neocortical neurons appear to be in their correct positions, and the brainstem is superficially normally formed. However, there have been isolated observations and some well-defined studies using special techniques to study neuronal structure and chemistry which identify some features which may represent faulty and/or delayed maturation.

Jellinger and Seitelberger (1986) noted microdysgenesis in three brains which exhibited persistence of small cells in the molecular layer of the frontal and the hippocampal cortex. These granular cells usually migrate into the cortex before birth (Friede 1989). The same authors compared the quantity and substructure of melanin in the substantia nigra of an 11 year old Rett brain and found it, in part, to resemble the substructure of melanin of a 5 year old control.

Belichenko (Armstrong 1997) observed fewer neurons in layers II and III than

V and VI. This suggested an arrest of cortical migration, with a decreased complement of neurons in the neocortex. The lack of gliosis argues against neuronal loss. The reduced branching of dendrites in the cortex (Armstrong et al. 1995) could also be interpreted to be the result of interrupted development. Kaufmann et al. (1995) demonstration of aberrant MAP2 expression may suggest an abnormal maturation of selected neuronal populations.

Poliakov (1961) has identified three time periods in the organization of the human cortex. The first, in utero, establishes the cortico-subcortical projections between the fifth layer of the cortex and the basal ganglia, brainstem and cord. At birth the second period of development involves an integration of layer III into the connections of layer V. In this period there is dendritic growth and identification of interneurons. This second period of cortical development which extends into the second year of life may be interrupted in Rett syndrome, resulting in the abnormalities of dendrites and interneurons that have been identified. The final stage of cortical ontogeny goes on for years and involves the associative cortical connections in the uppermost layers. These have not been studied anatomically in Rett sdyndrome.

In our examination of serotonin receptor binding in the Rett brainstem (see below), we have observed, in some of the nuclei concerned with autonomic control, an increased receptor binding which resembles the levels seen in an immature brain. This provides data from another technique which suggests that there may be an abnormal development in Rett syndrome.

3.5 The chemical anatomy of the Rett brain

Nomura et al. (1984) were among the first to suggest that neurotransmitter abnormalities could be the chemical basis for Rett syndrome. They defined abnormalities of muscle tone, eye movement, and sleep in their polygraph recordings of Rett girls and postulated that these abnormalities could be related to a deficiency of brainstem serotonin and dopamine. They relate the sleep abnormalities to serotonin deficiency, and the presence of muscle twitches to a dopamine abnormality. They also speculated that a brainstem deficiency could be responsible for a defective development and functioning of higher brain regions.

This idea that deficiency of a neurotransmitter could produce an effect on brain function and/or development in Rett syndrome is appropriate. The Rett disorder is first manifest in infancy, a critical period in brain development when many neurotransmitters show a changing pattern of expression and act as growth factors (Kinney et al. 1993, 1995; Zec et al. 1996).

There are many limited studies of neurotransmitters in Rett syndrome, using tissues from various sites or CSF. There have been various techniques utilized, such as spectroscopy and immunocytochemical assays. The biogenic amines, dopamine, norepinephrine, and serotonin were studied first (Riederer *et al.* 1986; Zoghbi *et al.* 1985; Brucke *et al.* 1987; Wenk *et al.* 1991, Zoghbi *et al.* 1989; Perry *et al.* 1988; Lekman *et al.* 1989, 1990; Nielsen *et al.* 1992; Percy 1992) (see Chapter 4). When opioids were found to be elevated in the CSF (Budden *et al.* 1990; Nielsen *et al.* 1991) a clinical trial of naloxone (Percy *et al.* 1994) was initiated. This was not successful in altering the function of the Rett girls. More recently, studies of acetylcholine (Wenk *et al.* 1991; Wenk 1997) and glutamate are underway (Hamberger *et al.* 1992; Lappalainen *et al.* 1996; Chapter 4). Other trophic factors, nerve growth factor (Lappalainen *et al.* 1996; Riikonen and Vanhala 1999) and substance P (Matsuishi *et al.* 1997) have been found to be deficient in the CSF. Wenk (1997) summarized the studies of neurotransmitters and peptides and concluded that only the acetylcholine markers are consistently reduced whereas all others show variable changes. He recently examined the ChAT immunoreactivity and p75 immunoreactivity (an NGF receptor) in the nucleus of Meynert in three Rett brains. He found decreased ChAT immunoreactivity, but normal p75 immunoreactivity. The disagreement about levels of specific markers may be related to different degrees of impairment in the Rett child (Percy 1992) or to the age at examination. (Leckman *et al.* 1989). There is also the real possibility that if some or all of the neurotransmitters do not develop appropriately, the responses expected in a normal system may not be present (Naidu 1997). It is noteworthy, though, that every system has had abnormalities recorded, particularly in the basal ganglia.

The chemoarchitecture of the brainstem in Rett syndrome has been incompletely studied. We have initiated an autoradiographic survey of receptor binding for three different types of neurotransmitters, (opioid, muscarinic cholinergic and serotoninergic) in the brainstem of Rett syndrome and have investigated the immunohistochemistry of the neuropeptide, substance P. We found elevated serotonin receptor binding and decreased substance P immunoreactivity in selected brainstem regions, and these studies are described below.

3.5.1 Serotonin studies in Rett syndrome

Nomura *et al.* (1984) first suggested a defect in the brainstem serotonin because of early autistic-like behaviour, and abnormal sleep patterns in the Rett infant. Riederer *et al.* (1986) examined brain tissue in an 11 year old Rett brain and reported decreased serotonin and 5IAA, a serotonin metabolite, in the caudate, putamen, globus pallidus, raphe and reticular region, and amygdala, with normal amounts in the cingulate cortex. Brucke (1987) examined brain tissue in an 11 year old Rett brain and compared it with a 5 year old control. In the Rett brain he found evidence of decreased serotonin and an increase in its metabolism in cingulate cortex, thalamus, hypothalamus, amygdala, nucleus basalis, substantia nigra and raphe/reticular region compared with a 5 year old control brain tissue.

It was normal in the occipital cortex and white matter. Lekman et al. (1989) examined brain tissue from five Rett brains ages 12, 17, 20, and 30. She found normal values for serotonin and 5HIAA in the frontal cortex, thalamus, hippocampus, caudate, putamen and globus pallidus, and decreases in the substantia nigra. Wenk et al. (1991) examined five Rett brains ages 4, 10, 12, 15, and 21 years in the frontal, temporal and occipital cortices, the putamen and amygdala and found no consistent changes in serotonin and 5HIAA. Harris et al. (1986) reported normal 5HIAA in the CSF of one 25 year old. Perry et al. (1988) found normal CSF serotonin and 5HIAA in five Rett girls (4, 6, 7, 10). Zoghbi et al. (1989) reported a reduction of CSF 5HIAA in 32 girls with RS (1.8–16 years). Budden et al. (1990) found normal values for 5HIAA in CSF of 12 Rett girls (2–15 years) and in all but the oldest girl. Nielsen et al. (1992) found that CSF levels of 5HIAA in 10 Rett girls (5.8–17.2 years) were less than the control, but the difference was not significant. He produced elevations of CSF values for 5HIAA in 11 Rett girls (6–17 years) with supplemental tyrosine and tryptophan (Nielsen et al. 1990).

3.5.2 Brainstem serotoninergic receptor binding studies in Rett syndrome

The brainstem is a major focus of research in Rett syndrome due to clinical irregularities in autonomic control and breathing (Chapters 1, 6), functions mediated in large part by the brainstem. Moreover, it has been postulated that autonomic control is immature in Rett syndrome, based upon specific patterns of autonomic dysfunction. For example, Peter Julu, using non-invasive neurophysiological investigation of brainstem autonomic control, has demonstrated the presence of apneustic breathing in young girls with RS, accentuating our interest in the role of serotonin in the Rett disorder (Julu et al. 1997; Kerr et al. 1998; Julu in Witt Engerström and Kerr 1998; Chapter 6). Given that serotonin is a key neurotransmitter involved in the modulation of brainstem autonomic control and breathing (Fornal and Jacobs 1998), as well as in neural development, it is a reasonable candidate molecule to analyse in relevant brainstem nuclei in Rett cases. In a pilot study of Rett brainstems, we postulated that 3H-lysergic acid diethylamide (LSD) binding to serotonergic receptors is altered (up or down-regulated) in brainstem nuclei related to autonomic control and/or to respiration, and is homologous to binding levels in immature, i.e. infant, brainstem nuclei. In this pilot study the relevant nuclei included: the nucleus of the solitary tract (visceral sensory input, dorsal respiratory group and central chemosensitivity), dorsal motor nucleus of the vagus (preganglionic parasympathetic outflow), hypoglossal nucleus (control of upper airway patency), nucleus raphe obscurus (central chemosensitivity, sympathetic inhibition or excitation via projection to interomedilolateral column, respiratory modulation via innervation of the phrenic nucleus), para-ambiguus region (ventral respiratory tract), arcuate nucleus (putative respiratory chemosensitive fields on the ventral medullary surface), periaqueductal grey (defence response) and nucleus paragigantocellularis (respiratory control). To test the specificity of altered serotonergic binding to cardiorespiratory related sites, analysis was performed in non-cardiorespiratory sites, e.g. principal, medial accessory, and dorsal accessory inferior olive (precerebellar relay), nucleus centralis (motor relay), inferior colliculus (auditory relay) and substantia nigra (motor relay) and in sites related to arousal, e.g. locus coeruleus, interpeduncular nucleus, nucleus pontis oralis, and median and dorsal raphe nuclei.

In the pilot study of serotonergic brainstem binding in Rett cases, we performed quantitative receptor autoradiography on glass mounted, standardized tissue sections according to our published methods (Zec et al. 1996).Quantitative densitometry of the autoradiograms was performed with an MCID imaging system (Imaging Research Inc., Ontario) and optical densities were converted to specific activity levels in femtomoles/milligram (fmol/mg) tissue with the use of 3H-standards. Tritiated-LSD was selected as the radioligand because it binds non-specifically to the subtypes of the serotonergic receptor (5HT1 1A-1D and 5HT2) and thus provides general information about multiple serotonin receptor subtypes. Three groups were compared: 'mature' Rett cases, $n=3$ (7, 7, and 35 years old), 'mature' controls, $n=4$ (4–68 years) and infant controls, $n=6$ (38–74 post-conceptional weeks). Note that the 'mature' Rett cases and controls consists of both children and adults, because in baseline studies we found no significant difference in brainstem serotonergic binding levels between these two age groups (Zec et al. 1996). Also note that the infant control values represent baseline, published data for comparison (Zec et al. 1996).

In this pilot study, we found a significant ($p<0.05$) increase in 3H-LSD binding to serotonergic receptors in Rett cases compared to 'mature' controls in seven brainstem nuclei (Table 3.1). The affected nuclei are not only restricted to brainstem cardiorespiratory control ($n=4$: nucleus of the solitary tract, dorsal motor nucleus of the vagus, hypoglassal nucleus, and nucleus raphe obscurus) as postulated in the study's hypothesis, but also include nuclei unrelated to brainstem cardiorespiratory control ($n=3$: nucleus centralis, dorsal accessory olive, medial accessory olive) (Table 3.1). In three nuclei there was a marginal difference ($0.05<p<0.10$) in serotonergic binding between the Rett cases and mature controls (principal inferior olive, nucleus gigantocellularis, and substantia nigra) (Table 3.1).

The finding of affected cardiorespiratory-related nuclei supports our hypothesis that such nuclei are involved in Rett pathology, but the finding of affected non-cardiorespiratory-related nuclei indicates that altered serotonergic binding in Rett brainstems is not specific to cardiorespiratory nuclei. The increase in receptor binding may reflect decreased serotonergic input into the affected nucleus, with a compensatory upregulation of receptor binding and/or binding affinity. Virtually all of the affected nuclei receive innervation from the caudal raphe complex (see

Table 3.1 Serotonergic receptor binding (fmol/mg tissue) in brainstem nuclei in Rett case, Rett controls and infant controls

	Rett cases	Mature controls	p value /M)	Infant controls	p value (M/I)
Cardiorespiratory-related nuclei					
1. NTS	33	16	*.0.4	43	0.05
2. DMX	26	14	*0.04	50	0.01
3. HG	31	9	*0.003	—	—
4. NROb	40	9	*0.006	41	0.01
5. ARC	8	5	0.43	9	NS
6. PAG	47	17	0.15	58	NS
7. NPGCL	13	9	0.21	34	0.05
Arousal-related nuclei					
8. LC	27	20	0.61	43	0.05
9. IPN	19	15	0.45	43	NS
10. NpoO	29	18	0.59	54	0.05
11. MR	52	48	0.72	147	0.01
12. DR	76	46	0.60	160	0.05
13. CUN	26	15	0.10	39	NS
Miscellaneous nuclei					
14. PIO	15	6	0.06	15	0.05
15. DAO	17	4	*0.01	27	0.05
16. MAO	17	5	*0.03	36	0.05
17. CENT	17	4	*0.06	30	0.05
18. IC	27	8	*0.01	30	NS
19. SN	86	17	0.06	—	—
20. BP	9	6	0.31	10	0.05

Abbreviations: NTS, nucleus of the solitary tract; DMX, dorsal motor nucleus of cranial nerve X; HG, hypoglossal nucleus; NROb, nucleus raphe obscurus; ARC, arcuate nucleus; PAG, periaqueductal grey; NPGCL, nucleus paragigantocellularis lateralis; LC, locus coeruleus; IPN, interpeduncular nucleus; PpoO, nucleus pontis oralis; MR, median raphe; DR, dorsal raphe; CUN, nucleus cuneiformis; PIO, principal inferior olive; DAO, dorsal accessory olive; MAO, medial accessory olive; CENT, nucleus centralis; IC, inferior colliculus; SN, substantia nigra; PB, basis pontis.
* significant.

below), suggesting the possibility that there is a loss/dysfunction of the serotonergic source neurons in this complex. Overall binding values in the infant controls are higher than in the 'mature' controls (Table 3.1), suggesting a decrease in receptor number and/or affinity between infancy and child/adulthood. Values in the Rett case are more 'infant-like' (high levels) than 'mature-like' (low levels) (Table 3.1, Fig. 3.3), supporting the hypothesis that there is delayed serotonergic maturation in selected Rett brainstem nuclei. Of interest in this regard, the binding pattern, in the subdivisions of the inferior olivary complex is likewise more 'infant-like' than 'mature-like' with higher binding in the DAO and MAO relative to the PIO in the Rett cases, like the infant cases, compared with higher binding in the PIO relative to the DAO and MAO in the 'mature-like' controls. Of note, all

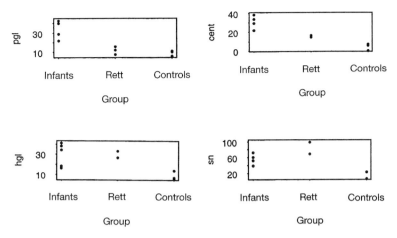

Fig. 3.3 The serotonin receptor binding in selected nuclei of Rett brainstems is compared with the binding present in these nuclei in infant and mature non-Rett control brainstems. In each graph the abscissa records the amount of receptor binding in fmol/mg of tissue. Along the ordinate the values for the infant, Rett and mature controls are presented in columns. In the nucleus paragigantocellularis lateralis (pgl) the binding in the Rett nuclei is similar to that of the mature controls. In the nucleus centralis (cent) and the hypoglossal nucleus (hgl) there is more binding in the Rett nuclei than in the mature control nuclei. In the substantia nigra (sn) there is more binding in the Rett nuclei than in either of the control groups. Note that the numbers of cases in each nuclei varied depending upon the availability of the tissue.

the statistically and marginally significantly affected nuclei in the Rett cases are involved in motor function, including the nucleus of the solitary tract which is not only visceral sensory, but also contains premotor neurons (dorsal respiratory group) that project to the phrenic nucleus in the spinal cord which is involved in the motor aspects of respiration.

The identification of potential abnormalities of serotonergic receptor binding in the Rett brainstem is worthy of further research involving a large number of Rett cases and mature controls. In the following paragraphs we consider the potential significance of altered brainstem serotonergic receptor binding in Rett syndrome, justifying further research of the serotonin/raphe system in this syndrome within and above the brainstem. Most of the CNS serotonin originates from serotonin-source neurons located in the midline raphe complex of the brainstem, with major ascending projections arising from the rostral raphe nuclei (nucleus raphe dorsalis, median raphe) to the forebrain, and descending projections arising from the caudal raphe nuclei (nucleus raphe obscurus, nucleus raphe pallidus, and nucleus raphe magnus) to the cerebellum, other brainstem nuclei and spinal cord. Serotonergic neurons also reside in nuclei of the reticular formation lateral to the midline, namely in the nucleus gigantocellularis, nucleus paragigantocellularis and intermediate reticular zone in the medulla and in the nucleus pontis oralis in the pons of the human infant.

A role for serotonin and the raphe complex has been proposed for multiple functions including motor activity, cardiovascular function, respiration, central chemoreception, cognition, mood, arousal, pain modulation, gut motility, and the regulation of cerebral blood flow and the blood brain barrier. A key feature of all serotonergic raphe neurons is their strong sleep state dependence in firing rates: the firing rates are increased during waking, reduced in NREM sleep, and fall nearly silent in REM sleep. Another general feature of brainstem serotonergic neurons is autoreceptor mediated feedback inhibition (Aghajanian *et al.*). Jacobs and co-workers point out however that, by itself, serotonin produces little or no change in neuronal activity: on the other hand, when it is combined with either direct application of excitatory amino acids (e.g. glutamate) or with electrical stimulation of dorsal roots or motor cortex, it facilitates motor output.

We have performed autoradiographic studies on the brainstems from three Rett syndrome cases ages 7, 7, and 35 years. Infant and mature controls consisted of six infants (mean age 56 post-conceptional weeks) and four mature controls (4, 20 and 68 years). Quantitative receptor autoradiography was performed on frozen tissue using our published methods for tissue preparation, sampling, establishment of controls for non-specific binding and generation of autoradiograms (Kinney *et al.* 1990, 1995; Zec *et al.* 1996). Quantitative densitometry of auto-

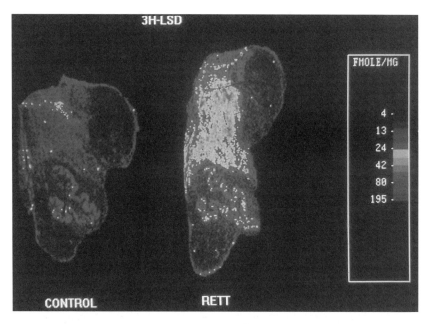

Fig. 3.4a Representative example of serotonin receptor binding in the medulla of a mature control brain (left) and a Rett brain (right). The photograph is colour-coded with a colour scale marking the specific binding activity levels in fmol/mg tissue. Note that there is a greater density of receptor binding in the regions of the nucleus of the solitary tract and the nucleus centralis in the Rett medulla. (See also colour plate section.)

radiograms was performed with an MCID imaging system (Imaging Research Inc., Ontario) and optical densities were converted to specific activities in fmol/mg tissue. The ligand used was 3H-LSD (5 nM) for which the putative binding sites are 5HT 1A–1D and $5HT_2$. Serotonin was used as displacer. The tissue was incubated for 60 minutes and the film exposed for 8 weeks.

Twenty-two nuclei of the brainstem were measured using standardized brainstem levels as defined in the Olszewski and Baxter (1954) atlas: the mid-medulla at the level of nucleus of Roler was used for measurements of hypoglossal nucleus, principal inferior olive, medial and dorsal accessory olive, nucleus of the solitary tract, dorsal motor nucleus of the vagus, raphe obscurus, arcuate nucleus and nucleus centralis medullae oblongata. Fig. 3.4*a*. The rostral medulla at the level of nucleus praepositus was used for measurement of nucleus gigantocellularis, nucleus paragigantocellularis lateralis, and nucleus raphe obscurus. The rostral pons at the level of the nucleus parabrachialis lateralis was used for the nucleus pontis oralis, basis pontis, medial raphe and locus ceruleus. The caudal midbrain at the level of the decussation of the superior cerebellar peduncle was used for measurements of nucleus cuneiformis, periaqueductal grey, nucleus raphe dorsalis, inferior colliculus, substantia nigra and interpeduncular nucleus. Fig. 3.4*b*. The significance of the differences in the mean binding values of the Rett and

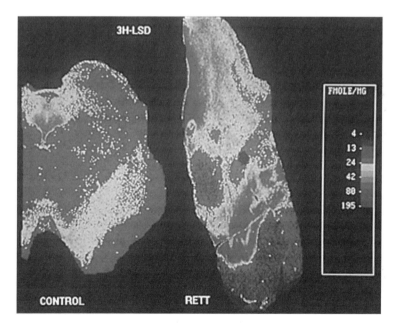

Fig. 3.4b Representative example of serotonin receptor binding in the midbrain of a mature control brain (left) and a Rett brain (right). The photograph is colour-coded with a colour scale marking the specific binding activity levels in fmol/mg tissue. Note that there is a greater density of receptor binding in the regions of the substantia nigra in the Rett midbrain. (See also colour plate section.)

the mature control group was compared for each nucleus using the appropriate version of the T test.

Twelve of the 22 nuclei analysed showed increased receptor binding for serotonin in the Rett cases compared to mature controls. For some of the nuclei tissue was only available for two Rett cases. In seven nuclei the increase was significant ($p<0.05$). These nuclei are the dorsal accessory olivary nucleus (5 times greater binding), the nucleus centralis (4 times greater binding), the raphe obscurus (4 times greater binding), the medial accessory olivary nucleus (4 times greater binding), the hypoglossal nucleus (3 times greater binding), the nucleus of the solitary tract (2 times greater binding), and the dorsal motor nucleus of the vagus (2 times greater binding). The substantia nigra exhibited 5 times greater binding with a p value of 0.059. These values, although significantly higher than the mature control values, are less than the values for the infant cases. More cases need to be analysed to verify the consistency of these pilot observations, and studies of specific serotonin receptors will need to be evaluated.

This identification of potential abnormalities of the serotonin receptors in Rett syndrome defines a brainstem pathology in Rett syndrome The serotonin neurons are located in the raphe system, and in cellular groups in the pontine and medullary reticular formation. They project to forebrain regions, cerebellum, spinal cord and to other brainstem nuclei. The elevation of serotonin receptors may indicate a decrease in the available serotonin with upregulation of the receptors, or it may reflect an incomplete maturation of this system, with levels remaining elevated, at the brainstem levels seen in the immature (i.e.infant) brainstem (Zec *et al.* 1996).

Serotonin is particularly worthy of consideration in relation to the pathoetiology of Rett syndrome because of its dual role in the neurophysiology of the autonomic system and in brain development. Serotonin has a diffuse functional role in the brain. It has a slow, prolonged effect and, following its release, (which may be under the control of locally acting neurotransmitters), it reinforces neuronal circuits by modulating the activity of amino acids and acetylcholine. Serotonin neurons are active in wakefulness inhibiting cholinergic neurons in the pons, and influencing noradrenergic neurons in the locus ceruleus. They are involved in the perception of pain and they influence the brainstem regulation of cardiorespiratory control. They influence cerebral circulation, the blood brain barrier and some of the neurons concerned with bowel motility via focal serotoninergic ganglion cells. Each of these spheres of serotonin influence is abnormal in Rett syndrome. These include the significant abnormalities concerned with body homeostasis: swallowing, gut motility (Motil *et al.* 1990), respiratory control (Witt Engerström and Kerr 1998), heart rate and EKG pattern (Sekul *et al.* 1994; Johnsrude *et al.* 1995), peripheral circulation, and pain perception (Hagberg *et al.* 1983). It seems probable that the abnormalities of serotonin receptor binding are related to these problems in neurophysiology.

A defective serotonin system could also be involved in producing the developmental defect in Rett syndrome. Serotonin is one of the first neurotransmitters to develop and its first function is as a growth factor influencing cell proliferation and maturation. The serotonin network requires specific serotonin receptors, each of which activate a transduction mechanism within the receptive cell. There are many types of serotonin receptors in the adult brain, but, because there are receptors which are expressed only during development, the elucidation of serotonin's possible role in altering brain development in Rett syndrome will be challenging to investigate.

3.5.3 Substance P in Rett syndrome

Substance P is a peptide which colocalizes with some serotonin neurons and functions as a neuromodulator in the central and the peripheral nervous system. It is decreased in the CSF of Rett girls (Matsuishi et al.1997). We have examined the immunocytochemistry of substance P (subP) in the brainstem, basal ganglia and frontal cortex in 14 Rett brains (6–35 years) and 10 control brains (2 months to 29 years). We used formalin fixed, paraffin embedded tissues, the peroxidase anti-peroxidase techniques employing the anti substance P antibody from Incstar. The degree of immunoreactivity was evaluated semiquantitatively using the control staining in the spinal cord dorsal horn as the maximum degree of staining.

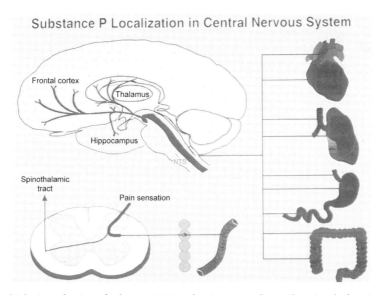

Fig. 3.5 Multiple sites of action of substance P. Note that in Rett syndrome there is a dysfunction of many of these sites, suggesting that the deficiency of substance P may be associated with the abnormality (illustrated by Kimiko Deguchi). (See also colour plate section.)

Substance P immunoreactivity in the dorsal horn of the spinal cord and the nucleus of the solitary tract in RS was compared with the staining of these regions in infants and young children. The degree of immunoreactivity of these regions in these non-Rett brains increased with age. The degree of staining in the Rett brains was similar to the youngest non-Rett brains.

In the spinal cord the Rett cases exhibited less staining in the dorsal horns, dorsal roots and intermediolateral column. Substance P was significantly reduced in the spinal trigeminal tract, the nucleus of the solitary tract, the reticular formation (at three levels, medulla, pons and midbrain) and the locus ceruleus. There was decreased subP in the frontal cortex and in the internal globus pallidus, but staining comparable to the controls in the hippocampus, the substantia nigra and the periaqueductal grey of the midbrain.

Many ganglia of the gastrointestinal tract, the heart and lungs contain subP and project sensory fibres to the central nervous system. There are substance P neurons and fibres in the spinal trigeminal nucleus, the dorsal motor nucleus of the vagus, the parvocellular reticular nucleus and the raphe obscurus and pallidus, the locus ceruleus, and the periaqueductal grey matter. Substance P containing fibres are present in many nuclei of the brainstem, striatum, pallidus and neocortex. Substance P neurons of the medulla project to the intermediolateral neurons of the cord and are important in blood pressure regulation (Pioro and Mai, 1990).

Substance P is a tachykinin which functions in pain transmission in the peripheral and central nervous systems, and in the excitation of the neurons involved in the control of respiratory and cardiovascular functions. It is involved in providing olfactory and visual information, controlling the calibre of pial blood vessels, salivation, gut motility, growth hormone and prolactin production. Experimentally it has been shown to influence neurite outgrowth and synapse stability (Dam *et al.* 1993). Thus, subP has a role in many of the specific functions which are defective in RS: respiratory control, heart rhythm and rate, peripheral circulation and sleep. There is a marked decrease of subP in Rett syndrome in the areas of spinal sensory input and integration (dorsal horn) and in the area of sympathetic output (intermediolateral cell column) which could influence pain perception and sympathetic outflow. In the Rett brainstem the marked decrease of subP immunoreactivity in the nucleus of the solitary tract, the major input of sensory information from the enteric nervous system and the site of integration of the cardiorespiratory reflexes presumably contribute to defects in these areas of autonomic functioning. The immunoreactivity for subP is also decreased in the locus ceruleus and the most of the reticular formation, nuclei concerned with arousal. The degree of substance P immunoreactivity was never greater than that observed in the 2 month brain. Thus the low levels of substance P in Rett syndrome resemble the levels normally present in an immature brain and could reflect an arrest of development of this peptide.

Substance P can be added to the increasing list of transmitters and growth factors that may be abnormally expressed at some time and at some specific brain site during the course of the Rett disorder: dopamine, acetylcholine, glutamate, serotonin, and nerve growth factor. The partial deficiencies of these neurotrophins can explain many of the characteristics of the Rett neurophysiology which resembles that of immaturity. Our challenge now is to define the mechanism for these deficiencies, so that appropriate treatment and prevention can be accomplished.

References

Aicardi, J. (1988). Rett syndrome. *International Pediatrics*, 3, 165–9.
Aghajanian, G.K., Sprouse, J.S., Sheldon, P., Rasmussen, K. (1990). Electrophysiology of the central serotonin system: Receptor subtypes and transducer mechanisms. In: *The neuropharmacology of serotonin* (eds Whittaker-Azmitia P.M. and Peroutka, S.J.) *Ann NY Acad Sc*, **600**, 93–103.
Amir, R.E., Van Den Veyver, I., Wan, M., Tran, C.Q., Francke, U., and Zoghbi, H.Y. (1999). Rett's syndrome is caused by mutations in X linked MECP2 encoding methyl-CpG-binding protein. *Nature genetics*. **23**, 185–8.
Armstrong, D.D. (1997). Recent developments in neuropathology-electron microscopy, brain pathology. *European Child and Adolescent Psychiatry*, **70**, 1997.
Armstrong, D.D., Dunn, K., and Antalffy, B. (1998). Decreased dendritic branching in frontal, motor, limbic cortex in Rett syndrome compared with trisomy 21. *Journal of Neuropathology and Experimental Neurology*. **57**, 1013–17.
Armstrong, D., Dunn, J.K., Antalffy, B., and Trivedi R. (1995). Selective dendritic alterations in the cortex of Rett syndrome. *Journal of Neuropathology and Experimental Neurology*, **54**, 195–201.
Armstrong, D.D., Dunn, J.K., Schultz, R.J., Herbert, D.A., Glaze, D.G., and Motil, K.J. (1999). Organ growth in Rett syndrome; a postmortem examination analysis. *Pediatric Neurology*, **20**, 125–29.
Bauman, M.L. and Kemper, T.K. (1982). Morphologic and histoanatomic observations of the brain in untreated human phenylketonuria. *Acta Neuropathologica*, **58**, 55063.
Bauman, M.L., Kemper, T. L., and Arin D.M. (1995). Microscopic observation of the brain in Rett syndrome. *Neuropediatrics*, **26**, 105–8.
Bauman, M.L., Kemper, M.D., and Arin, D.M. (1995). Pervasive neuroanatomic abnormalities of the brain in three cases of Rett's syndrome. *Neurology*, **45**, 1581–6.
Belichenko, P.V. and Dahlstrom, A. (1995). Studies on the 3-dimensional architecture of dendritic spines and varicosities in human cortex by confocal laser scanning microscopy and Lucifer Yellow microinjections. *Journal of Neuroscience Methods*, **57**, 55–61.
Belichenko, P.V., Oldfors, A., Hagberg, B., and Dahlstrom, A. (1994). Rett syndrome: 3-D confocal microscopy of cortical pyramidal dendrites and afferents. *Neurology Report*, **5**, 1509–13.
Belichenko, P.V., Hagberg, B. and Dahlstrom, A. (1997). Morphological study of neocortical areas in Rett syndrome. *Acta Neuropathol*, **93**, 50–61.
Brucke, T., Sofic, E., Killian, W., Rett, A., and Riederer, P. (1987). Reduced concentration and increased metabolism of biogenic amines in a single case of Rett-Syndrome: a postmortem brain study. *Journal of Neural Transmission*, **68**, 315–24.
Budden, S.S., Myer, E.C., and Butler, I.J. (1990) Cerebrospinal fluid studies in the Rett syndrome: biogenic amines and beta-endorphins. *Brain and Development*, **12**, 81–4.

Burd, L., Martsolf, J.T., and Randall, T. (1990). A prevalence study of Rett syndrome in an institutionalized population. *American Journal of Medical Genetics*, **36**, 33–6.

Casanova, M.F., Naidu, S., Goldberg, T.E., Moser, H.W., Khoromi, S., Kumar, A., Kleimnan, J.E., and Weinberger, D.R. (1991). Quantitative magnetic resonance imaging in Rett syndrome. *Journal of Neurophysiology*, **3**, 66–71.

Coker, S.B. and Melynk, A.R. (1991). Rett syndrome and mitochondrial enzyme deficiencies. *Journal of Child Neurology*, 166.

Cooke, D.W., Naidu, S., Plotnick, L., and Berkovitz, G.D. (1995). Abnormalities of thyroid function and glucose control in subjects with Rett syndrome. *Hormone Research*, **43**, 273–8.

Cornford, M.E., Philippart, M., Jacobs, B., Scheibel, A.B., and Vinters, H.V. (1994). Neuropathology of Rett syndrome: case report with neuronal and mitochondrial abnormalities in the brain. *Journal of Child Neurology*, **9**, 424–31.

Cronk, C.E. (1978). Growth of children with Down's syndrome: birth to age 3 years. *Pediatrics*, **61**, 564–8.

Dam, T.V., Handelmann, G.E., Quirion, R. (1993). Neurokinin and substance P receptors in the developing rat central nervous system. In: *Receptors in the developing nervous system* (eds Zagon and Mclaughlin) PP Chapman & Hall, London.

Ellaway, C.J., Sholler, G., Leonard, H., and Christodoulou, J. (1999). Prolonged QT interval in Rett syndrome. *Archives of Diseases of Childhood*, **80**, 470–72.

FitzGerald, P.M., Jancovic, J., and Percy, A.K. (1990). Rett syndrome and associated movement disorders. *Movement Disorders*, 202.

Fornal, C.A. and Jacobs, B.L. (1988). Physiologic and behavioral correlates of serotonergic single-unit activity. In: *Neuronal Serotonin* (ed. Osborne N.N. and Hamon M.) John Wiley & Sons, Chichester, England, 305–45.

Friede, R.L. (1989). Gross and microscopic development of the nervous system. In *Developmental neuropathology*, Springer, Berlin.

Galbraith, G.C., Philippart, M., and Stephen, L.M. (1996). Brain stem frequency-following responses in Rett syndrome. *Pediatric Neurology*, **15**, 26–31.

Glaze, D.G., Frost, J.D., Zoghbi, H.Y., and Percy, A.K. (1987). Rett's syndrome: correlation of electroencephalographic characteristics with clinical staging. *Archives of Neurology*, **44**, 1053–56.

Glaze, D.G., Frost, J.D, Zoghbi, H.Y., and Percy, A.K. (1987). Rett's syndrome: characterization of respiratory patterns and sleep. *Annals of Neurology*, **21**, 377–82.

Glaze, D.G., Schultz, R.J., and Frost, J.D. (1998). Rett syndrome: characterization of seizures versus non-seizures. *Electroencephalography and Clinical Neurophysiology*, **106**, 79–83.

Haas, R.H., Light, M., Rice, M., and Barshop, B.A. (1995). Oxidative metabolism in Rett syndrome. 1. Clinical studies. *Neuropediatrics*, **26**, 90–4.

Hagberg, B. (1985). Rett's syndrome: prevalence and impact on progressive severe mental retardation in girls. *Acta Paediatrics Scandinavia*, **74**, 405–8.

Hagberg, B. (1995). Clinical delineation of Rett syndrome variants. *Neuropediatrics*, **26**, 1–20.

Hagberg, B., Aicardi, J., Dias, K., and Ramos, O. (1983). A progressive syndrome of autism, dementia, ataxia, and loss of purposeful hand use in girls: Rett's Syndrome: report of 35 cases. *Annals of Neurology*, 471–9.

Hamberger, A., Gillberg, C., Palm, A., and Hagberg, B. (1992). Elevated CSF glutamate in Rett syndrome. *Neuropediatrics*, **23**, 212–3.

Hanefeld, F., Christen, H.J., Kruse, B., Frahm, J., and Hanicke,W. (1995). Cerebral proton magnetic resonance spectroscopy in Rett syndrome. *Neuropediatrics*, **26**, 126–7.

Harris, J.C., Wong, D.F., Wagner, H.N., Rett, A., Naidu, S., Dannals, R.F., Links,J.M., Batshaw, M.L. and Moser, H. (1986). Positron emission tomographic study of D2 dopamine receptor binding and CSF biogenic amine metabolites in Rett syndrome. *American Journal of Medical genetics*, **24**, 201–10.

Holm, V.A. (1986). Physical growth and development in patients with Rett syndrome. *American Journal of Medical Genetics*, **24**, 119–26.

Huttenlocher, P.R. (1974). Dendritic development in neocortex of children with mental defect and infantile spasms. *Neurology*, **24**, 203–10.

Jagadha, V. and Becker, L.E. (1989). Dendritic pathology: an overview of Golgi studies in man. *Canadian Journal of Neurological Science*, **16**, 41–50.

Jellinger, K. and Seitelberger, F. (1986). Neuropathology of Rett syndrome. *American Journal of Medical Genetics*, **24**, 259–88.

Jellinger, K., Grisold, W., Armstrong, D., and Rett, A. (1990). Peripheral nerve involvement in the Rett Syndrome. *Brain and Development*, **12**, 109–14.

Johnsrude, C., Glaze, D., Schultz, R., and Friedman, R. (1995). Prolonged QT intervals and diminished heart rate variability in patients with Rett syndrome. *Pacing Clinical Electrophysiology*, **18**, 889.

Julu, P.O.O., Kerr, A.M., Hansen, S., and Apartopoulos, F. (1997). Functional evidence of brain stem immaturity in Rett Syndrome. *European Child and Adolescent Psychiatry*, **6**, 47–54.

Kaufmann, W.E., Naidu, S., and Budden, S. (1995). Abnormal expression of microtubule-associated protein 2 (MAP-2) in the neocortex in Rett syndrome. *Neuropediatrics*, **26**, 109–13.

Kaufmann, W.E., Worley, P.F., Taylor, C.V., Bremer, M., and Isakson, P.C. (1997). Cyclooxygenase-2 expression during rat neocortical development and in Rett syndrome. *Brain and Development*, **19**, 25–34.

Kerr, A.M. (1992). A review of the respiratory disorder in the Rett syndrome. *Brain and Development*, **14(Suppl.)**, S43–5.

Kerr, A.M. (1995). Early clinical signs of the Rett disorder. *Neuropediatrics*, **26**, 67–71.

Kerr, A.M. and Stephenson, J.B.P. (1986). A study of the natural history of Rett's syndrome in 23 girls. *American Journal of Medical Genetics*, **24**, 77–83.

Kerr, A.M., Julu, P., Hansen, S., and Apartopoulos, F. (1998). Serotonin and breathing dysrhythmia in the Rett Syndrome. New developments in child neurology, presentations from the *VIII International Child Neurology Congress*, Llubljana, Slovenia, 13–17 September, Milivoj Velickovic Perat. 191195. Moduzzi Editore, Bologna.

Kinney, H.C., O'Donnell, T.J., Krieger, P., and White, W.F. (1993). Early developmental changes in 3H-nicotine binding in the human brainstem. *Neuroscience*, **55**, 1127–38.

Kinney, H.C., Ottoson, C.K., and White, W.F. (1990). Three-dimensional distribution of 3H-naloxone binding to opiate receptors in the human fetal and infant brainstem. *Journal of Comparative Neurology*, **291**, 55–78.

Kinney, H.C., Panigrahy, A., Rava, L.A., and White, W.F. (1995). Three dimensional distribution of 3H-quinuclidiinyl benzilate binding to muscarinic cholinergic receptors in the developing human brain stem. *Journal of Comparative Neurology*, **362**, 350–67.

Kitt, C.A. and Wilcox, B.J. (1995). Preliminary evidence for neurodegenerative changes in the substantia nigra of Rett syndrome. *Neuropediatrics*, **25**, 114–118.

Kozinetz, C.A., Skender, M.L., MacNaughton, N., Almes, M.J., Schultz, R.J., Percy A.K., and Glaze, D.G. (1993). Epidemiology of Rett Syndrome: a population-based registry. *Pediatrics*, **91**, 445–50.

Lappalainen, R., and Riikonen, R.S. (1996). High levels of cerebrospinal fluid glutamate in Rett syndrome. *Pediatric Neurology*, **15**, 213–6.

Lappalainen, R., Lindholm, D., and Riikonen, R. (1996). Low levels of nerve growth factor in cerebrospinal fluid of children with Rett syndrome. *Journal of Child Neurology*, **11**, 296–300.

Lekman, A., Witt Engerström, I., Gottfries, G., Hagberg, B.A., Percy, A.K., and Svennerholm, L. (1989). Rett syndrome: biogenic amines and metabolites in post mortem brain. *Pediatric Neurology*, **5**, 357–62.

Lekman, A., Witt Engerström, I., Holmber, B., Percy A.K., Svennerholm, L., and Hagberg, B. (1990). CSF and urine biogenic amine metabolites in Rett syndrome. *Clinical Genetics*, **37**, 173–8.

Marin-Padilla, M. (1976). Pyramidal cell abnormalities in the motor cortex of a child with Down's syndrome. A Golgi study. *Journal of Comparative Neurology*, **167**, 63–82.

Matsuishi, T., Nagamitsu, S., Yamashita, Y., Murakami, Y., Kimura A., Sakai T., Shoji, H., Kato, H., and Percy, A.K. (1997). Decreased cerebrospinal fluid levels of substance P in patients with Rett syndrome. *Annals of Neurology*, **42**, 978–81.

McArthur, A., and Budden, S. (1998). Sleep dysfunction in Rett syndrome: a trial of exogenous melatonin treatment. *Developmental Medicine and Child Neurology*, **40**, 186–92.

Morton, R.E., Bonas, R., Minford, J., Kerr, A., and Ellis, R.E. (1997). Feeding ability in Rett Syndrome. *Developmental Medicine and Child Neurology*, **39**, 331–5.

Motil, K., Schultz, R.J., Browning, B., Troliak, L., and Glaze, D.G. (1999). Oral pharyngeal and gastroesophageal dysmotility are present in girls and women with Rett Syndrome. *Pediatric Journal of Nutrition and Gastroenterology*, **29**, 31–7.

Motil, K.J., Schultz, R.J., Wong, W.W., and Glaze, D.G. (1998). Increased energy expenditure associated with repetitive involuntary movement does not contribute to growth failure in girls with Rett syndrome. *Journal of Pediatrics*, **132**, 228–33.

Murakami, J.W., Courchesne, E., Haas, R.H., Press, G.A., and Yeung-Courchesne, R. (1992). Cerebellar and cortical abnormalities in Rett syndrome. A quantitative MR analysis. *American Journal of Radiology*, **159**, 177–83.

Naidu, S. (1997). Rett syndrome: a disorder affecting early brain growth. *Annals of Neurology*, **42**, 3–10.

Nielsen, J.B., Friberg, L., Lou, H., Lassen, N.A. and Sam, I.L.K. (1990). Immature pattern of brain activity in Rett syndrome. *Archives of Neurology*, **47**, 982–6.

Nielsen, J.B., Lou, H.C., and Andresen, J. (1990). Biochemical and clinical effects of tyrosine and tryptophan in the Rett syndrome. *Brain and Development*, **12**, 143–7.

Nielsen, J.B., Bertelsen, A., and Lou, H.C. (1992). Low CSF HVA levels in Rett syndrome: a reflection of restricted synapse formation?. *Brain and Development* (**Suppl.**), S63–5.

Nielsen, J.B., Toft, P.B., Reske-Nielsen, E., Jensen, K.E., Chrisiansen, P., Thomsen, C., Hendriksen, O, and Lou, H.C. (1993). Cerebral magnetic resonance spectroscopy in Rett syndrome. Failure to detect mitochondrial disorder. *Brain and Development*, **15**, 107–12.

Nomura, Y., and Segawa, M. (1990). Characteristics of motor disturbances in the Rett syndrome. *Brain and Development*, **12**, 27–30.

Nomura, Y., Segawa, M., and Hasegawa, M. (1984). Rett syndrome; pathophysiological consideration. *Brain and Development*, **6**, 475–86.

Oldfors, A., Hagberg, B., Nordgren, H., Sourander, P., and Witt Engerström, I. (1988). Rett syndrome: spinal cord pathology. *Pediatric Neurology*, **4**, 172–4.

Oldfors, A., Sourander, P., Armstrong, D.L., Percy A.K., Witt Engerström, I., and Hagberg, B.A. (1990). Rett Syndrome: cerebellar pathology. *Pediatric Neurology*, **6**, 310–4.

Olszewski, J. and Baxter, D. (1954). *Cytoarchitecture of the human brain stem*. J.B. Lippincott, Montreal.

Percy, A.K. (1992). Neurochemistry of the Rett syndrome. *Brain and Development*, **14**(**Suppl.**), S57–62.

Percy, A.K., Glaze, D.G., Schultz, R.J., Zoghbi H.Y., Williamson, D., Frost, J.D., Jankovic, J.J., del Junco D., Skender M., Waring, S., et al. (1994). Rett syndrome; controlled study of an oral opiate antagonist, naltrexone. *Ann Neurol*, **35**, 464–70.

Percy, A.K., Zoghbi, H.Y., Lewis, K.R., and Jankovic, J. (1988). Rett syndrome: qualitative and quantitative differentiation from autism. *Journal of Child Neurology*, **3**(**Suppl.**), S63–5.

Perry, T.L., Dunn, H.G., Ho, H.H., and Crichton, J.U. (1988). Cerebrospinal fluid values for monoamine metabolites, gamma-aminobutyric acid, and other amino acid compounds in Rett syndrome. *Journal of Pediatrics*, **112**, 234–8.

Piazza, C.C., Fisher, W., Kiesewetter, K., Bowman L., and Moser, H. (1990). Aberrant sleep patterns in children with Rett syndrome. *Brain and Development*, **12**, 488–93.

Pioro, E.P., and Mai, J.K. (1990). Distribution of substance P- and enkephalin-immunoreactive neurons and fibers. In *The human nervous system* (ed. G. Paxinos), pp. 1051–94. Academic Press, San Diego, California.

Poliakov, G.I. (1961). Some results of research into the development of the neuronal structure of the cortical ends of the analyzers in man. *Journal of Comparative Neurology*, 117, 197–217.

Reiss, A.L., Faruque, F., Naudy, S., Abrams, M., Beaty, T., Bryan, N.R.N., and Moser, H. (1993). Neuroanatomy of Rett syndrome: a volumetric imaging study. *Annals of Neurology*, 34, 227–43.

Rett, A. (1977). Cerebral atrophy associated with hyperammonemia. In: *Handbook of clinical neurology*,Vol. 29 (ed. P.W. Vinken and G.W. Bruyn), pp. 305–25.

Riederer, P.,Weiser, M., Wichart, I., Schmidt, B., Killian, W., and Rett A. (1986). Preliminary brain autopsy findings in prodgredient Rett syndrome. *American Journal of Medical Genetics*, 24, 305–15.

Riikonen, R. and Vanhala, R. (1999). Levels of cerebrospinal fluid nerve-growth factor differ in infantile autism and Rett syndrome. *Developmental Medicine and Child Neurology*, 41, 148–52.

Schultz, R.J., Glaze, D.G., Motil, K.J., Armstrong, D.D., del Junco D.H.J., Hubbard, C.R., and Percy, A.K. (1993). The pattern of growth failure in Rett syndrome. *American Journal of Diseases of Children*, 147, 633–7.

Schultz, R., Glaze, D., Motil, K., Herbert, D., and Percy, A. (1998). Hand and foot growth in Rett syndrome. *Journal of Child Neurology*, 13, 71–4.

Sekul, E.A., Moak, J.P.,Schultz, R., and Percy, A.K. (1994). Electrocardiographic findings in Rett syndrome: an explanation for sudden death?. *Journal of Pediatrics*, 125, 80–2.

Stenbom,Y., Witt Engerström, I., and Hagberg, B. (1995). Gross motor disability and head growth in Rett syndrome— a preliminary report. *Neuropediatrics*, 26, 85–6.

Strach, B.A., Stoner, W.R., Smithe, S.L., and Jerger, J.F. (1994). Auditory evoked potential in Rett syndrome. *Journal of Academic Audiology*, 5, 226–30.

Subramaniam, B., Naidu, S., and Reiss, A.L. (1997). Neuroanatomy in Rett Syndrome: cerebral cortex and posterior fossa. *Neurology*, 48, 399–407.

Takashima, M., Becker L.E., Armstrong, D., and Chan, F. (1981). Abnormal neuronal development in the visual cortex of the human fetus and infants with Downs' syndrome. A quantitative and qualitative Golgi study. *Brain Research*, 225, 1–21.

Thommessen, M., Kase, B.F., and Heiberg, A., (1992). Growth and nutrition in 10 girls with Rett syndrome. *Acta Paediatrica*, 81, 686–90.

von Tetzchner, S., Jacobsen, K.H., Smith, L., Skjeldal, O.H., Heiberg, A., and Fagan, J.F., (1996). Vision, cognitive and developmental characteristics of girls and women with Rett syndrome. *Developmental Medicine and Child Neurology*, 38, 212–25.

Wenk, G.L. (1997). Rett syndrome: neurobiological changes underlying specific symptoms. *Progress in Neurobiology*, 51, 383–91.

Wenk, G.L. and Hauss-Wegrzyniak, B. (1999). Altered cholinergic function in the basla forebrain of girls with Rett syndrome. *Neuropediatrics*, 30, 125–9.

Wenk, G.L., Naidu, S., Casanova, M.F., Kitt, C.A., and Moser, H. (1991). Altered neurochemical markers in Rett's syndrome. *Neurology*, 41, 1753–6.

Wenk, G.L., Naidu, S., and Moser, H. (1989). Altered neurochemical markers in Rett syndrome. *Annals of Neurology*, 26, 467.

Witt Engerström, I. (1991). Rett syndrome in Sweden. *Acta Paediatric Scandinavia Goteborg*, S369.

Witt Engerström, I. (1992). Age related occurrence of signs and symptoms in the Rett syndrome. *Brain and Development*, 14(**Suppl.**), S11–120.

Witt Engerström, I. and Forslund, M. (1992). Mother and daughter with Rett syndrome (letter). *Developmental Medicine and Child Neurology*, 34, 1022–3.

Witt Engerström, I. and Kerr, A. (1998). Workshop on Autonomic Function in Rett Syndrome. Swedish Rett Center, Frosen, Sweden, May 1998. *Brain and Development*, **20**, 326.

Woodyatt, G. and Ozanne, A. (1992). Communication abilities and Rett syndrome. *Journal of Autism and Developmental Disorders*, **22**, 155–73.

Yamashita, Y., Matsuishi, T., Ishibashi, M., Kimura, A.,Onishi, Y., Yonekura,Y., and Kato, H. (1998). Decrease in benzodiazepine receptor binding in the brains of adult patients with Rett Syndrome. *Journal of Neurological Science*, **154**, 146–50.

Yoshikawa, H., Fueki, N., Suzuki H., Sakuragawa N., and Masaaki, I. (1991). Cerebral blood flow and oxygen metabolism in Rett syndrome. *Journal of Child Neurology*, **6**, 237–42.

Zappella, M. (1992). The Rett girls with preserved speech. *Brain and Development*, **14**, 98–101.

Zec, N., Filiano, JJ., Panigrahy, A., White, W.F., and Kinney, H.C. (1996). Developmental changes in 3H-lysergic acid diethylamine binding to serotonin receptors in the developing human brainstem. *Journal of Neuropathology and Experimental Neurology*, **55**, 114–25.

Zoghbi, H.Y. Percy, A.K., Glaze, D.G., Butler, I.J.N., Riccardi, V.M. (1985). Reduction of biogenic aminic levels in the Rett syndrome. *New England Journal of Medicine*, **313**, 921–4.

Zoghbi, H.Y., Milstien, S., Butler, I.J., Smith, O.B., Kaufman, S., Glaze. D.G., and Percy, A.K. (1989). Cerebrospinal fluid biogenic amines and biopterin in Rett syndrome. *Annals of Neurology*, **25**, 56–60.

4 Cortical development in Rett syndrome: molecular, neurochemical, and anatomical aspects

Walter E. Kaufmann

Summary

This chapter reviews changes in the cerebral cortex in Rett syndrome (RS), covering anatomical, neurochemical, and molecular aspects. In RS there is a severe and global reduction in cortical volume that seems to affect both grey and white matter. These changes are correlated with reductions in neuronal size and dendritic length. Some cortical areas, such as the prefrontal cortex, may be more affected. Immunochemical data demonstrate selective dendritic protein abnormalities, which suggest an early cortical disturbance in neuronal differentiation. The latter may be related to specific neurotransmitter system abnormalities, including moderate cholinergic deficit and relative increase in glutamate and some of its receptors. Finally, the recently reported 'Rett gene', *MECP2* may lead to dendritic anomalies by way of abnormal gene expression of the cholinergic gene, neurotrophins, and other regulatory proteins.

4.1 The cerebral cortex in Rett syndrome: general changes

The cerebral cortex is probably the brain region studied in greatest detail in Rett syndrome (RS) (Chapter 3 of this volume presents an overview of RS neuropathology). The interest in the cerebral cortex in RS is due to both the prominent role that the neocortex seems to play in the RS neurologic phenotype (cognitive and motor dysfunction) and the relative accessibility of this structure. This chapter presents a comprehensive overview of the changes affecting the cerebral cortex in RS, ranging from molecular to macroscopic levels. Interestingly RS is one of the few developmental disorders in which such a wide range of approaches has been applied, making the study of the cerebral cortex a model for mental retardation-associated syndromes.

One of the earliest and most distinctive clinical features of RS is deceleration in head growth that is detected by the middle of the first year of life (Naidu *et al.* 1986, 1995). For more details, see Chapter 1 that discusses the clinical features of RS. Although this reduction in head circumference seems to be part of a more global growth impairment, since height and then body weight follow a similar trend (Schultz *et al.* 1993), studies of brain weight suggest the specific nature of this abnormality. Armstrong *et al.* (1996, 1999) calculated relative organ weight values, by adjusting organ weight to body length, demonstrating that only the brain is absolutely and relatively reduced in RS. As the cerebral cortex, particularly the neocortex, is the main contributor to total brain weight (or volume), the deceleration in head growth is probably the first index of cortical pathology in RS.

Correlating with the reduced head circumference, early neuropathological evaluations demonstrated that brain weight was substantially reduced in RS (12–34%), in an age- and disease stage-dependent fashion (Jellinger *et al.* 1988). These preliminary data contrast with more recent and comprehensive studies. Armstrong and colleagues (1995) reported the largest series (22 subjects) of RS subjects, analysed in terms of brain weight. These authors showed a range of brain weight, with an average of approximately 900 g (below the lower 95% confidence limits of a normative sample), that remained relatively stable after the fourth postnatal year (Armstrong 1995; Armstrong *et al.* 1995). This lack of relationship between age and brain weight contrasted with the slight increase in brain weight in the control group, as evidenced by this cross-sectional analysis (Armstrong *et al.* 1995). Several normative studies of brain weight, including the most recent by Dekaban (1978), demonstrate that in agreement with head circumference 90% of the adult (defined as such between 20–50 years) brain size is reached by age 4, and 95% by the sixth postnatal year. It is assumed that, in humans, most of the postnatal increase in brain size is the consequence of neocortical expansion. Based on animal data and direct synaptic counting in the human neocortex (Huttenlocher and de Courten 1987), stabilization of neocortical volume is reached when the process of dendritic outgrowth and synaptogenesis become less prominent, and synaptic pruning, neuronal death, and axonal branching and myelination are prominent processes. Consequently, early impairment in brain growth in RS could be interpreted as either atrophy or reduced dendritic/synaptic formation. As delineated below, available neuroimaging and histologic data support the latter explanation.

Initial neuroimaging studies, employing qualitative computed tomography (CT) scans, reported global decreases in brain size (Nomura *et al.* 1984; Nihei and Naitoh 1990). These observations were followed by two morphometric analyses using magnetic resonance imaging (MRI). The first study by Casanova *et al.*

(1991) showed a significant reduction in whole hemispheric area. Reiss and colleagues (1993) carried out the first volumetric analysis in RS. They found a 30% decrease in total cerebral volume that affected predominantly grey matter (GM) (total GM: 59.9% of controls; total white matter (WM): 72.2% of controls). As stated above, neocortical volume is the most significant contributor of total cerebral volume. Therefore, these data indicate that the neuronal somata/dendritic component is the most affected in RS neocortex. In a follow-up study comprising a larger sample (20 subjects vs 11 in the 1993 publication), Reiss and colleagues confirmed their original results although the reduction in brain volume was more modest (~25%) and affected cerebral GM and WM almost equally (Subramaniam *et al.* 1997). The reduction in cortical GM volume was virtually identical to that of total cerebral GM (72.1% vs 72.2% of controls). In a preliminary study of 56 girls with stage II/III RS, using a semi-automatic method (based on stereotactic principles) and higher resolution (thinner) images than those employed in previous studies (for method, see Fig. 4.1 and Appendix), we confirmed the ~25% decrease in brain volume at the expense of the cortex (Abrams *et al.* 1999). Again, as in the study by Subramaniam *et al.* (1997), GM and WM seemed to be equally involved in RS. The latter is a puzzling observation since neuroanatomic and neuropathologic studies, which are described in detail below and preceded these neuroimaging analyses, clearly demonstrated that there was a reduction in neuronal size and dendritic arborizations (Bauman *et al.* 1995*a,b*; Armstrong *et al.* 1995) but no major qualitative changes in axons or myelin (Jellinger *et al.* 1988) in RS cortex. We have recently shown further evidence of significant changes in the cortical WM in RS. In a study of 17 girls at relatively early stages of RS (mean age: 6 years) by magnetic resonance spectroscopic imaging (MRS), a technique that provides information about concentrations of metabolites, we found that the neuronal marker *N*-acetyl-aspartate (NAA) was reduced not only in GM but also in the WM in most cortical regions, including the insular cortex. Moreover, only in the frontal lobe the decrease was greater in the GM as expected in a process affecting predominantly neuronal somas and dendrites (Horská *et al.*, in press). Another recent report, using a localized measure method in contrast with our whole slice approach, also demonstrated NAA reduction in the WM but not in the GM (Pan *et al.* 1999). As the only source of NAA in the WM is the axon, our data suggests that the decrease in cortical WM volume in RS is the result of decrease in axonal numbers and/or volume. Whether the nature of these axonal abnormalities is a primary defect or reduced complexity associated with smaller neuronal somas cannot be determined by these investigations. It will require the application of complementary *in vivo* imaging techniques, such as diffusion tensor imaging (Mori *et al.* 1999), which delineate axonal bundle architecture and volume and more sophisticated neuroanatomic methods than those previously employed. These studies would necessarily have to include individuals affected by other syndromes in which dendritic reduction is a major feature (e.g. Down's syndrome), in order to clarify the relationship between axonal and dendritic changes in RS.

The histologic substrate of the macroscopic global changes, delineated above, began to emerge with the pioneering work of Jellinger and collaborators (1986, 1988). These authors attempted first to determine whether RS was a malformative or degenerative disorder. A variety of non-specific changes, which included

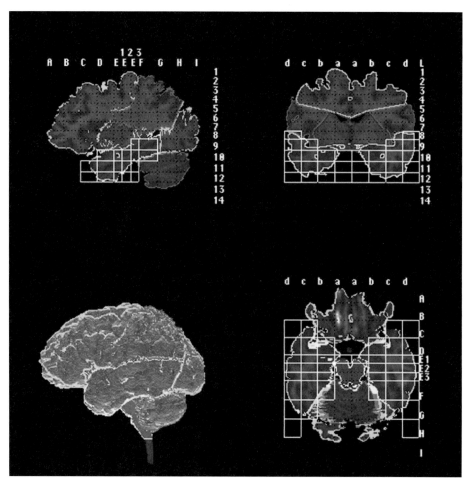

Fig. 4.1 Tri-planar view of the Talairach stereotaxic grid as applied on a brain. The brain has been positionally normalized and Talairach sectors designated as representing the temporal lobe are shown superimposed over manually derived sulcal-based, 'gold standard' regions. In this illustration, the gold standard temporal lobe, frontal lobe, parietal lobe, and occipital lobe boundaries are designated in yellow, blue, red, and green, respectively. The Talairach sectors appear as white boxes in the three orthogonal views. The figure on the upper left corresponds to a midsagittal view. The coronal slice (upper right) corresponds to the level of the amygdala/third ventricle and includes anterior levels of the posterior insula. The figure on the lower right presents an axial view. Finally, a rendered three-dimensional display, without the grid, is illustrated on the lower left. Reproduced with permission from Kates *et al.* (1999). (See also coloured plate section).

increased neuronal lipofuscin and mild gliosis, were noted (Jellinger *et al.* 1988). They demonstrated that in RS the neocortex does not show aberrant neuronal migration or storage, or significant atrophy. Abnormalities of uncertain significance, such as changes in the quality of neuronal chromatin staining, in several limbic cortices have been reported as characteristic of RS (Leontovich *et al.* 1999). Nevertheless, the nature of the diffuse cortical changes in RS was disclosed by the cytoarchitectonic evaluations performed by Bauman and collaborators (1995*a*, *b*). These authors demonstrated reduced neuronal size associated with increased neuronal cell packing density throughout the neocortex, limbic regions, and centroencephalic structures (basal ganglia and thalamus). Consequently, the decrease in cortical GM volume would be the result of smaller perikarya and more compact neuronal arrangements. Recent data on similar changes in language-related cortical regions is reported by Belichenko in Chapter 8. Unfortunately, the stereologically based quantitations of neuronal size and density reported by Bauman *et al.* (1995*b*) were confined to the hippocampus and entorhinal cortex. Therefore, it is not possible to estimate, from cytoarchitectonic data, the contribution of the reductions in perikarya and dendrites to the neocortical volumetric changes or the magnitude of the process in different cortical areas. The initial description of astrocytic reaction is important since gliosis is a marker of 'acquired' injury. We examined this issue in a comprehensive survey of three subjects representative of the age and clinical spectrum of RS. Our data showed that gliosis, evaluated by immunocytochemistry, is a variable feature although its severity can be greater than originally estimated (Kaufmann *et al.* 1995*b*). We expanded these observations in two recent studies. Using MRS we found that young RS girls with seizures had overall significantly higher choline (Cho) levels than RS patients without seizures (Horská *et al.*, in press). Considering that Cho is a metabolite whose concentration increases in gliosis and demyelination, and that gliosis is frequently associated with long-term seizures, the reported elevation in Cho is most likely due to gliosis. In another preliminary molecular study, using the new cDNA microarray technique that allows determinations of levels of expression of multiple genes in a single sample, we demonstrated that glial fibrillary acidic protein (GFAP, a characteristic astrocytic/gliosis marker) was upregulated in conjunction with other astrocytic but not oligodendrocytic genes (Colantuoni *et al.* 1999). These data indicate that, at least in some patients with RS, there is selective astrocytic upregulation or proliferation. At this point, it is unclear whether this is primary astrocytic defect or is part of a typical gliotic response.

Morphometric analyses by neuroimaging have shown that, in both sexes, between the ages of 4 and 18 there is an age-dependent increase in cerebral WM volume and a concomitant reduction in cortical GM (Giedd *et al.* 1996; Reiss *et al.* 1996). This normal pattern of brain development with relative 'loss' of GM and 'gain' of WM seems to be preserved in RS. In their two publications, Reiss and colleagues reported that their cross-sectional RS cohort showed the same positive correlation between age and WM volume as in controls. A slightly less significant (than controls) inverse relationship between GM volume and age was also found (Reiss *et al.* 1993; Subramaniam *et al.* 1997). We have recently provided additional evidence for preservation of normal cortical growth in RS. In a preliminary investigation that included, in addition to cross-sectional, longitudinal data on 19 patients with RS, we found similar age-dependent changes in GM and WM volumes in RS and normal controls (Abrams *et al.* 1999). These data support the hypothesis that the basic disturbance in cortical development in RS occurs early, and does not affect substantially subsequent cortical growth. Clinically, this anatomical feature may explain the relative stabilization of the neurologic symptoms after the second stage of the illness (Naidu 1997) and, neurobiologically, it suggests that only early phases of dendritic/synaptic formation are being affected since excessive pruning would have led to exaggerated decreases in GM volumes that were not observed.

In conclusion, in RS there is a severe and global reduction in cortical volume that seems to affect both GM and WM. Reductions in neuronal size and dendritic length would explain the GM abnormality. At present, no microscopic correlate of WM changes is available. Despite its decreased volume, the cortex appears to grow normally after the third year in RS.

4.2 Selective involvement of the cerebral cortex in Rett syndrome

Initial neuroanatomical and neuroimaging studies suggested a greater involvement of the frontal lobe, by reporting the presence of frontal or fronto-temporal 'atrophy' (Jellinger *et al.* 1988; Nomura *et al.* 1984; Nihei and Naitoh 1990; Yano *et al.* 1991). As discussed in the previous section, the diagnosis of atrophy in developmental disorders requires the demonstration of volumetric reduction due to neuronal loss. No neuroanatomical evidence supports atrophy, particularly in the cerebral cortex, as the basis for decreased brain size in RS. The changes in neuronal size and cell packing density, reported by Bauman *et al.* (1995*a*), rather suggest a growth arrest. Therefore, a more appropriate term to describe RS microencephaly is global hypodevelopment or hypoplasia. With respect to the greater severity in the frontal region, it is important to state that qualitative evaluations of either postmortem specimens or scans tend to overestimate frontal and anterior temporal lobe changes. The latter is due to the prominence of the anterior portions (poles) of these two lobes, contrasting with the 'enclosed' nature of the parietal lobe. Thus, modest changes in the volume or appearance of the frontal and temporal lobes are readily interpreted as 'atrophy'. Moreover as the frontal lobe accounts for approximately half of the cortical volume, it is easier to detect reductions in this structure (e.g. by inspecting the distance between central sulcus and frontal pole) than in other cortical regions. For all these reasons, an accurate characterization of selectivity in volumetric changes requires unbiased analyses. Stereological and other quantitative approaches, using neuropathological or neuroimaging data (Barta *et al.* 1997; Kates *et al.* 1999), would be the best way to elucidate this important question in RS pathology. Such studies of high–resolution MRI scans are currently ongoing in our centre; preliminary analyses using a semi-automatic method, described in the preceding section, indicate that no cortical lobe volume is preferentially reduced in RS (Abrams *et al.* 1999).

Though no volumetric comparisons among specific neocortical regions (lobar subdivisions) have been carried out in RS, systematic analyses of relative proportions (percentages) of each cortical tissue class (GM, WM, and CSF) were performed by Reiss and colleagues in their two investigations. These investigators used 5 mm slices, oriented in the anterior commissure–posterior commissure plane, to which they applied a coordinate system that divided the cerebral cortex into eight regions per hemisphere. Calculations of the percentages of each tissue class were made in each one of these regions. As in other conditions with reduced cortical volume, decreases in GM and/or WM were accompanied by increases in CSF proportions (Fox *et al.* 1996). Both studies (with a total of 20 subjects) showed a significant reduction in GM proportion throughout the cortex, with greater reductions in prefrontal, posterior frontal, and anterior temporal regions (>3.5% of total volume). Relative preservation was observed in posterior temporal lobe and posterior occipital regions (Reiss *et al.* 1993; Subramaniam *et al.* 1997). Investigations measuring specific cortical regions are absolutely essential in order not only to confirm these initial observations, but also for determining the neurobiological bases of the RS neurologic phenotype. We have begun a re-evaluation of regional cortical pathology in RS in a two-step approach: in an initial phase, we are carrying out a comprehensive survey of the entire cortex by semi-automatic protocols. The latter that are exemplified in Fig. 4.1 allow the study of a large number of subjects, and will disclose regions of interest in RS. In a second phase, these volumetrically abnormal regions will be confirmed by measurements using more precise manual-tracing techniques (Kates *et al.* 1997). As an example of these initial survey approaches, this chapter includes an appendix— a proposal for the study of the insular cortex, an area of great interest for the understanding of sudden death in RS.

To date no cytoarchitectonic correlates of the fronto-occipital imaging differences are yet available. However, quantitative studies of neuronal dendrites by Golgi impregnations have disclosed regional cortical changes. Armstrong and collaborators (1995) demonstrated that basal, and in some instances apical, branches of pyramidal cells from prefrontal and motor cortices were significantly reduced, when compared to normal controls. In agreement with the MRI data, these decreases were not found in the occipital cortex (Armstrong 1995; Armstrong *et al.* 1995 and Chapter 3). A more recent investigation, by the same group, provided additional evidence for the specificity of the dendritic abnormalities in RS cerebral cortex. When compared with cells from individuals with Down's syndrome (DS), dendritic arborizations from RS subjects showed the greatest reductions again in premotor, motor, and inferior temporal cortices (Armstrong *et al.* 1998). Considering that DS is one of the first developmental disorders in which dendritic anomalies—specifically reductions in dendritic branching—were described, these findings in RS underscore the severity and topographic specificity of the neuronal pathology in RS. Based on the significant contribution that dendritic length makes to GM volume, it is likely that more severe decreases in dendritic trees are the bases for greater involvement of anterior frontal and temporal regions. Nevertheless, in order to determine with certainty the degree of neuronal involvement of certain cortical regions, neuroimaging volumetric analyses of specific cortical regions as well as cytoarchitectonic stereological quantitations are needed.

Additional evidence of the regional selectivity comes from the stereologically based quantitative studies of the hippocampus, carried out by Bauman and collaborators (1995*a*, *b*). These investigators showed that although neuronal soma size was reduced throughout the hippocampus, greater changes were found in the CA3 and CA4 sectors of the pyramidal layer. Another parameter, cell packing density, was consistently elevated in the pyramidal layer in the three subjects studied by these authors, with again CA4 showing the larger values (Bauman *et al.* 1995*a,b*). Belichenko reported decreased neuronal staining in the entorhinal cortex (Belichenko *et al.* 1997). Armstrong and colleagues (1995, 1998) measured dendritic arborizations from different hippocampal neuronal populations. In this case, the subiculum seemed to be the most affected hippocampal region. Unfortunately, no dendritic evaluations were performed on the neuronal populations shown to be most affected on cytoarchitectonic evaluations (e.g. CA4).

In summary, neuroanatomical and neuroimaging studies of the cerebral cortex in RS indicate that this disorder may affect certain neuronal populations more severely. The data on regional cortical pathology, described above, are limited and consistent with greater involvement of the newest (phylogenetically and ontogenetically) cortical areas (prefrontal, anterior temporal). A comprehensive *in vivo* re-evaluation of regional involvement in RS is an essential complement to the postmortem dendritic analyses.

4.3 Molecular pathology in RS neocortex

Most of the data on cortical histopathology in RS come from studies using traditional methods, such as Nissl and Golgi techniques. In order to gain insight into the mechanism by which dendritic abnormalities take place in RS, we used a combined immunochemical approach. The latter allows a characterization of the molecular composition of somas and dendrites, the two neuronal components known to be morphologically affected in RS. Cytoskeletal proteins are stable molecules (suitable for studies of postmortem specimens) which are characterized by a distinctive ontogenetic profile. The onset of their expression coincides and serves as substrate for specific phases of dendritic and axonal development. Finally, cytoskeletal protein levels decline to an adult steady level shortly after their initial expression. Consequently, examining a particular panel of cytoskeletal proteins may help to delineate not only dendritic composition, but also the timing of the dendritic disturbance. In our first investigation (Kaufmann et al. 1995a,b), we found a selective reduction in immunostaining for microtubule-associated protein (MAP)-2, a marker of the period of dendritic branching and expansion. This finding that involved exclusively pyramidal excitatory neurons (markers of inhibitory GABAergic neurons were unaltered) was generalized throughout the neocortex. A follow-up study (Kaufmann et al. 1997c) demonstrated no clear cortical regional specificity. A striking result of these investigations was the observation that MAP-2 immunoreactivity in WM neurons was virtually absent. This contrasted with both normal controls (Kaufmann et al. 1995b) and DS subjects (Kaufmann and Naidu 1995), which showed a distinctive immunostained neuronal population in superficial WM. Neurons in neocortical WM are a small population of spindle-shaped or modified pyramidal cells, of unknown function. Nonetheless, they constitute the remainder of the subplate layer in the adult brain (essentially after the fourth postnatal year). The subplate layer or zone is one of the first neocortical layers, located at the GM–WM junction. It serves as an early cortical organizer by interacting with migrating neuroblasts and incoming afferents (Allendoerfer and Shatz 1994). Of relevance to RS is the hypothesis proposed by Kostovic and Rakic (1990) that states that cortical expansion (growth, gyral formation), particularly of association cortices as those affected in RS, is dependent on a well-developed (thick) subplate layer. The fact that WM neurons are present, but do not express MAP-2, suggests a maturational disturbance that can have its origin in anomalous subplate development.

Immunoblotting (Western blotting) assay is the standard technique for quantifying the levels of a protein in a tissue sample. Its only disadvantage when compared with immunocytochemistry is the lack of spatial and, therefore, cell type resolution. Therefore, protein levels should not only be expressed in reference to amounts of tissue, but also to markers that indicate tissue composition (e.g., the neuronal marker neuron specific enolase or NSE). Consequently, we developed an immunoblotting assay for specific measurements of dendritic protein levels (Kaufmann et al. 1997b). When applied to frontal cortex homogenates from individuals with RS and DS, it showed that absolute and relative levels of cytoskeletal proteins were dramatically different in both conditions. In RS all surveyed proteins were reduced, although the most severe decreases involved MAP-5, a marker of early dendritic differentiation, and MAP-2, a protein associated with dendritic branching (Kaufmann *et al.* 1997*a*). Higher molecular weight non-phosphorylated neurofilaments, markers of late dendritic development, were only minimally affected (Kaufmann *et al.* 1997*a*) as previously demonstrated by immunocytochemical data (Kaufmann *et al.* 1995*b*). In contrast, all cytoskeletal proteins were globally elevated per neuron in DS.

The complexity of dendritic abnormalities in RS neocortex is underscored by our studies of cyclooxygenase 2 (COX-2) immunoreactivity. *COX-2* is one of the earliest reported non-transcription factor immediate early genes (Yamagata *et al.* 1993; Kaufmann and Worley 1999). COX-2 is the inducible form of cyclooxygenase, the first enzyme in the prostanoid synthetic pathway. It is expressed selectively in the cell bodies and dendrites of neurons in neocortical and limbic regions (Kaufmann *et al.* 1996). Its expression, particularly targeting to distal dendrites, is a late event that coincides with dendritic/synaptic pruning. We examined the pattern of COX-2 immunostaining in different neocortical regions, observing that the intensity of COX-2 immunoreactivity was decreased in frontal and temporal regions whereas it was relatively preserved in the occipital cortex. Contrasting the findings on MAP-2, COX-2 distribution better parallels the dendritic quantitations by Golgi-based analyses.

In summary, the immunochemical analyses of dendritic proteins provide a complementary view to Golgi (Armstrong *et al.* 1995, 1998) and dye labelling (Belichenko *et al.* 1994) analyses of dendrites in RS. It appears to be a selective reduction of proteins associated with early phases of dendritic development. These decreases do not seem universal to all conditions with decrease in dendritic arborizations. In fact, in DS there appears to be an accumulation of proteins in shorter dendrites. The molecular findings in RS are in agreement with the observations that brain/cortical volume remains relatively stable after the fourth year. An increase in pruning will probably lead to a reduction in cortical GM that could span, at least, part of this period. Nevertheless, the possible involvement of the late dendritic/synaptic phase cannot be ruled out in RS considering the abnormalities in COX-2 immunoreactivity, a molecular marker of this late period of dendritic development.

4.4 Neurotransmitter systems in the neocortex in RS

Hypopigmentation of the substantia nigra in RS, which resembles the morphological changes seen in Parkinson disease, was one of the first neuropathological features described in RS (Jellinger and Seitelberger 1986; Jellinger *et al.* 1988). It suggested an involvement of, at least, one of the dopaminergic pathways in this condition. The numerous studies, which have evaluated markers of different neurotransmitter systems in fluid and tissue samples in RS, have reported inconsistent findings. These contradictory data could be due to a number of factors, including sample size and characteristics and methodology employed in the analyses. This review is limited to studies evaluating the cerebral cortex.

Among the monoamines, the best characterized is dopamine (DA). After initial studies by Riederer *et al.* (1985) and Brucke *et al.* (1987) in a single RS case, which demonstrated reduced DA levels and increased DA turnover (increased ratios of metabolites to neurotransmitter), Wenk and colleagues examined several cortical regions in five cases with RS and found variable but marked reduction of DA endogenous levels (Wenk *et al.* 1991). The metabolite 3,4-dihydroxyphenylacetic acid (DOPAC) was essentially unchanged (Wenk *et al.* 1991). In an expanded sample of 12 RS subjects and 14 female controls, Wenk (1997) was not able to reproduce the reduction in DA previously reported. Moreover, other dopaminergic markers that included the metabolite homovanillic acid, the DA reuptake site, and D2 receptors (by ligand binding) did not differ between both groups (Wenk 1997). These data contrast with similar assessments in the basal ganglia where both DA and reuptake sites are markedly reduced (Riederer *et al.* 1985; Brucke *et al.* 1987; Lekman *et al.* 1989; Wenk 1995). In summary, the status of the dopaminergic innervation to the cerebral cortex in RS is still unclear. Discrepancies between evaluations of cortex and basal ganglia could be explained by the fact that these regions receive afferents from two different pathways: nigrostriatal and mesocortical (originating in the ventral tegmental area). On the other hand, the preliminary quantitations of neuronal numbers in the ventral tegmental area and substantia nigra by Kitt and Wilcox (1995) indicated an approximately equal 30% decrease in both regions.

With the exception of the study by Wenk and collaborators (1991), which examined frontal, temporal, and occipital cortices and found no changes in serotonin, norepinephrine, and their metabolites, no other systematic evaluation of these monoamines has been carried out. Corroborating data on this lack of cortical serotoninergic and noradrenergic changes in RS would be of great importance, since abnormalities in brainstem function linked to these two monoamines have long been recognized in this disorder (for an overview on clinical features, see Chapter 1 by Kerr and Witt Engerström). Nomura and Segawa in Chapter 7, and also Segawa in Chapter 8, review the 'monoamine hypothesis' in RS. These authors suggest that the sleep abnormalities that characterize RS specifically, irregularity in the time of waking up and falling asleep at night and profound daytime sleep, are most likely the consequence of noradrenergic and serotoninergic hypofunction, which develops between late gestation and the early postnatal period. Another functional evidence of serotonin disturbance has been provided by the studies of respiratory abnormalities by Julu and Kerr, which are discussed in detail in Chapter 6. These evaluations of breathing function, and its autonomic correlates, demonstrated poor autonomic integration and multiple breathing dysrhythmias. Such findings suggest that in RS there is immaturity in medullary function, and that breath holding (a typical feature of stage III) may represent lack of serotoninergic modulation of the brainstem respiratory oscillators (Julu et al. 1997). Recently, neurochemical evidence of serotoninergic dysfunction has been reported by Armstrong and Kinney (see Chapter 3). These authors showed that in young individuals with RS there is an increase in several brainstem nuclei in serotoninergic receptors (Chapter 3), as demonstrated by postmortem (3H)lysergic acid diethylamide binding autoradiography (Panigraphy et al. 1998). These results suggest again immaturity in this monoaminergic system since this pattern is normally observed between gestational week 25 and the neonatal period. The relevance of these findings for RS cortical development is still unclear, since the affected nuclei are innervated by the caudal raphe complex that has relatively few ascending projections. Nevertheless, as experimental data show that serotoninergic afferents play a role in neuronal maturation and organization in the cerebral cortex (Goldberg 1998; Gonzalez-Burgos et al. 1996; Osterheld-Haas and Hornung 1996), this monoaminergic system deserves further examination in RS.

Wenk and colleagues (Wenk et al. 1991, 1993; Wenk and Mobley 1996; Wenk 1997) also studied the cholinergic system in consecutive studies. Examination of the cortical cholinergic afferents was stimulated by the neuropathological observation by Kitt et al. (1990) in one subject with RS of the decrease in the number of basal forebrain neurons (the source of cholinergic afferents to cortex). Wenk and collaborators demonstrated a variable, but consistent, decrease in the activity of the synthetic enzyme choline acetyltransferase (ChAT) in several brain regions. However, the reductions were only significant in the hippocampus, basal ganglia, and thalamus. In contrast, changes in the neocortex were rather modest in the 10–18% range (Wenk et al. 1991, 1993). A follow–up study compared ChAT activity with density of binding to the cholinergic vesicular transporter (using the ligand vesamicol), the reuptake mechanism for acetylcholine. There was a non-significant decline in both ChAT and vesamicol binding in frontal and cingulate cortices (Wenk and Mobley 1996). These contrasted with significant but again parallel reductions in the putamen, in the RS sample, and with previous reports on Alzheimer disease that demonstrated an inverse correlation between decreased ChAT activity and preserved vesamicol (Ruberg et al. 1990). The reduction in vesamicol binding in RS differs also from experimental cholinergic denervation. In young (3 months) and old (24 months) rats with basal forebrain lesions, vesamicol binding is preserved in the presence of reduced ChAT activity (Wenk and Mobley 1996). These data suggest a regulatory mechanism by which deficiency in synthesis of acetylcholine is compensated by increased 'recycling' of the neurotransmitter. As a single gene codes for both ChAT and vesicular transporter, an analysis of changes in gene expression may disclose a potential therapeutic target in conditions such as RS.

For the purpose of evaluating changes in the level of expression of the ChAT gene, we are developing quantitative immunoblotting assays for both proteins coded for by the gene: the enzyme ChAT and the vesicular transporter. Our preliminary data on ChAT demonstrates that, in cytosolic fractions of frontal cortex, in RS there is a 29% reduction in protein levels when compared to normal controls. This difference is very similar to the 23% decrease in ChAT activity in midfrontal cortex found by Wenk and Mobley in 12 RS subjects. As our measurements were done in 'pure' cytosolic fractions, without the detergent (Triton) treatment used in the ChAT activity assay, we also measured ChAT levels in membrane pellets that would contain enzyme that is solubilized by Triton. We found that ChAT levels in membrane fractions are lower than in cytosol and that, in this case, RS subjects showed a reduction of only 12%. Our ChAT level data suggest that in RS the reduction in ChAT activity would be the consequence of decreased ChAT protein levels, particularly of the most soluble form of the enzyme. The distinct effect on two different forms of the enzyme is puzzling, since it supports the notion that the reduction in ChAT levels is not simply the consequence of fewer functional cholinergic neurons but it may also involve abnormal regulation of ChAT gene expression. A recent study by Wenk and Hauss-Wegrzyniak (1999) provides further evidence in this direction. These authors found that, although in RS there are normal nerve growth factor (NGF) levels in the cortex, there is a decrease in the number of ChAT immunoreactive neurons in the basal forebrain. This reduction in immunostaining is not due to neuronal loss as originally concluded from the report by Kitt *et al.* (1990), since there are no changes in the number of neurons stained with an antibody against the low affinity (p75) NGF receptor. As basal forebrain neurons co-express both ChAT and p75, Wenk and Hauss-Wegrzyniak (1999) postulated that in RS basal forebrain neurons are not capable of producing ChAT protein despite appropriate NGF and NGF receptor levels.

Data on the postsynaptic aspect of the cholinergic system are more limited. Wenk (1997) reported preliminary studies on nicotinic subtype of cholinergic receptors, in which he found decreases in frontal and temporal cortices. He also examined indirectly postsynaptic and signal transduction changes secondary to cholinergic transmission, by evaluating Na/K-ATPase activity. Na/K-ATPase sites, measured by the binding of the ligand ouabain, and these were not altered in RS.

Glutamate is the main excitatory neurotransmitter in the cerebral cortex. Several studies have reported an increase in glutamate in CSF (Hamberger *et al.* 1992; Lappalainen and Riikonen 1996). Although direct evaluations of glutamate in brain parenchyma by immunochemical techniques have not yet been published, a recent MRS study reported elevated glutamate/NAA ratio in the cortical GM (Pan *et al.* 1999). Glutamate receptors were evaluated by ligand binding in cortical homogenates by Wenk *et al.* (1993). Both adenosine monophosphate acid (AMPA) and N-methyl-D-aspartate (NMDA) subtypes of glutamate receptors were unchanged in four RS subjects. Recently Blue and colleagues (1999) studied the same receptors, as well as the kainate and metabotropic subtypes, by autoradiography, in the superior frontal gyrus. Although there were no group differences, when compared with controls, there was a trend towards higher densities of all but the kainate type of glutamate receptors in younger (<10 years) RS subjects. Older RS individuals showed levels below those of controls (Blue *et al.* 1999). These data suggest that the significantly higher density of NMDA receptors in the cortex of RS girls may be related to some of the neurologic features that characterize stages II and III (e.g. epileptic activity). Changes in the glutamatergic system in RS are most likely secondary in nature since related candidate genes, such as an enzyme that metabolizes this neurotransmitter glutamate dehydrogenase-2 (GLUD2) that is located in Xq25, show no mutations in RS (Wan and Francke 1998).

Other neurotransmitter systems have not been comprehensively examined in the cerebral cortex. Nevertheless, μ-opioid, neurotensin, and GABAergic receptors seem to be unaffected, though the latter showed the same ontogenetic profile as that of glutamate receptors (Wenk *et al.* 1993; Blue *et al.* 1999). Calbindin immunoreactive subtype of GABAergic neurons is also preserved in RS (Kaufmann *et al.* 1995*b*). Neuropeptides have been examined in a limited fashion. In our initial investigation of the neocortex in RS, we showed that neuropeptide Y (NPY) immunostaining was unchanged particularly in the deep cortex and white matter (Kaufmann *et al.* 1995b). These data in conjunction with that on calbindin suggested that GABAergic neurons, which frequently co-express neuropeptides, were selectively preserved in RS. A recent study by Armstrong and colleagues (Chapter 3), carried out in a relatively large sample covering a wide age spectrum, showed that contrasting with NPY another neuropeptide—substance P—is reduced in expression. Substance P immunostaining was decreased in frontal cortex, globus pallidus, and several brainstem and spinal cord regions. The specificity of the change was underscored by the lack of involvement of the hippocampus, substantia nigra, and periaqueductal grey matter. The pattern of substance P immunoreactivity rather resembled that of a young infant in all RS subjects (see Chapter 3). Considering that substance P is involved in multiple sensory and regulatory functions, these abnormalities may explain many features of the RS phenotype. Again, more systematic studies of neuropeptidergic neurons would clarify the role of these interneurons in the pathogenesis and manifestations of RS. Finally, Yamashita *et al.* (1997) found a decrease in benzodiazepine binding sites in frontotemporal cortex, by SPECT, in subjects with stage IV RS.

In conclusion, although many studies have reported contradictory data in regard to neurotransmitter systems in RS, a consistent picture has begun to emerge in the cortex. There are abnormalities involving the dopaminergic, cholinergic, and glutamatergic systems. The former seem to involve the nigrostriatal and not the mesocortical/limbic systems, therefore, sparing the cerebral cortex. The cholinergic dysfunction consists, at least, of an impairment in basal forebrain ChAT expression that leads to a moderate reduction in cortical cholinergic innervation without appropriate compensation. The concentration of the neurotransmitter glutamate is increased and associated with a relative elevation in the density of some subtypes of glutamate receptors (e.g. NMDA) in young subjects with RS.

4.5 Potential pathogenetic mechanisms: MeCP2 and the RS neurologic phenotype

A major breakthrough in the understanding of RS has been recently reported. In support of the hypothesis that RS is a genetic disorder (Thomas 1996; Sirianni *et al.* 1998), Zoghbi and colleagues have demonstrated that in a significant proportion of subjects with sporadic RS, and in some familial cases, there is a mutation in the coding region of the *MECP2* gene (Amir *et al.* 1999). This gene encodes a transcriptional regulatory protein, termed methyl-CpG-binding protein 2 or MeCP2. MeCP2 binds in a selective manner methylated cytosine residues, in symmetrically positioned CpG dinucleotides. As CpG clusters, a common configuration of CpG dinucleotides also termed islands, are preferentially located in the promoter regions of genes silenced by DNA methylation, it is postulated that MeCP2 represses tissue-specific gene transcription (Nan *et al.* 1997). Further evidence about MeCP2's role in repressing transcription was provided by Coffee *et al.* (1999), who showed that silencing of the abnormally methylated Fragile X syndrome gene (*FMR1*) is mediated by MeCP2. For more details about MeCP2 and its mutations in RS, see Chapter 2 in this volume.

Although the frequency of *MeCP2* mutations in RS is still under investigation, the demonstration of mutations involving the two functional domains of MeCP2 supports the hypothesis that a decrease in MeCP2 function is a primary event in RS pathogenesis. Consequently a major challenge in RS research is the identification of MeCP2 targets, the genes that are being regulated by MeCP2, and of the mechanism by which abnormal levels of these target proteins lead to the RS neurologic phenotype. With regard to the cerebral cortex, the demonstration of a characteristic and severe reduction in neuronal soma size and dendritic arborizations suggests that an impairment in neuronal differentiation and growth is the essential process underlying the RS cortical phenotype. Additional evidence of decrease in the levels of dendritic proteins associated with early dendritic formation, namely MAP-5 and MAP-2, suggests that MeCP2 deficit influences directly or indirectly the expression of proteins that are essential for early dendritic development. The demonstration in RS of abnormal MAP-2 immunoreactivity in WM neurons is highly suggestive of aberrant subplate formation, since MAP-2 expression is one of the first signs of neuronal differentiation in these cells (Allendoerfer and Shatz 1994). A disruption in maturation of subplate neurons would occur immediately after neuronal migration, reinforcing the hypothesis that cortical abnormalities in RS arise early, most likely, during midgestation.

Based on these data, we could postulate the following sequence of events: MeCP2 deficit leads to downregulation or upregulation of early dendritic proteins, particularly in pioneer neuronal populations. As these early neurons influence maturation of later developing neurons (layers II–VI) as well as cortical connectivity in general, abnormally differentiated subplate neurons lead to a global disturbance in dendritic/synaptic organization. Superimposed on this secondary abnormality affecting most cortical neurons would also be the direct effect of MeCP2 deficit on neuronal gene expression.

There is considerable anatomical, neurochemical, and molecular evidence to support the notion that abnormal MeCP2 expression does not influence *directly* dendritic protein expression and, therefore, dendritic development in RS. Most of these data concern MAP-2, a highly dynamic protein which is critical for dendritic expansion and is regulated by a variety of neurotransmitter systems in the adult brain (Johnson and Jope 1992). We have focused on MAP-2 because of its multi-regulation and the selectivity of its changes in RS (Kaufmann *et al.* 1995*b*). In collaboration with Dr Christine Hohmann, we have found that early and transient cholinergic deficit results in selective long-term MAP-2 downregulation in the cerebral cortex (Kaufmann *et al.* 1995*a*, 1997*a*). For these studies, we used a model developed by Hohmann and collaborators (1988) that consists of lesioning unilaterally the mouse basal forebrain, shortly after birth, which prevents the arrival of cholinergic afferents to the cortex. These mice exhibit a profound but reversible deficit in ChAT activity for 2–3 weeks (Hohmann *et al.* 1988). Despite the transient nature of the ChAT deficit, cortical neurons show reductions in dendritic arborizations and abnormal thalamo-cortical connections (Hohmann *et al.* 1991*a*, *b*). These relatively moderate dendritic changes are correlated, in adult mice, with a selective decrease in MAP-2 immunostaining (Kaufmann *et al.* 1995*a*) that resembles the one observed in RS (Kaufmann *et al.* 1995*b*). Although the dendritic tree changes in cholinergic-deprived mice are of a lesser magnitude than those described in RS (Armstrong *et al.* 1995), they suggest that a marked cholinergic deficiency at the time when these afferents arrive to the subplate (15–18 weeks according to Kostovic and Rakic 1990) is sufficient to have long-term abnormalities in neuronal differentiation as those found in RS. At present, there is no information about perinatal neurotransmission in RS. However, the moderate reductions in cortical ChAT activity reported by Wenk and colleagues (Wenk *et al.* 1991, 1993; Wenk and Mobley 1996; Wenk 1997) seem to be present since early childhood. Hence, it is possible that in RS there is an early but not as severe deficit in cortical cholinergic innervation. The persistence of this deficiency, probably in combination with other factors, may explain the more severe reduction in dendritic arborizations present in RS.

As stated above, the cholinergic-dendritic correlative data suggest that MeCP2 deficit may influence dendritic development through reductions in ChAT expression. This raises the question of whether decreases in ChAT levels are directly caused by MeCP2 deficiency or not. In support of a direct relationship is the recent study by Wenk and Hauss-Wegrzyniak (1999) that showed a selective impairment in ChAT expression in basal forebrain neurons, despite preservation of NGF and NGF receptors, which is in agreement with our preliminary immunoblotting data. Moreover, data on the vesicular transporter that is coded for by the same ChAT gene indicate a lack of compensatory upregulation in RS (Wenk and Mobley 1996). The latter suggests that in RS there is no reduction in cortical cholinergic afferents but a major disruption in the regulation of both components of the ChAT gene. An alternative hypothesis is that abnormal ChAT expression and, at least in some extent, decreased dendritic growth are the consequence of disturbances in growth factors and their receptors. Neurotrophins, such as NGF, are known to regulate the expression of specific neurotransmitters (Eiden 1998). However, neurotrophins also play a complex role in dendritic development in the cerebral cortex. Studies by Katz and collaborators (McAllister *et al.* 1997; Horch *et al.* 1999) demonstrated that brain-derived neurotrophic factor (BDNF) and NT-3 maintain a complex balance of dendritic growth of pyramidal neurons in a layer-specific manner. Of especial interest for RS is the action of NT-3, which inhibits BDNF-dependent dendritic growth in supragranular cortical layers (McAllister *et al.* 1997) since the latter seem to be most affected in RS neocortex (Kaufmann *et al.* 1995a,b). Furthermore, the same investigators have recently shown that BDNF overexpression leads to dendritic growth and instability (Horch *et al.* 1999) that resemble anomalies found in developmental disorders (Kaufmann 1996).

In conclusion, the profound disturbance in cortical development that characterizes RS would be the result of abnormal regulation in gene expression, at least, during the period of early neuronal differentiation. MeCP2 deficit would influence cholinergic gene expression, directly, or via the neurotrophins system. Impairment in dendritic development would be the consequence of several factors, mainly cholinergic deficiency and neurotrophin imbalance. MeCP2 effects seem to be time-specific since cortical growth follows normal patterns after early childhood. Although this hypothesis does not exclude other mechanisms, including other neurotransmitter systems, we postulate that the search for MeCP2 targets should focus on regulatory genes that influence early cortical differentiation.

Acknowledgements

Preparation of this chapter was supported by grants from the National Institutes of Health HD 24448 and HD 24061 and by a grant from the Research for Rett Syndrome Foundation.

References

Abrams, M.T., Mazur-Hopkins, P., Pearlson, G.D., Kaufmann, W.E., and Naidu, S. (1999). Brain MRI changes in Rett syndrome: cross-sectional and serial data. *Society for Neuroscience Abstracts*, **25**, 488.

Allendoerfer, K.L. and Shatz, C.J. (1994). The subplate, a transient neocortical structure: its role in the development of connections between thalamus and cortex. *Annual Review of Neuroscience*, **17**, 185–218.

Amir, R.E., Van den Veyver, I.B., Wan, M., Tran, C.Q., Francke, U., and Zoghbi, H.Y. (1999). Rett syndrome is caused by mutations in X-linked MECP2, encoding methyl-CpG-binding protein 2. *Nature Genetics*, **23**, 185–8.

Andreasen, N.C., Rajarethinam, R., Cizadlo, T., Arndt, S., Swayze, V.W. 2nd, Flashman, L.A., O'Leary, D.S., Ehrhardt, J.C., and Yuh, W.T. (1996). Automatic atlas-based volume estimation of human brain regions from MR images. *Journal of Computed Assisted Tomography*, **20**, 98–106.

Armstrong, D.D. (1995). The neuropathology of Rett syndrome–overview 1994. *Neuropediatrics*, **26**, 100–4.

Armstrong, D.D., Dunn, K., and Antalffy, B. (1998). Decreased dendritic branching in frontal, motor and limbic cortex in Rett syndrome compared with trisomy 21. *Journal of Neuropathology and Experimental Neurololgy*, **57**, 1013–7.

Armstrong, D., Dunn, J.K., Antalffy, B., and Trivedi, R. (1995). Selective dendritic alterations in the cortex of Rett syndrome. *Journal of Neuropathology and Experimental Neurololgy*, **54**, 195–201.

Armstrong, D.D., Dunn, J.K., Schultz, R.J., Herbert, D.A., Glaze, D.G., and Motil, K.J. (1999). Organ growth in Rett syndrome: a postmortem examination analysis. *Pediatric Neurology*, **20**, 125–9.

Armstrong, D., Kearney, D.L., Dunn, J.K., Hebert, D., Schultz, R., Chapieski, L., Motil, K., Zoghbi, H., and Glaze, D. (1996). Morphologic studies of selective developmental arrest in Rett syndrome. In *Hand in hand with Rett syndrome*, pp. 50. Goteburg, Sweden.

Augustine, J.R. (1985). The insular lobe in primates including humans. *Neurological Research*, **7**, 2–10.

Barta, P.E., Dhingra, L., Royall, R., and Schwartz, E. (1997). Improving stereological estimates for the volume of structures identified in three-dimensional arrays of spatial data. *Journal of Neuroscience Methods*, **75**, 111–8.

Bauman, M.L., Kemper, T.L., and Arin, D.M. (1995a). Pervasive neuroanatomic abnormalities of the brain in three cases of Rett's syndrome. *Neurology*, **45**, 1581–6.

Bauman, M.L., Kemper, T.L., and Arin, D.M. (1995b). Microscopic observations of the brain in Rett syndrome. *Neuropediatrics*, **26**, 105–8.

Belichenko, P.A., Hagberg, B., and Dahlström, A. (1997). Morphological study of neocortical areas in Rett syndrome. *Acta Neuropathologica (Berlin)*, **93**, 50–61.

Belichenko, P.V., Oldfors, A., Hagberg, B., and Dahlström, A. (1994). Rett syndrome: 3-D confocal microscopy of cortical pyramidal dendrites and afferents. *NeuroReport*, **5**, 1509–13.

Blue, M.E., Naidu, S., and Johnston, M.V. (1999). Development of amino acid receptors in frontal cortex from girls with Rett syndrome. *Annals of Neurology*, **45**, 541–5.

Brucke, T., Sofic, E., Killian, W., Rett, A., and Riederer, P. (1987). Reduced concentrations and increased metabolism of biogenic emmins in a single case of Rett syndrome. *Journal of Neural Transmission*, **68**, 315–29.

Casanova, M.F., Naidu, S., Goldberg, T.E., Moser, H.W., Khoromi, S., Kumar, A., Kleinman, J.E., and Weinberger, D.R. (1991). Quantitative magnetic resonance imaging in Rett syndrome. *Neuropsychiatry and Clinical Neuroscience*, **3**, 66–72.

Cechetto, D.F. and Saper, C.B. (1987). Evidence for a viscerotopic sensory representation in the cortex and thalamus in the rat. *Journal of Comparative Neurology*, **262**, 27–45.

Coffee, B., Zhang, F., Warren, S.T., and Reines, D. (1999). Acetylated histones are associated with FMR1 in normal but not fragile X-syndrome cells. *Nature Genetics*, 22, 98–101.

Colantuoni, C., Yu, J., Kaufman, W., Hyder, K., Chenchik, A., Killian, J., Khimani, A., Garlick, R., Naidu, S., and Pevsner, J. (1999). Abnormal glial gene expression in human Rett syndrome brain revealed by high-density cDNA microarrays. *Society for Neuroscience Abstracts*, 25, 489.

Crosby, E.C., Humphrey, T., and Lauer, E.W. (1962). *Correlative anatomy of the nervous system*. Macmillan, New York.

Cukiert, A., Forster, C., Andrioli, M.S., and Frayman, L. (1998). Insular epilepsy. Similarities to temporal lobe epilepsy. Case report. *Arquivo de Neuropsiquiatria*, 56, 126–8.

Dekaban, A.S. (1978). Changes in brain weights during the span of human life: relation of brain weights to body heights and body weights. *Annals of Neurology*, 4, 345–56.

Eiden, L.E. (1998). The cholinergic gene locus. *Journal of Neurochemistry*, 70, 2227–40.

Fox, N.C., Warrington, E.K., Freeborough, P.A., Hartikaine, P., Kennedy, A.M., Stevens, J.M., and Rossor, M.N. (1996). Presymptomatic hippocampal atrophy in Alzheimer's disease. A longitudinal MRI study. Brain, 119, 2001–7.

Giedd, J.N., Snell, J.W., Lange, N., Rajapakse, J.C., Casey, B.J., Kozuch, P.L., Vaituzis, A.C., Vauss, Y.C., Hamburger, S.D., Kaysen, D., and Rapoport, J.L. (1996). Quantitative magnetic resonance imaging of human brain development: ages 4–18. *Cerebral Cortex*, 6, 551–60.

Glaze, D.G., Schultz, R.J., and Frost, J.D. (1998). Rett syndrome: characterization of seizures versus non-seizures. *Electroencephalography and Clinical Neurophysiology*, 106, 79–83.

Goldberg, J.I. (1998). Serotonin regulation of neurite outgrowth in identified neurons from mature and embryonic Helisoma trivolvis. *Perspectives in Developmental Neurobiology*, 5, 373–87.

Gonzalez-Burgos, I., del Angel-Meza, A.R., Barajas-Lopez, G., and Feria-Velasco, A. (1996). Tryptophan restriction causes long-term plastic changes in corticofrontal pyramidal neurons. *International Journal of Developmental Neuroscience*, 14, 673–9.

Hamberger, A., Gillberg, C., Palm, A., and Hagberg, B. (1992). Elevated CSF glutamate in Rett syndrome. *Neuropediatrics*, 23, 212–3.

Hohmann, C.F., Brooks, A.R., and Coyle, J.T. (1988). Neonatal lesions of the basal forebrain cholinergic neurons result in abnormal cortical development. *Brain Research*, 470, 253–64.

Hohmann, C.F., Kwiterovich, K.K., Oster-Granite, M.L., and Coyle, J.T. (1991a). Newborn basal forebrain lesions disrupt cortical cytodifferentiation as visualized by rapid Golgi staining. *Cerebral Cortex*, 1, 143–57.

Hohmann, C.F., Wilson, L., and Coyle, J.T. (1991b). Efferent and afferent connections of mouse sensory-motor cortex following cholinergic deafferentation at birth. *Cerebral Cortex*, 1, 158–72.

Horch, H.W., Kruttgen, A., Portbury, S.D., and Katz, L.C. (1999). Destabilization of cortical dendrites and spines by BDNF. *Neuron*, 23, 353–64.

Horská, A., Naidu, S., Herskovits, E.H., Wang, P.Y., Kaufmann, W.E., and Barker, P.B. (2000). Quantitative proton MR spectroscopic imaging in early Rett syndrome. *Neurology*, 54, 712–22.

Huttenlocher, P.R. and de Courten, C. (1987). The development of synapses in striate cortex of man. *Human Neurobiology*, 6, 1–9.

Jellinger, K. and Seitelberger, F. (1986). Neuropathology of Rett syndrome. *American Journal of Medical Genetics*, 24, 259–88.

Jellinger, K., Armstrong, D., Zoghbi, H.Y., and Percy, A.K. (1988). Neuropathology of Rett syndrome. *Acta Neuropathologica (Berlin)*, 76, 142–58.

Johnson, G.V. and Jope, R.S. (1992). The role of microtubule-associated protein 2 (MAP-2) in neuronal growth, plasticity, and degeneration. *Neuroscience Research*, 33, 505–12.

Kaplan, D.M., Liu, A.M.C., Abrams, M.T., Warsofsky, I.S., Kates, W.R., White, C.D., Kaufmann, W.E., and Reiss, A.L. (1997). Application of an automated parcellation method to the analysis of pediatric brain volumes. *Psychiatry Research Neuroimaging*, 76, 15–27.

Kates, W.R., Abrams, M.T., Kaufmann, W.E., Breiter, S.N., and Reiss, A.L. (1997). Reliability and validity of MRI measurement of the amygdala and hippocampus in children with fragile X syndrome. *Psychiatry Research (Neuroimaging)*, **75**, 31–48.

Kates, W.R., Warsofsky, I.S., Patwardhan, A., Abrams, M.T., Liu, A.M.C., Naidu, S., Kaufmann, W.E., and Reiss, A.L. (1999). Automated Taliarach atlas-based parcellation and measurement of cerebral lobes in children. *Psychiatry Research (Neuroimaging)*, **91**, 11–30.

Kaufmann, W.E. (1996). Mental retardation and learning disabilities: a neuropathologic differentiation. In *Developmental disabilities in infancy and childhood* (ed. A.J. Capute and P.J. Accardo), Vol. 2, pp. 49–70. Paul H. Brookes, Baltimore.

Kaufmann, W.E. and Naidu, S. (1995). Is Rett syndrome a subplate disease? *Society for Neuroscience Abstracts*, **21**, 735.

Kaufmann, W.E. and Worley, P.F. (1999). The role of early neural activity in regulating immediate early gene expression in the cerebral cortex. *Mental Retardation and Developmental Disabilities Research Reviews*, **5**, 41–50.

Kaufmann, W.E., Hohmann, C.F., Israel, J.J., and Naidu, S. (1995a). Microtubule-associated protein 2 is abnormally expressed in the neocortex of Rett syndrome subjects and in a related animal model. *Annals of Neurology*, **38**, 500.

Kaufmann, W.E., Naidu, S., and Budden, S. (1995b). Abnormal expression of microtubule-associated protein 2 (MAP-2) in neocortex in Rett syndrome. *Neuropediatrics*, **26**, 109–13.

Kaufmann, W.E., Taylor, C.V., Hohmann, C.F., Sanwal, I.B., and Naidu, S. (1997a). Abnormalities in neuronal maturation in Rett syndrome neocortex: preliminary molecular correlates. *European Child and Adolescent Psychiatry*, **6**(**Suppl. 1**), 75–7.

Kaufmann, W.E., Taylor, C.V., and Lishaa, N.A. (1997b). Immunoblotting patterns of cytoskeletal dendritic protein expression in human neocortex. *Molecular and Chemical Neuropathology*, **31**, 235–44.

Kaufmann, W.E., Worley, P.F., Pegg, J., Bremer, M., and Isakson, P. (1996). Cox-2, a synaptically induced enzyme, is expressed by excitatory neurons at postsynaptic sites in rat cerebral cortex. *Proceedings of the National Academy of Sciences (USA)*, **93**, 2317–21.

Kaufmann, W.E., Worley, P.F., Taylor, C.V., Bremer, M., and Isakson, P.C. (1997c). Cyclooxygenase 2 expression during rat neocortical development and in Rett syndrome. *Brain and Development*, **19**, 25–34.

Kerr, A.M., Armstrong, D.D., Prescott, R.J., Doyle, D., and Kearney, D.L. (1997). Rett syndrome: analysis of deaths in the British survey. *European Child and Adolescent Psychiatry*, **6**(**Suppl. 1**), 71–4.

Kitt, C.A. and Wilcox, B.J. (1995). Preliminary evidence for neurodegenerative changes in the substantia nigra of Rett syndrome. *Neuropediatrics*, **26**, 114–8.

Kitt, C.A., Troncoso, J.C., Price, D.L., Naidu, S., and Moser, H.W. (1990). Pathological changes in substantia nigra and basal forebrain neurons in Rett syndrome. *Annals of Neurology*, **28**, 416–7.

Kostovic, I. and Rakic, P. (1990). Developmental history of the transient subplate zone in the visual and somatosensory cortex of the macaque monkey and human brain. *Journal of Comparative Neurology*, **297**, 441–70.

Lappalainen, R. and Riikonen, R.S. (1996). High levels of cerebrospinal fluid glutamate in Rett syndrome. *Pediatric Neurology*, **15**, 213–6.

Lekman, A., Witt Engerström, I., Gottfries, J., Hagberg, B., Percy, A.K., and Svennerholm, L. (1989). Rett syndrome: biogenic amines and metabolites in postmortem brain. *Pediatric Neurology*, **5**, 357–62.

Leontovich, T.A., Mukhina, J.K., Fedorov, A.A., and Belichenko, P.V. (1999). Morphological study of the entorhinal cortex, hippocampal formation, and basal ganglia in Rett syndrome patients. *Neurobiology of Disease*, **6**, 77–91.

McAllister, A.K., Katz, L.C., and Lo, D.C. (1997). Opposing roles for endogenous BDNF and NT-3 in regulating cortical dendritic growth. *Neuron*, **18**, 767–78.

Mesulam, M.-M. (1985). *Principles of behavioral neurology*. F.A. Davis, Philadelphia.

Mori, S., Kaufmann, W.E., Pearlson, G.D., Crain, B.J., Stieltjes, B., Solaiyappan, M., and van Zijl, P.C.M. (2000). *In vivo* visualization of human neural pathways by MRI. *Annals of Neurology*, **47**, 412–4.

Naidu, S. (1997). Rett syndrome: a disorder affecting early brain growth. *Annals of Neurology*, **42**, 3–10.

Naidu, S., Hyman, S., Harris, E.L., Narayanan, V., Johns, D., and Castora, F. (1995). Rett syndrome studies of natural history and search for a genetic marker. *Neuropediatrics*, **26**, 63–6.

Naidu, S., Murphy, M., Moser, H.W., and Rett, A. (1986). Rett syndrome: natural history in 70 cases. *American Journal of Medical Genetics*, **24**, 61–72.

Nan, X., Campoy, F.J., and Bird, A. (1997). MeCP2 is a transcriptional repressor with abundant binding sites in genomic chromatin. *Cell*, **88**, 471–81.

Nihei, K. and Naitoh, H. (1990). Cranial computed tomographic and magnetic resonance imaging studies on the Rett syndrome. *Brain and Development*, **12**, 101–5.

Nomura, Y., Segawa, M., and Hasegawa, M. (1984). Rett syndrome–clinical studies and pathophysiological consideration. *Brain and Development*, **6**, 475–86.

Oppenheimer, S. (1993). The anatomy and physiology of cortical mechanisms of cardiac control. *Stroke*, **24**(**Suppl. 12**), 13–5.

Osterheld-Haas, M.C. and Hornung, J.P. (1996). Laminar development of the mouse barrel cortex: effects of neurotoxins against monoamines. *Experimental Brain Research*, **110**, 183–95.

Pan, J.W., Lane, J.B., Hetherington, H., and Percy, A.K. (1999). Rett syndrome: 1H spectroscopic imaging at 4.1 Tesla. *Journal of Child Neurology*, **14**, 524–8.

Panigraphy, A., Zec, N., Frost White, W., Filiano, J.J., and Kinney, H.C. (1998). 3-Dimensional anatomic relationship of serotonergic and muscarinic receptor binding in the pontine reticular formation of the human infant brainstem. *Clinical Neuropathology*, **17**, 318–25.

Reiss, A.L., Abrams, M.T., Singer, H.S., Ross, J.L., and Denckla, M.B. (1996). Brain development, gender and IQ in children. A volumetric imaging study. *Brain*, **119**, 1763–74.

Reiss, A.L., Faruque, F., Naidu, S., Abrams, M., Beaty, T., Bryan, R.N., and Moser, H. (1993). Neuroanatomy of Rett syndrome: a volumetric imaging study. *Annals of Neurology*, **34**, 227–34.

Riederer, P., Brucke, T., Sofic, E., Kienzl, E., Schnecker, K., Schay, V., Kruzik, P., Killian, W., and Rett, A. (1985). Neurochemical aspects of the Rett syndrome. *Brain and Development*, **7**, 351–60.

Ruberg, M., Mayo, W., Brice, A., Duyckaerts, C., Hauw, J.J., Simon, H., LeMoal, M., and Agid, Y. (1990). Choline acetyltransferase activity and [3H]vesamicol binding in the temporal cortex of patients with Alzheimer's disease, Parkinson's disease, and rats with basal forebrain lesions. *Neuroscience*, **35**, 327–33.

Schultz, R.J., Glaze, D.G., Motil, K.J., Armstrong, D.D., del Junco, D.J., Hubbard, C.R., and Percy, A.K. (1993). The pattern of growth failure in Rett syndrome. *American Journal of Diseases of Children*, **147**, 633–7.

Sekul, E.A., Moak, J.P., Schultz, R.J., Glaze, D.G., Dunn, J.K., and Percy, A.K. (1994). Electrocardiographic findings in Rett syndrome: an explanation for sudden death?. *Journal of Pediatrics*, **125**, 80–2.

Sirianni, N., Naidu, S., Pereira, J., Pillotto, R.F., and Hoffman, E.P. (1998). Rett syndrome: confirmation of X-linked dominant inheritance, and localization of the gene to Xq28. *American Journal of Human Genetics*, **63**, 1552–8.

Subramaniam, B., Naidu, S., and Reiss, A.L. (1997). Neuroanatomy in Rett syndrome: cerebral cortex and posterior fossa. *Neurology*, **48**, 399–407.

Talairach, J. and Tournoux, P. (1988). *Co-planar stereotaxic atlas of the human brain*. Thieme, New York.

Thomas, G.H. (1996). High male:female ratio of germ-line mutations: an alternative explanation for postulated gestational lethality in males in X-linked dominant disorders. *American Journal of Human Genetics*, **58**, 1364–8.

Wan, M. and Francke, U. (1998). Evaluation of two X chromosomal candidate genes for Rett syndrome: glutamate dehydrogenase-2 (GLUD2) and rab GDP-dissociation inhibitor (GDI1). *American Journal of Medical Genetics*, **78**, 169–72.

Wenk, G.L. (1995). Alterations in dopaminergic function in Rett syndrome. *Neuropediatrics*, **26**, 123–5.

Wenk, G. (1997). Selective changes in Rett syndrome neurochemistry: findings of normal dopaminergic and decreased cholinergic function. *European Child and Adolescent Psychiatry*, **6**(**Suppl. 1**), 87–8.

Wenk, G.L. and Hauss-Wegrzyniak, B. (1999). Altered cholinergic function in the basal forebrain of girls with Rett syndrome. *Neuropediatrics*, **30**, 125–9.

Wenk, G.L. and Mobley, S.L. (1996). Choline acetyltransferase activity and vesamicol binding in Rett syndrome and in rats with nucleus basalis lesions. *Neuroscience*, **73**, 79–84.

Wenk, G.L., Naidu, S., Casanova, M.F., Kitt, C.A., and Moser, H. (1991). Altered neurochemical markers in Rett's syndrome. *Neurology*, **41**, 1753–6.

Wenk, G.L., O'Leary, M., Nemeroff, C.B., Bissette, G., Moser, H., and Naidu, S. (1993). Neurochemical alterations in Rett syndrome. *Developmental Brain Research*, **74**, 67–72.

Yamagata, K., Andreasson, K.I., Kaufmann, W.E., Barnes, C.A., and Worley, P.F. (1993). Expression of a mitogen-inducible cyclooxygenase in brain neurons: regulation by synaptic activity and glucocorticoids. *Neuron*, **11**, 371–86.

Yamashita, Y., Matsuishi, T. Kimura, A., Ishibashi, M., Onishi, Y., Kato, H., and Yonekura, Y. (1997). Decreased benzodiazepine receptor binding in the brain of adult Rett patients. *European Child and Adolescent Psychiatry*, **6**(**Suppl 1**), 88.

Yano, S., Yamashita, Y., Matsuishi, T., Abe, T., Yamada, S., and Shinohara, M. (1991). Four adult Rett patients at an institution for the handicapped. *Pediatric Neurology*, **7**, 289–92.

Yasui, Y., Breder, C.D., Saper, C.B., and Cechetto, D.F. (1991). Autonomic responses and efferent pathways from the insular cortex in the rat. *Journal of Comparative Neurology*, **303**, 355–74.

Zhang, Z. and Oppenheimer, S.M. (1997). Characterization, distribution and lateralization of baroreceptor-related neurons in the rat insular cortex. *Brain Research*, **760**, 243–50.

APPENDIX. Study of the insular cortex in Rett syndrome: a proposal for neuroimaging analyses

Introduction

Considering that the present book is focussed on the autonomic dysfunction in RS (see Chapters 1 and 2, 6 to 10), this chapter includes an appendix that outlines a proposal for the study of the insular cortex (IC). The IC is a neocortical region that, despite its isocortical (six layers) organization, is closer related to the limbic system than to the rest of the neocortex (Mesulam 1985). As such it seems to play an important role in cardiovascular regulation, constituting one of the highest levels of neural processing of autonomic information. Based on this, the IC may be involved in the pathogenesis of autonomic dysfunction and sudden death in RS. The latter is a major cause of decreased life expectancy in RS; sudden death occurs throughout life, typically during sleep, and without obvious causes (Naidu 1997). Abnormal anatomy and function of the cardiac conduction system have been postulated as a base for this phenomenon (Kerr *et al.* 1997; Sekul *et al.* 1994). Nonetheless, a central mechanism for sudden death in RS, involving specifically the IC, has also been hypothesized on the bases of the relatively high prevalence of non-seizure paroxysmal events with autonomic component in RS (Glaze *et al.* 1998; insular autonomic seizures: Cukiert *et al.* 1998) and on the well-established association between insular lesions and cardiac injury and arrhythmias (reviewed by Oppenheimer 1993).

At present, the only data on the IC in RS come from our *in vivo* spectroscopic study (Horská *et al.*, 2000). We found that there was a significant reduction in the concentration of the neuronal marker NAA, while the glial/myelin metabolite Cho was unchanged. Because of technical constraints, we could not differentiate the relative contribution of GM and WM to these abnormalities. Compared with other cortical regions, the insular changes were of similar magnitude to those involving frontal GM or temporal and parietal WM. For this reason, we propose a comprehensive investigation of the IC, which should include all strategies already applied to other cortical regions. The analyses must comprise, at least, volumetric evaluations by structural imaging, cytoarchitectonic and Golgi histologic studies, neurochemical and immunochemical evaluations of neurotransmitter systems and other neural proteins, and functional analyses by electrophysiologic and imaging techniques.

As a first approach for characterizing abnormalities in the IC in RS, here we propose a neuroimaging protocol for characterizing volumetric changes. It is based on the semi-automatic technique that employs the Talairach atlas (Talairach and Tournoux 1988) as referential system. This approach that divides the brain into 1232 three-dimensional rectangular sectors was pioneered by Andreasen et al. (1996) for the analysis of brains from adult subjects, particularly those affected by psychiatric disorders. Given the differences in sulcal/gyral anatomy between children and adults, and the potential effect of disease processes on major landmarks, we validated this parcellation approach in normal children and groups with Fragile X and Rett syndromes by comparing atlas-based divisions with 'gold standards' manually traced (Kaplan et al. 1997; Kates et al. 1999). Figure 4.1 demonstrates a tri-planar view of the Talairach grid on a brain, applied in this case to the temporal lobe. This atlas-based system has the advantage, when compared to manual tracing techniques, of allowing multiple measurements in large samples. However, it shows high sensitivity and specificity only for the measurement of large structures, such as cerebral lobes (Abrams et al. 1999; Kates et al. 1999). This is due to the fact that this referential system does not take into consideration individual variations in sulcal and gyral architecture. Despite its limitations, Talairach-based cortical subdivisions represent an adequate system for surveying volumetric changes, when anatomical or clinical information is unable to more precisely delineate regional involvement or when general trends in patient populations are being investigated. For these reasons, these regional surveys should necessarily be followed by manual tracing-based protocols, as those we reported for hippocampal and amygdala volumes in subjects with Fragile X syndrome (Kates et al. 1997).

Insular cortex protocol

Background:

The IC is an 'island', in the medial aspect of the Sylvian fissure, beneath the opercular region of the frontal lobe. It has a triangular shape, with a vertex extending anterolaterally, being separated from the neighbouring cortical regions by the circular or limiting fissure (Crosby et al. 1962). The two main components of the IC are delineated by the mediolaterally extending central fissure. An anterior portion comprising, in general, the two gyri breves and the precentral gyrus of island, corresponds histologically to agranular isocortex (with relatively narrow recipient layer IV and more prominent pyramidal neuron-rich layers V and VI, such as the motor cortex) towards the orbitofrontal cortex. The posterior region includes the two gyri longi and cytoarchitectonically is granular cortex (with broad layer IV, as primary sensory cortices) (Crosby et al. 1962; Oppenheimer 1993). The IC connects with both typical limbic regions, such as the amygdala, and other neocortices that have strong limbic 'affiliation' including orbitofrontal and cingulate areas (Mesulam 1985). Other brain regions that connect with the IC, in humans, are parietal (somatosensory) and temporal neocortices, caudate (tail), putamen, claustrum, and the dorsal thalamus. Functionally, the IC appears to be involved in visceral sensory (taste) and visceromotor functions, vestibular function, movement generation (supplementary motor region), and certain aspects of language (Augustine 1985). With regard to cardiac function, studies in rats indicate that the posterior (granular) IC has both sensory and motor areas (Cechetto and Saper 1987; Yasui *et al.* 1991; Zhang and Oppenheimer 1997). It contains neurons that respond to changes in blood pressure as well as cells that can elicit pressor and depressor responses. Both groups of cells have similar, but distinct, connections in the rat. For instance, pressor and depressor sites connect with the amygdala and lateral hypothalamus while only the latter sites connect with the locus ceruleus and spinal trigeminal nucleus. Data on direct insular stimulation in epileptic patients, undergoing temporal lobotomy, showed that the right IC originates pressor responses and tachycardia while responses in the opposite direction (parasympathetic effects) are produced by left insular stimulation (Oppenheimer 1993; Oppenheimer *et al.* 1996).

Protocol:

After brains are oriented in the anterior commissure–posterior commissure plane and the Talairach grid has been applied, the IC is measured in the horizontal (axial) plane. In this plane, the IC is measured beginning in the first slice showing claustrum (and putamen) in the dorso-ventral direction. The stopping slice is the most ventral one showing again these two basal ganglia nuclei. Only sectors of the Talairach atlas that contain 50% or higher proportions of IC are defined as IC components (between parentheses: IC and grey matter (GM) proportions). The first two letters represent the sector, and L or R the hemisphere:

Anterior insula (gyri breves and precentral gyrus of island)
DbL6 (100%), EbL6 (100% cortex, 50% GM), CbL7 (100%), DbL7 (100% cortex, 50% GM), CbL8 (50%), DcL8 (100%), DbL9 (100% cortex, 50% GM), DbR6 (100%), EbR6 (100% cortex, 50% GM), CbR7 (100%), DbR7 (100% cortex, 50% GM), CbR8 (50%), DcR8 (100%), DbR9 (100% cortex, 50% GM).

Posterior insula (gyri longi):
FbL6 (100% cortex, 75% GM), *EcL7* (50%), FbL7 (100% cortex, 25% GM), *EcL8* (100%), FbR6 (100% cortex, 75% GM), EcR7 (50%), FbR7 (100% cortex, 25% GM), EcR8 (100%).

Since the parcellation method is applied after tissue has been segmented into three classes (GM, WM, CSF), volumes are obtained for each tissue class. Values for IC WM should be taken with caution, since appropriate delineation from adjacent extreme capsule (containing association fibres for the IC; Crosby *et al.* 1962) with this method is not possible. The variables to calculate are the following:

(1) Total insular volume.
(2) Ratio of insular volume to total cortical grey volume.
(3) Total anterior insular volume.
(4) Total posterior insular volume, hypothesized as abnormal in autonomic dysfunction/sudden death.
(5) Proportion of anterior and posterior regions to total insular volume. It is postulated that posterior/total ratio will be more informative in RS subjects with autonomic dysfunction.
(6) Parasympathetic/sympathetic insular ratio, by calculating left posterior insula (underlined sectors) to right posterior insula ratios.

In summary, a method for 'screening' for volumetric differences in the IC in RS is proposed. Different morphometric variables of potential functional significance, in terms of cortical control of cardiac function, are also defined. Implementation of this protocol may lead to future studies focusing on the role of IC in several aspects of the RS neurologic phenotype.

5.1 The Rett syndrome: a proposed mechanism of genetic origin and inheritance

M.A. Hulten

There can be no doubt that the Rett syndrome (RTT, McKusick Catalogue No. 312750) affects females primarily, occurring with an incidence of around 1 per 10 to 15 000 new-born girls (Akesson *et al.* 1996). In the British Survey, conducted by Kerr, of 640 recorded Rett cases, 531 (83%) were classic and 109 (17%) atypical (in 1999) (see Chapter 1). In congruence with observations elsewhere, the majority of these RTT cases are sporadic, and there are only a few families having more than one affected RTT child. Nevertheless, not only RTT concordance between identical twin sisters and the occurrence of RTT in sisters, half sisters and cousins, but in particular the report of a mother and daughter, both having Rett syndrome (Witt Engerström and Forslund 1992), points to this severe neurological disorder being a single gene condition, which is either X-linked or sex limited in its expression— although more complex models have also been postulated (Johnson 1980; Buhler *et al.* 1990).

Strict X-linkage of a dominant RTT gene mutation would imply lethality of hemizygous males, and lack of male to male inheritance in families. To date there is no indication of a reduction in birth rates of males in the majority of RTT families, having a single affected female (Martinho *et al.* 1990). Such sporadic RTT females are thus expected to either represent a new mutation or result from maternal germinal mosaicism (Thomas 1996). No relevant data in respect of male lethality are available in the families with more than one affected female, as numbers are so few. Genealogical studies in Sweden, using church book data to trace the biological relationships between current RTT cases, indicate male to male transmission of asymptomatic carriers (Åkesson *et al.* 1996). This is also apparent in the UK family, the pedigree of which is illustrated in Fig. 5.1.1. What then is the most likely mechanism of genetic origin and inheritance for Rett Syndrome, which could explain these circumstances? Recently a proportion of RTT females have been found to have mutations in the X-linked gene MECP2 (see Chapter 2). My vision, conceived before this discovery, is aimed to understand, in particular,

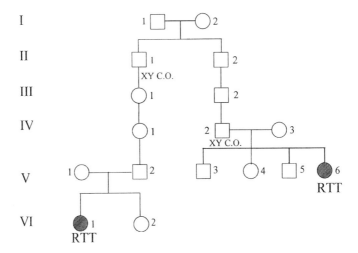

Fig. 5.1.1 Pedigree of RTT family S, proposed to exemplify the PAR XqYq repeat amplification model.

The founder male I:1 carries a permissive Yq amplification of DNA repeats adjacent to the postulated RTT gene, located within the homologous XqYq segment. He transmits this Y chromosome to his two sons II:1 and II:2.

An unequal XY crossing over (C.O.) occurs at meiosis in II:1, leading to the transferral of a moderately increased repeat to his daughter III:1, who becomes an asymptomatic carrier. This X in turn is inherited by her daughter IV:1 and her grandson V:2. An expansion of the Xq repeat takes place in some cells during meiosis in V:2. This X is inherited by his daughter VI:1. She has the RTT phenotype as the expanded repeat is leading to a disturbance in gene expression of the putative RTT gene.

The second son II:2 of the founder male I:1 transmits the permissive Yq DNA repeat amplification to his son III:2 and grandson IV:2. An unequal crossing over (C.O.) in an occasional spermatocyte of IV:2 leads to a large expansion of the repeat, and impaired gene function in his RTT daughter V:6.

the male to male transmission, as exemplified by family S (Fig. 5.1.1) on the assumption that the two RTT cases in this family are not coincidental.

I presume that one RTT gene mutation concerns an X-linked gene, which has a homologue on the Y. The RTT gene on the X chromosome is normally expressed, while the Y homologue is not, as is the case with e.g. the recently discovered SYBL1 gene, mapped to the XqYq pairing (PAR) segment (D'Esposito *et al.* 1997). It seems likely that the silencing of the SYBL1 gene is due to its position adjacent to the heterochromatic block Yqh (Hulten *et al.* 1995). The postulated RTT gene is located in the same XqYq segment, and is supposed to be silenced in the same way. The net result of this situation is that normal males and females would each have one copy of the RTT gene expressed, i.e. from their single active X chromosome.

My second assumption is that in some cases the Rett syndrome is due to a disturbance in gene expression akin to that in the Fragile X syndrome and other disorders involving amplification of repeated DNA sequences (Reddy and Housman 1997). Such amplification is expected to be permissive on the Y, but over a certain threshold frequency impairs the expression of its counterpart on the X. The implication of this hypothesis is that an original RTT premutation may have taken place many generations ago on the Y chromosome in a founder male (I:1 of family S), and any DNA repeat instability and amplification would go unnoticed with male to male transmission, having no phenotypic implications in carrier sons (II:1 and II:2).

My third assumption is that male to female transmission may occur via XqYq recombination in occasional spermatocytes, perhaps provoked by DNA repeat amplification in a carrier male (II:1 and IV:2). Crossing over within the XqYq pairing segment is normally rare (Kvaloy *et al.* 1994), but it seems likely a 'hot spot' for unequal recombination may be created by DNA repeat amplification. A moderate repeat Yq to Xq transfer may be expected to give rise to a phenotypically normal, asymptomatic carrier daughter (III:1), while a transfer large enough to disturb the expression of the presumptive RTT(X) gene would lead to a daughter having the Rett syndrome (V:6). Paternal transmission might thus be expected to be common in sporadic cases.

Any affected RTT female would have a 1:1 risk of having an RTT daughter, although this result would not normally be realized, as RTT females, due to their mental handicap, only very rarely reproduce (Witt Engerström and Forslund 1992). An asymptomatic female carrier of a moderate DNA repeat amplification is likewise expected to transmit the RTT premutation to both her sons and daughters with a 1:1 risk. Female repeat instability in the germ line is not required to explain the pattern of inheritance in family S (Fig. 5.1.1). However, on this model, female germ line instability and amplification would seem obligate in other families with RTT half sisters or cousins with transmission via an asymptomatic mother. It remains to be ascertained in such families whether there are any indications of the expected male lethality of hemizygous sons.

In conclusion, I have presented a model for the genetic origin and inheritance of the Rett syndrome, based on the classical concept of partial sex linkage, where DNA repeat amplification impairs expression of a presumptive RTT gene, located at the tip of Xq, but is of no consequence on its homologue on the Yq, as this is not normally expressed. The size of the homologous XqYq segment is estimated to be around 320 Kb (Kvaloy *et al.* 1994), creating new hopes for the identification of the relevant DNA sequences including the presumptive RTT gene. The identification of a foolproof biological marker for the Rett syndrome is not only of diagnostic significance, but will also become a most important tool for evaluation of recurrence risks in families, who are already burdened by having a child with this devastating disease.

Acknowledgements

This paper is dedicated to my brother Pontus in memory of our diseased sister Ingrid. I am grateful to family S for their help in compiling the family tree of Fig. 5.1.1, and Dr A. Kerr for introducing this family to me. I am also most thankful for the inspiration provided by the UK Rett Syndrome Association, and in particular to members, who have provided blood samples for our Genetic Bank, which has recently become a useful resource for diagnosis and risk estimates Cheadle *et al.* 2000; Vacca *et al.* 2000. During my long-standing contact with the Association, I have been impressed by the vitality and dedication of its members, so many of whom have been able to turn a difficult situation into a most positive, sharing and sometimes even joyful experience.

References

Akesson, H.O. Hagberg, B., and Wahlstrom, J. (1996). Rett syndrome, classical and atypical: genealogical support for common origin. *J. Med. Genet.*, **33**, 764–6.

Buhler, W.M., Malik, N.J., and Aljan, M. (1990). Another model for the inheritance of Rett syndrome. *Am. J. Med. Genet.*, **36**, 126–31.

Cheadle, J.P., Gill, H., Fleming, N., Maynard, J., Kerr, A.M., Leonard, H., Krawczak, M., Cooper, D.N., Lynch, S., Thomas, N., Hughes, H., Hulten, M., Sampson, J.R., and Clarke, A. (2000). Long-read sequence analysis of the MECP2 gene in Rett syndrome patients: correlation of disease severity with mutation type and location. *Molecular Genetics*, 9, 7, 1119–29.

D'Esposito, M. *et al.* (1997). Differential expression pattern of XqPAR-linked genes SYBL1 and IL9R correlates with the structure and evolution of the region. *Hum. Mol. Genet.*, **6**, 1917–23.

Hagberg, B. (1985). Rett Syndrome: Swedish approach to analysis of prevalence and cause. *Brain Dev.*, 7, 277–80.

Hulten, M.A., Stacey, M., and Armstrong, S. (1995). Does junk DNA regulate gene expression in humans?. *J. Clin. Mol. Pathol.*, **48**, 118–23.

Johnson, W.F. (1980). Metabolic interference and the +/− heterozygote: a hypothetical form of simple inheritance which is neither dominant nor recessive. *Am. J. Hum. Genet.*, **32**, 374–86.

Kvaloy, K., Galvagni, F., and Brown, W.R.A. (1994). The sequence organisation of the long arm pseudoautosomal region of the human sex chromosomes. *Hum. Mol. Genet.*, **3**(5), 771–8.

Martinho, P.S., *et al.* (1990). In search of a genetic basis for the Rett syndrome. *Hum. Genet.* **86**, 131–4.

Reddy, P.S. and Housman, D.E. (1997). The complex pathology of trinucleotide repeats. *Curr. Opin. Cell Biol.*, **9**, 364–72.

Thomas, G.H. (1996). High male:female ratio of germ-line mutations: an alternative explanation for postulated gestational lethality in males in X-linked dominant disorders. *Am. J. Hum. Genet.*, **58**, 1364–8.

Vacca, M., Filippini, F., Budillon, A., Rossi, V., Mercadante, G., Manzati, E., Gualandi, F., Bigoni, S., Trabbanelli, C., Pini, G., Calzolari, E., Ferlinin, A., Meloni, I., Hayek, G., Zappella, M., Renieri, A., D'Urso, M., D'Esposito, M., MacDonald, F., Kerr, A.M., Dhanjal, S. and Hulten, M. (accepted 2000). Mutation analysis of the MECP2 gene in British and Italian Rett sysdrome families. *Journal of Molecular Medicine*.

Witt Engerström, I. and Forslund, M. (1992). Mother and daughter with Rett Syndrome. *J. Child. Neurol. Suppl.*, **3**, S76–8.

5.2 Amino acid receptor studies in Rett syndrome

Mary E. Blue and Michael V. Johnson

For several years we have hypothesized that Rett syndrome (RS) involves a defect in genetic programs that regulate neuronal differentiation and the establishment of synaptic connections. Our first autoradiographic experiments determined whether RS altered the developmental expression of receptors for the amino acid neurotransmitters glutamate and GABA. Glutamate and GABA are the neurotransmitters for the majority of excitatory and inhibitory synapses in the CNS. Based on the clinical features of RS, we chose the superior frontal gyrus (SFG) and basal ganglia regions for our studies comparing the distribution and density of glutamate and GABA receptors in postmortem brain slices from 9 RS girls and 10 control females. Our results showed regional, receptor subtype, and age-specific alterations in amino acid neurotransmitter receptors in RS (Blue *et al.* 1999*a, b*). By dividing the cases into younger (8 years old or younger) and older age groups, we showed that the density of NMDA, AMPA, GABA, and metabotropic glutamate receptors in the SFG and of GABA receptors in the caudate tended to be higher in younger RS girls than controls while the densities in older patients fell below controls (see Fig. 5.2.1). The biphasic pattern of developmental differences in receptor binding was statistically significant for NMDA receptors in the SFG, which demonstrated the greatest disparity between the older and younger groups (Blue *et al.* 1999*b*). We also found significant reductions in AMPA and NMDA receptor density in the putamen and in KA receptor density in the caudate of older RS cases compared to controls (Blue *et al.* 1999*a*). In contrast, the density of metabotropic glutamate receptors was not altered significantly in the basal ganglia of RS patients. In terms of age-related changes in receptor density, we generally found more striking reductions in older RS patients; control subjects showed more limited changes in receptor density with age.

The recent discovery of mutations in the MeCP2 protein in girls with Rett syndrome (Amir *et al.* 1999) fits nicely with a hypothesis of aberrant gene expression in synapses in RS. Confirmation that transcriptional regulation of

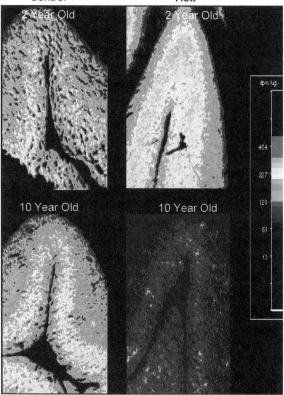

Fig. 5.2.1 Pseudocolor images of [3H] CGP39653 binding of N-methyl-D-aspartate (NMDA) receptors in 2-year-old (upper panel) and 10-year-old (lower panel) Rett syndrome (RS) patients and controls. The density of NMDA receptors appears markedly higher in the 2-year-old RS patient compared to her age-matched control. In contrast, the density of NMDA receptors is lower in the 10-year-old RS patient than in her age-matched control. Reprinted from Blue *et al.* (1999b), with permission of Lippincott Williams & Wilkins, Inc. (See also colour plate section.)

multiple genes is the key defect in RS makes examining expression of synaptic neurotransmitter related genes all the more important. Our findings that NMDA glutamate receptors were expressed at higher than control levels in young RS girls but underexpressed in older patients (Blue *et al.* 1999b), suggest that the major transcriptional regulation disorder is manifest in the early postnatal period of childhood, during the encephalopathy phase of RS. These studies are the first to report neurobiological markers that have a biphasic age-related expression that correlates with the biphasic clinical transition from the early encephalopathy phase to the later plateau or 'burn-out' phase of the disorder. This early phase of brain development appears to be a critical one for the expression of RS and it will be important to focus gene expression studies on this period. It is possible that gene expression abnormalities will be less apparent in studies that use samples from older girls.

It is interesting to note that the dendritic pathology in RS (Bauman *et al.* 1995; Belichenko *et al.* 1997) parallels the stunted development of neuropil in disorders such as cretinism and Rubinstein-Taybi syndrome (Pogacar *et al.* 1973; Rosman 1972). Both disorders involve defects in proteins that regulate the transcription of multiple genes: in cretinism unliganded nuclear thyroid receptors silence gene expression while in Rubinstein-Taybi, CREB binding protein, a transcriptional co-activator, is defective (Engelkamp and van Heyningen 1996; Oike *et al.* 1999; Petrij *et al.* 1995; Taine *et al.* 1998). MeCP2, a transcription factor that links methylated CpG sequences with transcriptional repressive protein complexes (Nan *et al.* 1998; Razin 1998), normally silences this same transcriptional machinery at sites in close proximity to nuclear thyroid receptors and CREB binding protein.

Our studies of neurotransmitter receptor expression in postmortem brain and studies in the neurobiological model in the mouse remain very important for understanding the disease and for designing therapeutic interventions. However, with the discovery of the role of MeCP2, we can focus even more sharply and try to understand the links between these synaptic markers and the role of MeCP2 in their expression. It is important to note that it is unknown whether the NMDA receptor or other neurotransmitter receptors are under direct control of MeCP2. It is also unknown whether mutations in MeCP2 discovered in RS are likely to have an effect to activate or silence gene expression.

References

Amir, R.E., Van den Veyver, I.B., Wan, M., Tran, C.Q., Francke, U., and Zoghbi, H.Y. (1999). Rett syndrome is caused by mutations in X-linked MECP2, encoding methyl-CpG-binding protein 2. *Nature Genetics*, **23**, 185–8.

Bauman, M.L., Kemper, T.L., and Arin, D.M. (1995). Microscopic observations of the brain in Rett syndrome. *Neuropediatrics*, **26**, 105–8.

Belichenko, P.V., Hagberg, B., and Dahlstrom, A. (1997). Morphological study of neocortical areas in Rett syndrome. *Acta Neuropathologica,* **93**, 50–61.

Blue, M.E., Naidu, S., and Johnston, M.V. (1999*a*). Altered development of glutamate and GABA receptors in the basal ganglia of girls with Rett syndrome. *Experimental Neurology*, **156**, 345–52.

Blue, M.E., Naidu, S., and Johnston, M.V. (1999*b*). Development of amino acid receptors in frontal cortex from girls with Rett syndrome. *Annals of Neurology*, **45**, 541–5.

Engelkamp, D. and van Heyningen, V. (1996). Transcription factors in disease. *Current Opinion in Genetics and Development*, **6**, 334–42.

Nan, X., Ng, H.H., Johnson, C.A., Laherty, C.D., Turner, B.M., Eisenman, R.N., and Bird, A. (1998). Transcriptional repression by the methyl-CpG-binding protein MeCP2 involves a histone deacetylase complex. *Nature*, **393**, 386–9.

Oike, Y., Hata, A., Mamiya, T., Kaname, T., Noda, Y., Suzuki, M., Yasue, H., Nabeshima, T., Araki, K., and Yamamura, K. (1999). Truncated CBP protein leads to classical Rubinstein-Taybi syndrome phenotypes in mice: implications for a dominant-negative mechanism. *Human Molecular Genetics*, **8**, 387–96.

Petrij, F., Giles, R.H., Dauwerse, H.G., Saris, J.J., Hennekam, R.C., Masuno, M., Tommerup, N., van Ommen, G.J., Goodman, R.H., Peters, D.J., and Breuning, M.H. (1995). Rubinstein-Taybi syndrome caused by mutations in the transcriptional co-activator CBP. *Nature*, **376**, 348–51.

Pogacar, S., Nora, N.F., and Kemper, T.L. (1973). Neuropathological findings in the Rubinstein-Taybi syndrome. *Rhode Island Medical Journal*, **56**, 114–21.

Razin, A. (1998). CpG methylation, chromatin structure and gene silencing—a three-way connection. *The EMBO Journal*, **17**, 4905–8.

Rosman, N.P. (1972). The neuropathology of congenital hypothyroidism. *Advances in Experimental Medicine and Biology*, **30**, 337–66.

Taine, L., Goizet, C., Wen, Z.Q., Petrij, F., Breuning, M.H., Ayme, S., Saura, R., Arveiler, B., and Lacombe, D. (1998). Submicroscopic deletion of chromosome 16p13.3 in patients with Rubinstein-Taybi syndrome. *American Journal of Medical Genetics*, **78**, 267–70.

5.3 Melatonin and the Rett syndrome disorder

Sarojini S. Budden

Rett syndrome is a neurological disorder resulting from an early arrest of brain development. The secondary impact of this has a devastating effect on brain functions including sleep disorders. Sleep disturbances often develop during the earlier stages of rapid deterioration in Rett syndrome and may continue throughout the individual's lifetime.

The earliest sleep studies in Rett syndrome done by Nomura *et al.* (1987) indicated the involvement of the noradrenergic and serotonergic systems which is consistent with the central involvement of the autonomic nervous system. Segawa and Nomura (1992) showed that sleep abnormalities increase with age involving disturbances in the different stages of sleep and the variations in the tonic and phasic components of nocturnal sleep and REM-NREM cycles. Unusual EEG ϕ rhythms over the central cortical region in the sleep-wake state have also been reported by Niedermeyer *et al.* (1997).

The basic synchronization of the sleep-wake cycle with the light-dark cycle is a complex neurobiological mechanism which is dependent on the hypothalamic circadian clock located in the suprachiasmatic nuclei (SCN). These nuclei regulate nearly all body functions that have a circadian rhythm such as sleep-wake cycles, hormonal secretion, and body temperature. The SCN are positioned just dorsal to the optic chiasm and receive direct innervation from the retina (Hendrickson *et al.* 1972; Moore and Lenn 1972). The SCN conveys photic information to the pineal gland via a multisynaptic pathway (Moore and Klein, 1974). Synthesis of the pineal hormone melatonin is under adrenergic control; it is produced through the night. Levels rise to 60–300 pg/ml, depending on the person's age and other factors (Attanasio *et al.* 1985; Waldauser *et al.* 1988; Cavallo 1991). During day, circulating melatonin levels are almost undetectable and influence the SCN timekeeping, thus forming a feedback loop (Redman *et al.* 1983; McArthur *et al.* 1991; Lewy *et al.* 1992).

It is not known whether the circadian system is dysfunctional in Rett syndrome. A postmortem examination of a single case with Rett syndrome revealed diminished hypothalamic levels of serotonin and norepinephrine (Brucke et al. 1987) which suggests that circadian rhythm regulation could have been compromised. Armstrong (Chapter 3) has also shown alterations of serotonin receptors in the brainstem resembling those of an immature brain which may also explain the lack of neuromaturational organization of sleep-wake cycles.

Miyamoto et al. (1999) have studied the circadian rhythm of serum melatonin in two females with Rett syndrome and showed that the peak time of melatonin secretion was not only delayed but that the peak value was at a lower limit. These findings would suggest that sleep disorders in individuals with Rett syndrome may relate to impaired phasic secretion of melatonin.

McArthur and Budden (1998) showed that exogenous melatonin significantly improved total sleep time, sleep efficiency, and decreased latency of sleep onset in nine individuals with Rett syndrome. Jan and O'Donnell (1996) have used melatonin successfully in the treatment of sleep disorders which are associated with blindness, deaf-blindness, mental retardation, autism and neurological diseases. Long-term effects of chronic melatonin use in pediatric patients are unknown at this time.

References

Attanasio, A., Borrelli, P., and Gupta, D. (1985). Circadian rhythms in serum melatonin from infancy to adolescence. *Journal of Clinical Endocrinology and Metabolism*, **61**, 388–9.

Brucke, T., Sofic, E., Killian, W., Rett, A., and Riederer, P. (1987). Reduced concentrations and increased metabolism of biogenic amines in a single case of Rett Syndrome: a postmortem brain study. *Journal of Neural Transmission*, **68**, 315–24.

Cavallo, A. (1992). Plasma melatonin rhythm in normal puberty: interaction of age and pubertal stage. *Neuroendocrinology*, **55**, 372–9.

Hendrickson, A.E., Waggoner, N., and Cowan, W.M. (1972). An autoradiographic and electron microscopic study of retino-hypoyhalamic connections. *Zeitschrift Fur Zellforschung Und Mikroskopische Anatomie*, **135**, 1–26.

Hunt, A.E. and Gillette, M.U. (1997). Melatonin action and signal transduction in the rat suprachiasmatic circadian clock: activation of protein kinase C at dusk and dawn. *Endocrinology*, **138**, 627–34.

Jan, J.E. and O'Donnell, M.E. (1996). Use of melatonin in the treatment of pediatric sleep disorders. *Journal of Pineal Research*, **21**(4), 193–9.

Lewy, A., Ahmed, S., Jackson, J., and Sack, R. (1992). Melatonin shifts human circadian rhythms according to a phase-response curve. *Chronobiology International*, **9**, 380–92.

McArthur, A.J. and Budden, S.S. (1998). Sleep dysfunction in Rett Syndrome: a trial of exogenous melatonin treatment. *Developmental Medicine and Child Neurology*, **40**(3), 186–92.

McArthur, A.J., Gillette, M.U., and Prosser, R. (1991). Melatonin directly resets the rat suprachiasmatic circadian clock *in vitro*. *Brain Research*, **565**, 158–61.

Miyamoto, A., Oki, J., Takahashi, S., and Okuno, A. (1999). Serum melatonin kinetics and long-term melatonin treatment for sleep disorders in Rett Syndrome. *Brain and Development*, **21**(1), 59–62.

Moore, R.Y. and Klein, D.C. (1974). Visual pathways and the central neural control of a circadian rhythm in pineal serotonin N-acetyl-transferase activity. *Brain Research*, **71**, 17–33.

Moore, R.Y. and Lenn, N.J. (1972). A retinohypothalamic projection in the rat. *Journal of Comprehensive Neurology*, **146**, 1–14.

Niedermeyer, E., Naidu, S.B., and Plate, C. (1997). Unusual theta rhythms over central region in Rett Syndrome: considerations of underlying dysfunction. *Clinical Electroencephalography*, **28**(1), 36–43.

Nomura, Y., Honda, K., and Segawa, M. (1987). Pathophysiology of Rett syndrome. *Brain and Development*, **9**(5), 506–13.

Redman, J., Armstrong, S., and Ng, K. (1983). Free-running activity rhythms in the rat: entrainment by melatonin. *Science*, **219**, 1089–91.

Segawa, M. and Nomura, Y. (1992). Polysomnography in Rett Syndrome. *Brain and Development*, **14**(**Suppl.**), S46–54.

Waldhauser, F., Weizenbacher, G., Tatzer, E., Gisinger, B., Waldhauser, M., Schemper, M., and Frisch, H. (1988). Alterations in nocturnal melatonin levels in human with growth and aging. *Journal of Clinical Endocrinology and metabolism*, **66**, 648–52.

5.4 Early abnormality in pterin levels in Rett syndrome

Souad Messahel, Anne E. Pheasant, Hardiv Pall, and Alison M. Kerr

Reports of altered neurotransmitter metabolism in Rett syndrome (particularly monoamines, see Chapters 7 and 8) have led investigators to study the pathways of their synthesis. Tetrahydrobiopterin (BH_4) is an essential cofactor for the aromatic amino acid hydroxylases and, as such, is necessary for the synthesis of noradrenaline, dopamine and serotonin. Neopterin is a naturally occurring pterin which is an intermediate in BH_4 biosynthesis. It is now well established that increased neopterin levels are associated with activation of the cellular immune system and that neopterin is a clinically useful, though non-specific, marker of immune activation in patients (Fuchs *et al.* 1993). There is increasing evidence that an abnormal immune response contributes to some neurological disorders and neopterin has been found to be raised in a number of these such as Alzheimer's disease, Down's syndrome and depression (Armstrong *et al.* 1995; Anderson *et al.* 1992).

Early studies on biopterin metabolism in Rett syndrome produced conflicting results. Bolthauser *et al.* (1986) and Sahota *et al.* (1985) found normal levels of biopterin derivatives in the serum and urine of patients with Rett syndrome whereas Zoghbi *et al.* (1989) found raised levels of total biopterins in CSF, thus raising the possibility of a localized CNS change in biopterin metabolism. Recently we measured urinary neopterin and biopterin in 40 subjects with Rett syndrome, 8 of their healthy sisters and 29 female control volunteers (age range 2–54 years). The results confirm earlier preliminary findings (Fuchs *et al.* 1996) that urinary neopterin levels are raised in a proportion of young girls (under 6 years) with Rett syndrome but not in the older women. In contrast, urinary biopterin levels are not different from controls in the youngest children but remain low while control values increase with age. These findings may indicate that immune activation occurs during the regression phase of Rett syndrome and that this may accompany, contribute to or cause the abnormalities observed. The results also raise the possibility that an inherited fault in tetrahydrobiopterin metabolism increases the risk of developing the disorder possibly via altered monoamine metabolism. For example, the observed increase in serotonin receptor density in the medulla (Witt Engerström and Kerr 1998) is suggestive of early lack of serotonin: a deficiency of BH_4 could cause a failure of serotonin synthesis.

The sisters of the Rett girls were found to have urinary pterin levels between those of the Rett subjects and the controls. It is possible that, in common with their Rett sisters, these healthy girls have inherited a mild abnormality of pterin metabolism which is not inevitably expressed as disease but nevertheless predisposes to the development of a disorder in the presence of an additional mutation, e.g. in the MECP2 gene (Amir *et al.* 1999). The nature of the disorder seen would vary with the nature of the other abnormality. Certainly an explanation must be found to explain a rather high incidence of a variety of other neurological disorders in the families of girls with Rett disorder (autism, schizophrenia, depression, epilepsy, see Chapters 1 and 15).

References

Amir, R.E, Van den Veyver, I.B., Wan, M., Tran, C.Q., Francke, U., and Zoghbi, H.Y. (1999). Rett syndrome is caused by mutations in X-linked MECP2, encoding methyl-CpG-binding protein 2. Nature Genetics, 23, 185–8.

Anderson, D.N., Abou-Saleh, M.T., Collins, J., Hughes, K., Cattell, R.J., Hamon, C.G.B., Blair, J.A., and Dewey, M.E. (1992). Pterin metabolism in depression: an extension of the amine hypothesis and possible marker of response to ECT. Psychological Medicine, 22, 863–9.

Armstrong, R.A., Cattell, R.J., Winspur, S.J., and Blair, J.A. (1995). The levels of neopterin, biopterin and the neopterin/biopterin ration in urine from control subjects and patients with Alzheimer's disease and Down's syndrome. Pteridines, 6, 185–9.

Bolthauser, E., Niederwieser, A., Kierat, L., and Haenggeli, C.A. (1986). Pterins in patients with Rett syndrome. American Journal of Medical Genetics, 24, 317–21.

Fuchs, D., Pheasant, A.E., Wachter, H., and Blair, J.A. (1996). In Increased urinary neopterin concentrations in the early phase of Rett syndrome. World Congress on Rett Syndrome, p. 52 (abstract).

Fuchs, D., Weiss, G., and Wachter, H. (1993). Neopterin, biochemistry and clinical use as a marker for cellular immune reactions. International Archives of Allergy and Immunology, 101, 1–6.

Sahota, A., Leeming, R., Blair, J., and Hagberg, B. (1985). Tetrahydrobiopterin metabolism in the Rett disease. Brain and Development, 7, 349–50.

Witt Engerström, I., and Kerr, A. (1998). Workshop on autonomic function in Rett syndrome. Brain and Development, 20, 323–6.

Zoghbi, H.Y., Milstien, S., Butler, I.J., Smith, E.O., Kaufman, S., Glaze, D.G., and Percy, A.K. (1989). Cerebrospinal fluid biogenic amines and biopterin in Rett syndrome. Annals of Neurology, 25, 56–60.

5.5 Neurotrophic factors in the pathogenesis of Rett syndrome

Raili Riikonen

Mutations on MECP2 now appear to be responsible for the disorder (Amir *et al.* 1999), although the precise pathogenesis is still to be worked out. Rett disorder (RD) is believed to be a neurodevelopmental rather than a neurodegenerative disease. It is characterized by early failure of brain growth, with small brains and dendritic abnormalities but no features characteristic of degenerative diseases (Armstrong 1995). The head circumference of the patient is normal at birth but early deceleration of brain growth occurs at 2–3 months. RD is characterized by a process of triggering factors at the time when vigorous brain growth with synapse formation and pruning should be at a peak. Timing seems to be important in Rett Syndrome (RS).

5.5.1 Nerve growth factors

The neurotrophic factors are important regulators of neuronal growth, differentiation, and survival during the developmental period of natural cell death. The pattern of expression of neurotrophic factors in the central nervous system and their actions may be quite distinct. Nerve growth factor β-NGF is the first and best-known of the neurotrophic factors. The other members of this group are brain-derived neurotrophic factor (BDNF), neurotrophin-3–4/5 (NT-3-/4/5), insulin-like growth factors (IGFs), ciliary neurotrophic factor (CNTF), fibroblast growth factor (FGF) and glial-cell-line-derived neurotrophic factor (GDNF). Neurotrophins bind to and activate specific cell surface transmembrane glycoproteins, tyrosine kinase (Trk) receptors. Trk A is a high-affinity receptor for NGF, Trk B for BDNF and NT-4/5, Trk C for NT-3, and Trk IGF-1 for IGF-1 and IGF-2. Ret-c is a functional receptor for GDNF. The NGF gene is located on the proximal short arm of chromosome 1, the BDNF gene on chromosome 11, the NT-3 gene on chromosome 12, and the IGF-1 gene on chromosome 12.

NGF acts especially on cholinergic cells of the basal forebrain, but it also has an effect on other neurons, for example in the striatum, thalamus, and brainstem. BDNF also acts on the basal cholinergic neurons, but it is an important survival factor for dopaminergic neurons in the substantia nigra, as is also GDNF. In animal models, NGF activates the gene expression of choline acetyltransferase (ChAT), the enzyme responsible for synthesizing acetylcholine. In the adult primate brain, human NGF is biologically active and prevents atrophy of the basal forebrain cholinergic neurons after injury (Hefti 1986).

5.5.2 Clinical disorders: neurotrophic factors

Neurotrophic factors have been suggested to be significant in neurodegenerative disorders, such as Alzheimer's and Parkinson's diseases and amyotrophic lateral sclerosis (Connor and Dragunow 1988).

There are few studies on the CSF NGF in humans. It has been shown that CSF NGF is elevated by inflammatory processes and in autoimmune disease (Laudiero *et al.* 1992; Riikonen *et al.* 1997, 1998), and also in patients with progressive brain atrophy (Suzaki *et al.* 1997) and initially in patients with brain injury (Patterson *et al.* 1993). Low CSF NGF levels were found in patients with symptomatic infantile spasms (Riikonen *et al.* 1997) and with severe neonatal asphyxia (Riikonen *et al.* 1999). Low CSF IGF-1 levels were found in patients with cerebellar degeneration (Riikonen *et al.*, 1999) and infantile neuronal lipofuscinosis (Riikonen *et al.* 2000). The research to date indicates a potential role for neurotrophic factors in the treatment of acute brain damage or neurodegenerative disorders (Sariola *et al.* 1994; Connor and Dragunow 1998).

5.5.3 Rett syndrome and neurotrophic factors

We have studied four neurotrophic factors from the CSF of patients with RS, i.e. NGF, BDNF, GDNF, and IGF-1, and also from the serum (except of GDNF) using the sensitive two-site ELISA method.

We found low concentrations of CSF NGF but normal serum levels in RS as compared with other patients (Fig. 5.5.1) (Riikonen and Vanhala 1999). Excitotoxic glutamate was high in the CSF of the same patients (Lappalainen and Riikonen 1996). Low CSF NGF could well fit for the evidence for loss of basal forebrain neurons in RS: (a) in volumetric studies, cortical forebrain volume, together with that of the nucleus caudatus and midbrain, is reduced (Reiss *et al.* 1993); (b) neuropathologic studies show reduced size and number of these cells (Belichenko and Hagberg 1997), and small amounts of ChAT (Wenk *et al.* 1991). SPECT studies have also shown hypometabolism of the frontal lobes (Uvebrandt

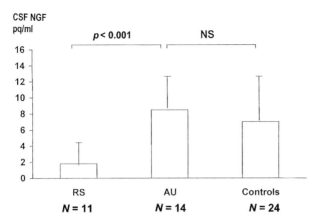

Fig. 5.5.1 Cerebrospinal fluid nerve growth factor (NGF) concentrations in patients with Rett syndrome (RS), in patients with autism (AU) and in other control patients. The levels of patients with RS were significantly lower than in patients with autism which were of the same levels as in the controls.

et al. 1993; Lappalainen *et al.* 1997). In RS, reduced pigmentation in the substantia nigra is a constant neuropathologic finding and dopaminergic dysfunction is suggested. Unfortunately, we could not confirm this by examining CSF BDNF and GDNF because our methods were not sufficiently sensitive. The levels of serum and CSF IGF-1 did not differ from the controls either (Vanhala *et al.*, 2000).

Low concentrations of CSF NGF could reflect the neuronal loss in general; they seem not to be specific for RS. Interestingly, however, we found that CSF NGF was grossly normal in autism and low to negligible in RS (Riikonen and Vanhala 1999). This is in agreement with different morphologic and neurochemical findings (brain growth, affected brain areas, neurotransmitter metabolism) in these two, in earlier stages often similar, disorders. Could CSF NGF be a biologic marker for differentiation?

Genes for BDNF and IGF-2, both located on chromosome 11, as well as the gene of the bcl-2 protein, which is essential for normal apoptosis and is located on chromosome 22, have also been studied, but no sequence abnormalities were found (Anvret *et al.* 1994).

We think that in the future it would be important to study (a) neurotrophic factors with more sensitive methods, (b) other nerve growth factors also, (c) genes influencing neurotrophic factors and their receptors and transporters as well as (d) brain tissues from autopsies for local changes in neurotrophic factors, and (e) clinical trials with neurotrophic factors (IGFs?) or drugs stimulating their production.

In conclusion, low CSF NGF and elevated glutamate concentrations, primary or secondary to the neuropathologic changes associated with RS, indicate that these factors may be involved in the pathogenesis of the disease.

References

Amir, R., Van den Veyver, I., Wan, M., Tran, C., Francke, U., and Zoghbi, H. (1999). Rett syndrome is caused by mutations in X-linked MECP2, encoding methyl-CpG-binding protein 2. *Nature Genetics*, **23**, 185–8.

Anvret, M., Zhang, Z., and Hagberg, B. (1994). Rett syndrome: the bcl-2 gene — a mediator of neurotrophic mechanisms? *Neuropediatrics*, **25**, 323–4.

Armstrong, D. (1995). The neuropathology of Rett syndrome — overview 1994. *Neuropediatrics*, **26**, 100–4.

Belichenko, P. and Hagberg, B. (1997). Morphological study of neocortical areas in Rett syndrome. *Acta Neuropathologica*, **93**, 50–61.

Connor, B. and Dragunow, M. (1998). The role of neuronal growth factors in neurodegenerative disorders of the human brain. *Brain Research Reviews*, **27**, 1–39.

Hefti, F. (1986). Nerve growth factor promotes survival of septal cholinergic neurons after fimbrial transsections. *Journal of Neuroscience*, **6**, 2155–62.

Lappalainen, R., Liewenthal, K., Sainio, K., and Riikonen, R. (1997). Brain perfusion SPECT and EEG findings in Rett syndrome. *Acta Neurologica Scandinavica*, **95**, 44–50.

Lappalainen, R. and Riikonen, R. (1996). High levels of cerebrospinal fluid glutamate in Rett syndrome. *Pediatric Neurology*, **15**, 213–16.

Laudiero, L., Aloe, L., Levi-Montalcini, R., Schilter, D., Gielssen, S., and Otten, U. (1992). Multiple sclerosis patients express increased levels of beta nerve growth factor in the cerebrospinal fluid. *Neuroscience Letters*, **147**, 91–2.

Patterson, S., Grady, M., and Bothwell, M. (1993). Nerve growth factor and fibroblast growth factor-like neurotrophic activity in cerebrospinal fluid of brain injured human patients. *Brain Research*, **605**, 43–9.

Reiss, A., Faruque, F., Naidu, S., Abrams, M., Beaty, T., Bryan, R., *et al.* (1993). Neuroanatomy of Rett syndrome: volumetric imaging study. *Annals of Neurology*, **34**, 227–34.

Riikonen, R., Korhonen, L., and Lindholm, D. (1999). Cerebrospinal fluid nerve growth factor — a marker of asphyxia? *Pediatric Neurology*, **20**, 137–41.

Riikonen, R., Söderström, S., Korhonen, L., and Lindholm, D. (1998). Overstimulation of nerve growth factors in postinfectious and autoimmune diseases. *Pediatric Neurology*, **18**, 231–5.

Riikonen, R., Söderström, S., Vanhala, R., Ebendal, T., and Lindholm, D. (1997). West syndrome: cerebrospinal fluid nerve growth factor and effect of ACTH. *Pediatric Neurology*, **17**, 224–9.

Riikonen, R., Somer, M., and Turpeinen, U. (1999). Low insulin-like growth factor (IGF-1) in the cerebrospinal fluid of children with PEHO syndrome (progressive encephalopathy, hypsarrhythmia and optic atrophy) and cerebellar degeneration. *Epilepsia (NY)*, **40**, 1642–48.

Riikonen, R., Vanhanen, S-L., Tyynelä, J., Santavuori, P. and Turpeinen, U. (2000). CSF insulin-like growth factor-1 in infantile ceroid lipofuscinosis. *Neurology*, **54**, 1828–32.

Riikonen, R. and Vanhala, R. (1999). Levels of cerebrospinal fluid nerve growth factor differ in infantile autism and Rett syndrome. *Developmental Medicine and Child Neurology*, **41**, 148–52.

Sariola, H., Sainio, K., Arumäe, U., and Saarma, M. (1994). Neurotrophins and ciliary factor: their biology and pathology. *Annals of Medicine*, **26**, 355–63.

Suzaki, I., Hara, T., Tanaka, C., Dejima, S., and Takeshita, K. (1997). Elevated nerve growth factor levels in cerebrospinal fluid associated with progressive cortical atrophy. *Neuropediatrics*, **28**, 268–71.

Uvebrandt, P., Bjure, J., Sixt, R., Engerström, I., and Hagberg, B. (1993). Regional cerebral blood flow: SPECT as a tool for localization of brain dysfunction. In *Rett syndrome — clinical and biological aspects* (ed. B. Hagberg), pp. 80–5. MacKeith Press, London.

Vanhala, R., Korhonen, L., Lindholm, D., and Riikonen, R. (1998). Neurotrophic factors in cerebrospinal fluid and serum of patients with Rett syndrome. *Journal of Child Neurology*, **13**, 420–33.

Vanhala, R., Turpeinen, U, and Riikonen, R. Insulin-like growth factor-1 (IGF-1) in the cerebrospinal fluid (CSF) and serum in Rett syndrome. *Ped Neurol*, in press, 2000.

Wenk, G., Naidu, S., Casanova, M., Kitt, C., and Moser, H. (1991). Altered neurochemical markers in Rett's syndrome. *Neurology*, **41**, 1753–6.

6 The central autonomic disturbance in Rett syndrome

Peter O.O. Julu

Summary

This chapter describes the important role of the central autonomic system in the developing brain and introduces Rett syndrome as a congenital dysautonomia. The chapter also examines evidence from the central autonomic system and cardiorespiratory neurons, which suggests that early brainstem dysfunction underlies the respiratory disturbance and may contribute to sudden deaths in the Rett disorder.

6.1 What is Rett syndrome?

Rett syndrome can be defined as a congenital neurodevelopmental disorder. Its clinical character is described in Chapter 1 and the causative mutations in MECP2 gene in Chapter 2. I will repeat certain clinical features of the disorder here in relation to autonomic dysfunction:

(1) Mental disability of variable severity, speech ranging from none to a few words. It is not clear if this is due to lack of growth factors leading to inadequate brainstem projections into the cerebral cortex in early intrauterine development; however brainstem autonomic nuclei do participate in the early projections into the cerebral cortex, making them relevant to any discussion of learning disability.
(2) Mood and movement disorder with features of hand stereotypy and agitation in the Rett disorder suggest poor coordination. This is probably due to meagre integrative inhibitions to be discussed later in this chapter. The brainstem functions that reveal lack of integrative inhibition will be described.
(3) EEG and sleep abnormalities include slow background waves lacking α-wave

activity during the alert periods and abnormal EEG during sleep, making staging difficult.

(4) Epilepsy and non-epileptic vacant spells are features of the disorder (Chapter 1). Immature, small, excitable neurons or lack of inhibitory signals are possible causes of epilepsy in the Rett disorder. Possible effects of epilepsy on brainstem function will be discussed further later. Some vacant spells appear to coincide with autonomic shutdowns at the level of the brainstem.

(5) Breathing dysrhythmia is a constant feature in the Rett disorder, each person showing more than one type of abnormal breathing rhythm, usually five or more. Thirteen types of abnormal breathing rhythm are described in Rett syndrome and their effects on autonomic function will be discussed later.

(6) Dysautonomia in the Rett disorder was suspected from the cold, blue feet and wide pupils suggesting sympathetic over-activity (Chapter 1). This is now confirmed by objective measurement of autonomic functions including baseline cardiac vagal tone, cardiac sensitivity to spontaneous baroreflex and the responses of the mean arterial blood pressure to the various breathing abnormalities. All the objective tests show evidence of a lack of restraint of sympathetic activity due to low levels of cardiovascular parasympathetic activity. We can therefore now regard the Rett disorder as one of the congenital dysautonomias.

These clinical features are all directly or indirectly connected to autonomic function. It is therefore reasonable to advocate that clinical autonomic assessment should be part of the procedure for diagnosis and follow-up in the management of the Rett disorder. Objective clinical autonomic measurements can provide reproducible results that can be used to monitor the progress of the disease.

From current knowledge of basic neuroscience we expect these clinical features of Rett syndrome to influence autonomic function.

6.2 Historical perspectives

The autonomic nervous system was described in detail by two Cambridge Physiologists in Trinity College. Although they were in the same department, they had diverse interests.

Vasomotor nerves: Gaskel was interested in the innervation of the vessels of the viscera. He stimulated a fierce debate among physiologists when he first suggested that the heart had its own pacemaker and can therefore generate its own rhythm of contraction, independent of nervous excitation. Mainstream physiologists at that time strongly believed that all muscles could only contract following nervous excitation and the heart is basically a muscle. Pacemaker property of the sino-atrial node of the heart is now well established. By studying the innervation of blood vessels of the viscera, Gaskel published a book in 1920 entitled *The involuntary nervous system*.

Secretomotor nerves: Professor Langley who was the head of the Department of Physiology at that time was interested in the mechanism of salivary secretion. He studied the nervous stimulation of various secretory glands and published a book in 1921 entitled *The autonomic nervous system*.

Sympathetic and parasympathetic nerves
Gaskel's vasomotor and Langley's secretomotor nerves are parts of the autonomic nervous system that supplies every organ in the body. Langley's book title was adopted by the scientific community to describe both vasomotor and secretomotor nerves. The main significance of this historical description of the autonomic nervous system is that it facilitates our understanding of the target-organs involved and the arrangement of this complex nervous system. From this historical perspective, it will be evident that secretomotor nerves will form the bulk of the parasympathetic branch of the autonomic nervous system. The target-organs of these nerves will be secretory glands in which they will innervate the secretory cells. There are of course exceptions to this general rule, where parasympathetic targets are specialized muscle cells in the iris, the heart and the bladder. In the iris, parasympathetic nerves innervate muscles for constricting the pupils (pupiloconstrictors), thereby performing a sphincter-like instead of a secretomotor function. In the heart, the main parasympathetic targets are specialised muscle cells called pacemakers in the sino-atrial node and conducting tissues, while in the bladder the parasympathetic targets are the detrusor muscles that initiate voiding.

Gaskel's vasomotor nerves are the sympathetic branch of the present autonomic nervous system. The main targets of these nerves are smooth muscles in the vascular wall and other organs serving sphincter-like functions. There are also exceptions to this generalization in the suprarenal glands and the skin. In the adrenal medulla, the sympathetic targets are chromaffin cells that release adrenaline and noradrenaline into the bloodstream, while in the skin, sympathetic targets in the sweat glands are secretory cells producing sweat. It follows that the sympathetic nerves are executing secretomotor instead of sphincter-like functions in the suprarenal glands and the skin and the targets here are not smooth muscle cells but secretory cells. Therefore both sympathetic and parasympathetic nerves can perform sphincter-like and secretomotor functions in different target-organs. However, parasympathetic nerves are largely secretomotor while sympathetic nerves are largely vasomotor, in other words, executing sphincter-like functions.

Reciprocal innervation
A feature of the autonomic nervous system is reciprocal innervation of target-organs by sympathetic and parasympathetic systems (see Chapter 9). The

physiological effect of sympathetic stimulation in a target-organ is usually the reverse of the effect of parasympathetic stimulation. For example, in the iris, sympathetic stimulation activates the pupillodilator muscles and widens the pupils while parasympathetic stimulation activates the pupilloconstrictor muscles and narrows the pupils. In salivary glands, sympathetic stimulation reduces output while parasympathetic stimulation increases output. In the heart, sympathetic stimulation increases the rate (positive chronotropic effect) and force (positive inotrophic effect) of contraction, while parasympathetic stimulation reduces the rate (negative chronotropic effect) of contraction. In the intestines, sympathetic stimulation reduces motility while parasympathetic stimulation increases motility. Thus the two branches of the autonomic system work in balance to achieve the required effect at a particular point in time, changing from time to time according to physiological need. There are exceptions to the reciprocal innervation of target-organs. The skin and the suprarenal glands have no reciprocal innervation, both are supplied only by the sympathetic branch of the autonomic nervous system.

It is evident that the discovery of the autonomic system was the result of interests in the neural controls of body fluid secretions and the regulation of blood vessel tones in the viscera.

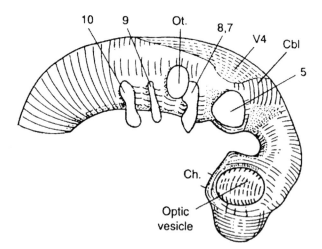

Fig. 6.1 Right lateral view of the brain at approximately 28 post-ovulatory days (embryonic stage 13) showing the primordia of various somatic and autonomic nuclei in the primitive brainstem. The brainstem makes up the bulk of the whole brain at this stage. Ch., chiasmatic plate; 5, 7, 8, 9 and 10, primordia of respective cranial nerves and nuclei; Cbl, primitive cerebellum; V4, fourth ventricle with a translucent roof; Ot., otic plate. Reprinted from *The embryonic human brain: an atlas of developmental stages*, R. O'Rahilly and F. Müller, Copyright © 1994, by permission of Wiley-Liss, Inc., a subsidiary of John Wiley & Sons Inc.

6.3 Intrauterine development of the brainstem and the central autonomic system

The brainstem is very important for the development of the rest of the nervous system, including the cerebral cortex and other higher functions. The neural disc

Supra-spinal	Week/Day	Spinal and peripheral
Myelination in pyramidals	40	
	38	
	36	
	34	
	32	
Sulci and gyri in cortex	30	
Intensive synaptic+cortical growth	28	
Subcortical fibres penetrate cortical plate	26	Normal vasomotor function
	24	Ganglia cells in rectum
Subcortical fibres wait in subplate	22	
Myelination begins in the brain	20	Observable heart rate variation
Dienceph & Hippo electric activity	18	Heart beat can be auscultated
Cortical fibres pass internal capsule	16	
Caudal growth of corpus collosum	14	Adrenergic neuroeffector + Meissner's Plexus
Increased brain synapses	12	Ach neuroeff + synchronous heart beat
Cortical plate reaches occipital area	10	Conduction system in heart + Auerbach's Plexus
Future insula appears	56	Catecholamine neurotransmitters
Glial + Schwann cells in Cr.N	54	
Cortical plate appears rostrally	52	
Interconnections of brain nuclei	50	
Somatic reflexes+brainstem activity	48	Heart responds to adr stimuli
	46	
4 nuclei of Amygd present	44	
Multiple integration tracts appear	42	Grey rami + Vagal Preg fibres
NTS + first Amygd nucleus appear	40	
Brain asymmetry noticed	38	
Neurohypophysis appears	36	
Spinal tracts of 7 and 8 nerves	34	Pregangl. neurons in IML-CC
Hypoth, Amygd & Hippo area seen	32	Vertebrae are well defined
Common afferent tract develops	30	
Cr.N nuclei + cerebellum appear	28	Heart responds to Ach stimuli
First N.fibre of embryo in brainstem	26	
Cr.N related to neural crests	24	
Neural tube formed	22	
Neural plate + major brain divisions	20	Neural plate
Neural grove appears	18	

Ovulation

Fig. 6.2 A chart of landmark features in the development of the autonomic nervous system. Only the approximate days and weeks are indicated. The heart was used to represent peripheral autonomic development because of its importance in clinical monitoring of the autonomic functions in general (see Section 6.3.2). Ach, acetylcholine; adr, adrenergic; Amygd, amygdaloid; CC, cell column; Cr.N, cranial nerves; Dienceph, diencephalon; Hippo, hippocampus; Hypoth, hypothalamus; IML, intermediolateral; neuroeff, neuroeffector; N.fibre, nerve fibre; NTS, nucleus of tractus solitarius; Pregangl and Preg, preganglionic; 7 and 8 nerves, facial and vestibular nerves. Note that the first nerve fibre in human life differentiates in the brainstem at approximately 26 post-ovulatory days.

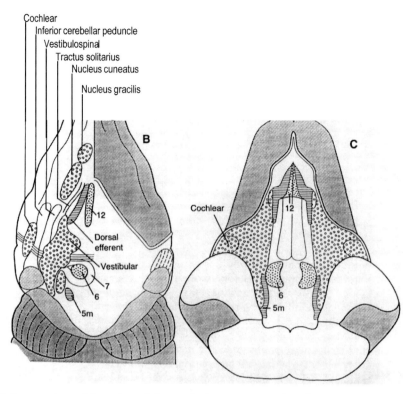

Fig. 6.3 A comparison of the embryonic human brainstem at approximately 56 post-ovulatory days (B) and the brainstem of a fullterm newborn baby (C) to illustrate the structural similarity. 6 and 12, nuclei of the respective cranial nerves; 7, genu of the facial nerve; 5m, motor fibres of the trigeminal nerve. Reprinted from *The embryonic human brain: an atlas of developmental stages*, R. O'Rahilly and F. Müller, Copyright © 1994, by permission of Wiley-Liss, Inc., a subsidiary of John Wiley & Sons Inc.

is derived from the ectodermal layer of the embryo in the third post-ovulatory week and curls up and fuses into the neural tube. By the end of the fourth week, the embryo is about 8 mm long, but most of the brainstem cranial nuclei are recognizable and the brainstem is the largest cell mass in the brain (Fig. 6.1). The development of autonomic structures proceeds as outlined in the chart in Fig. 6.2. The brainstem develops so rapidly between the fifth to the eighth week that during an increase from 8 to 22 mm of the maximum body length, the embryonic brainstem at eight weeks is already structurally comparable to that of a newborn baby (Fig. 6.3). The brainstem in the eighth week, the end of the embryonic period and start of the foetal period, is the largest cell mass in the brain, followed by the thalamus and cerebellum (Fig. 6.4). A thin layer of cells known as the cortical plate represents the cerebral cortex at this stage of development and the rest of the intracranial space is filled with fluid (Fig. 6.4). The most advanced histological part of the forebrain at this stage of development is the amygdaloid nucleus.

6.3.1 Neural projections from the brainstem provide the mainstay of nervous integration

It is most important to recognize that most of the neuronal integration during the foetal stage of development throughout up to birth is achieved by caudo-cranial projections from the brainstem to the developing cortex. Descending tracts project from the brainstem to the spinal cord and to cranial nerves and ganglia. It is therefore imperative that the brainstem and its nuclei should develop early during the embryonic stage of intrauterine life if they are to play leading roles in further development of the brain during the foetal stage of intrauterine life that follows. Groups of neuronal projections from the brainstem that use similar neurotransmitters appear at the same time. Serotonergic cranial projections from the brainstem are the earliest to appear.

6.3.2 The heart offers a means of studying brainstem development

The heart is one of the earliest autonomic target-organs to develop peripherally. It is a single most important site for clinical evaluation of the autonomic function

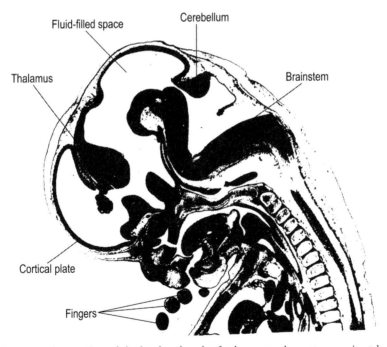

Fig. 6.4 A near median section of the head and neck of a human embryo at approximately 52 post-ovulatory days illustrating the major cell masses of the brain. A thin layer of cells, the cortical plate, represents the future cerebral cortex. Reprinted from *The embryonic human brain: an atlas of developmental stages*, R. O'Rahilly and F. Müller, Copyright © 1994, by permission of Wiley-Liss, Inc., a subsidiary of John Wiley & Sons Inc.

and especially brainstem autonomic function. Both sympathetic and parasympathetic functions of the brainstem can be evaluated non-invasively by monitoring the characteristics of cardiac cycles. There are some rudimentary and asynchronous heartbeats and the myocardium can respond to cholinergic stimuli by the fourth post-ovulatory week, indicating that the heart already has functional cholinergic receptors before it can beat synchronously. The heart will not respond to adrenergic stimuli until the seventh post-ovulatory week, three weeks later than it can respond to cholinergic stimuli. Since the foetal stage of intrauterine life starts at the eighth post-ovulatory week, this means the embryo enters the foetal stage with functional adrenergic and cholinergic receptors in the heart. However there is no evidence of neuroeffector cholinergic or adrenergic transmissions in any tissue in the embryo at this stage of development. Although the receptors of these autonomic neurotransmitters are present and are functional in the heart there is no neural communication through them during the embryonic stage. Somatic reflex responses have been reported at seven post-ovulatory weeks (O'Rahilly et al. 1990); it is therefore likely that somatic neuroeffector transmission starts earlier than its autonomic counterpart.

Cholinergic neuroeffector transmission starts at 11 post-ovulatory weeks, one week after myocardial conductive tissue has developed (Fig. 6.2). The heart starts to beat synchronously a week later following the initiation of cholinergic neuroeffector. It is therefore evident that a synchronous heartbeat cannot be achieved until myocardial conducting tissues and cholinergic neuroeffector transmissions are in place. These two processes may be required for synchronous heartbeats to occur. When the heart beats synchronously, the whole myocardial excitation is under the control of the pacemaker in the sino-atrial node. Although catecholamine neurotransmitters appear between eight and nine post-ovulatory weeks, there is no evidence of adrenergic neuroeffector transmission until 14 post-ovulatory weeks, two weeks later than the initiation of synchronous heartbeats. It is therefore unlikely that adrenergic neuroeffector transmission is a prerequisite for synchronous heartbeats.

The earliest reported observable change in heart rate caused by change in the autonomic tone is at 20 post-ovulatory weeks (Papp 1988; Walker 1974). We have recorded foetal heart rate and cardiac vagal tone simultaneously in utero as early as 16 post-ovulatory weeks using a combination of the NeuroScope method (described later) and magnetocardiography. Vagal deceleration of the heart could be clearly identified in a 35-week foetus using the same methodology (Fig. 6.5). It is theoretically possible to measure foetal cardiac vagal tone by 12 post-ovulatory weeks when cholinergic neuroeffector transmission has begun and the heart is under synchronous excitation by the sino-atrial node. This would require a combination of the NeuroScope method and magnetocardiography. By 25 post-ovulatory weeks, the cardiovascular responses that regulate vasomotor tone are already in place and functional (Gootman and Gootman 1983), indicating that the

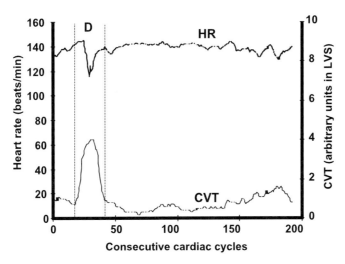

Fig. 6.5 Simultaneous and synchronized recordings of both heart rate (HR) and cardiac vagal tone (CVT) in a 35-week old human foetus inside the womb using the non-invasive NeuroScope method in combination with magnetocardiography. There was clear vagal deceleration of the foetal heart rate in the zone marked D. The resting foetal CVT was kept below 2 arbitrary units in the Linear Vagal Scale (LVS) except during the period of deceleration. There was increased HR variability towards the end of the records due to the upward drift of the CVT. Obtained from Julu et al. (manuscript submitted).

essential cardiovascular functions of the autonomic nervous system are fully operational by 25 post-ovulatory weeks. Cardiovascular responses to cold stress are normal and mature in a newborn baby(Gootman and Gootman 1983). This may be a sign of the maturity of the cardiovascular sympathetic and the baroreceptor systems.

The baroreceptor system may be mature at term, but other autonomic systems continue to mature after birth and through the first five years of life (Kissel et al. 1981). Although all the adrenergic compounds are present at birth, their concentrations in the body are very low and only approach the adult levels at 5 years of age, reaching them at adolescence. The vas deferens is innervated after birth and there are presumed to be interactions of intrinsic and extrinsic factors during autonomic development after birth (Kissel et al. 1981). The iris and the pineal gland are not substantially innervated until after birth, and the possible external factors required for these two organs are light and the light–dark cycles respectively.

Thus the brainstem develops early in embryonic life and plays a major role in the subsequent development of the foetal brain, and the function of the foetal brainstem can be monitored non-invasively inside the womb by studying consecutive cardiac cycles using appropriate methods.

6.4. Functional organization of the mature autonomic nervous system

6.4.1 Medullary sympathetic centres

The basic organization of the autonomic nervous system is discussed in Chapter 9, so here I will outline the relevant central organization beginning with the presympathetic vasomotor neurons (PSVMN) in the rostral part of the ventro-lateral medulla oblongata. It is now well recognized that the neuronal mass that actually drives the autonomic target-organs in the rest of the body is situated in the brainstem and the rostral ventrolateral medulla (VLM) is probably the main site of the sympathetic driver neurons (Guyenet et al. 1996). It is also now apparent that the spatial arrangement of the neuronal mass in the rostral VLM is not random but is ordered according to the target-organs being innervated (Damsey and McAllen 1988; Guyenet et al. 1996; Jordan 1995). If we accept this relatively new concept of central autonomic organization, then we can appreciate that the powerhouse of the autonomic nervous system is in the brainstem. The partial segregation of the sympathetic neuronal drivers in the brainstem allows them to function independent of each other (Guyenet et al. 1996; Jordan 1995) and stimulation of a specific group of the sympathetic drivers at the level of the brainstem will activate only specific target-organs. For example, skeletal muscle vasoconstrictors all over the body can be activated by stimulation of their discrete and partially segregated neuronal drivers in the brainstem (Jordan 1995). This is 'organotopic arrangement'(Guyenet et al. 1996).

How do the PSVMN drive the sympathetic system? There are three hypotheses. In the first, a distributed afferent network with a wide range of excitatory inputs from the ponto-medullary reticular formation and in the second, a local network within the rostral VLM, is available to drive the PSVMN. These two hypotheses require inter-neuronal communication through synapses to maintain sympathetic activity. However experimental exclusion of synaptic transmissions only affects known reflexes like baroreflex and chemoreflex without abolishing baseline sympathetic tone, and this would suggest that inter-neuronal communications through synapses are not crucial for the generation of baseline sympathetic tone within the rostral VLM, reviewed in detail by Guyenet et al. (1996). The third and more probable hypothesis is that pacemaker neurons within the rostral VLM maintain the baseline sympathetic tone. There is electrophysiological and anatomical evidence to support this hypothesis (Guyenet et al. 1996). If pacemaker neurons maintain the baseline sympathetic tone then the activity of these pacemakers ought to be modulated by other means in order to change the tone. The modulation of sympathetic tone, both up and down by different centres in the brain, is achieved through G-protein dependent receptor agonists of various kinds. Peptides like thyrotrophin releasing hormone (TRH), arginine vasopressin (AVP), neuropeptide-Y (NPY), calcitonin gene related peptide (CGRP), or β-adrenergic agonist, opioids like enkephalins, amino acids like γ-aminobutyric acid-β (GABA$_β$) agonist and purinergic agonist like adenosine are all active in the rostral VLM. The polypeptide angiotensin-II does not act through G-protein receptor agonist, but if injected directly into the rostral VLM will increase sympathetic tone probably by activation of the adrenergic system (Guyenet et al. 1996). So the rostral VLM has the facility for the integration of sympathetic activity to suit the needs of the rest of the body and the higher centres in the brain actually use the facility for this purpose.

6.4.2 Supra-medullary centres that affect sympathetic activity

There are areas of the brain higher than the rostral VLM, which modulate autonomic responses when they are stimulated. The areas include the parabrachial nuclei in the pons, periaqueductal grey matter in the midbrain and the hypothalamus being a major site of autonomic modulation. The limbic nuclei and their cortices, notably the medial nucleus of the amygdala, the cingulate gyrus and the insular cortex also evoke autonomic responses when stimulated or they may respond to autonomic stimulation. The responses evoked by stimulation of supra-medullary centres are stereotyped due to differential activation of the driver neurons in the brainstem (Guyenet et al. 1996). Stimulation of specific sites of the supra-medullary nuclei tends to activate or inhibit a fixed set of brainstem driver neurons, hence the stereotyped responses (Guyenet et al. 1996). However, the autonomic representation in the insular cortex and possibly the cingulate gyrus appears to be according to the different parts of the body for example, head, arms, hands, lower limbs or the abdomen have separate groups of neurons; it is therefore 'somatotopic' (Cechetto and Chen 1992). It appears that stereotyped autonomic responses would involve the activation of at least one specific site of a supra-medullary nucleus. For example, the defence response elicited by the stimulation of the anterior hypothalamic defence area in the supraoptic nucleus would invariably cause retraction of nictitating membrane, widening of the pupils, piloerection, withdrawal of the cardiac vagal tone, tachycardia and vasoconstriction in the cat (Jordan 1995). Autonomic responses limited to only one part of the body, for example the lower limb, will probably involve the activation of a specific site in the autonomic cortex where there is evidence of somatotopic representation. Generalized organotopic excitation, for example of all sweat glands in the body, can be achieved at the brainstem level where the driver neurons are partially segregated and packed together in organotopic arrangement.

6.4.3 Brainstem parasympathetic centres

With the exception of the sacral outflow, parasympathetic functions are executed by specialized cranial nerve nuclei. The brainstem parasympathetic system comprises the autonomic nuclei of the third (oculomotor), seventh (facial), ninth (glossopharyngeal) and tenth (vagus) cranial nerves. These are discrete nuclei and are widely separated from each other, quite a different arrangement from the sympathetic driver neurons in the rostral VLM.

The autonomic motor nucleus of the oculomotor nerve is called the Edinger–Westphal nucleus in the periaqueductal grey matter of the midbrain; it drives the pupilloconstrictor muscles of the iris serving a sphincter-like function in the light reflex. The autonomic motor nuclei of the facial nerve consist of the superior salivatory and the lacrimatory nuclei in the pons. The superior salivatory nucleus is secretomotor to the sublingual and submandibular salivary glands, and the lacrimatory nucleus is secretomotor to the lacrimal glands in the production of tears.

The autonomic motor nucleus of the glossopharyngeal nerve is the inferior salivatory nucleus in the medulla oblongata, which is secretomotor to the parotid salivary gland. The motor nuclei of the vagus nerve are in the dorsal vagus nucleus and the nucleus ambiguus (Fig. 6.6). Autonomic motor nuclei of the vagus nerve are secretomotor to most part of the gastrointestinal tract up to the descending colon and they are also secretomotor in the lower airways. Neurons in the dorsal nucleus of the vagus nerve facilitate gut motility. Both the vagus nerve and the sympathetic nervous system affect the functions of the gut through two local nervous networks. The Meissner's plexus is a submucosal network of nerves and ganglia spread throughout the gut, and Auerbach's plexus is a myenteric network (situated between the two muscle layers of the gut) also spread throughout the gut. The vagus nerve and sympathetic nerve fibres synapse extensively with the ganglia in the two local nervous networks (Chapter 9). The cardiovagal motor neurons, the only parasympathetic input to the heart, are situated in the caudal part of the nucleus ambiguus (Fig. 6.6).

How does the brainstem parasympathetic system work?
It is generally true that baseline parasympathetic activity is maintained by reflex action in which the afferent arm of the reflex arc may or may not be in the same cranial nerve as the efferent arm of the same reflex. There is no evidence to date, to suggest that pacemaker activity maintains any of the parasympathetic tone anywhere in the central nervous system. In the light reflex of the eye, the afferent arm of the reflex arc is in the optic nerve, which is the second cranial nerve, and the efferent arm of the reflex arc is in the oculomotor nerve. The size of the pupil is maintained in inverse proportion to the ambient light intensity by the activity of this reflex. The pupilloconstrictor reflex can also be evoked as the eye accommodates near objects, where a different mechanism from that of the light reflex is used, this time involving the cerebral cortex, or it can be modulated by stimulation of specific sites in the supra-medullary autonomic nuclei as was discussed above.

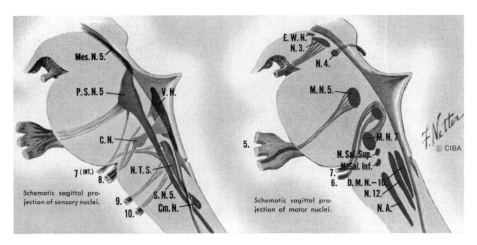

Fig. 6.6 Schematic sagittal projections of the mature human brainstem to illustrate the autonomic sensory and motor nuclei. Sensory nuclei: C.N., cochlear nucleus; Cm.N., commissural nucleus; Mes.N.5, mesencephalic nucleus of trigeminal nerve; N.T.S., nucleus of tractus solitarius; P.S.N.5, principal sensory nucleus of trigeminal nerve; S.N.5., spinal nucleus of trigeminal nerve; V.N., vestibular nucleus. Motor nuclei: D.M.N.10, dorsal motor nucleus of vagus; E.W.N., Edinger–Westphal nucleus; M.N.5., motor nucleus of trigeminal nerve; M.N.7., motor nucleus of facial nerve; N.A., nucleus ambiguus; N.11., nucleus of spinal accessory; N.12., nucleus of hypoglossal; N.Sal.Inf., inferior salivatory nucleus; N.Sal.Sup., superior salivatory nucleus; Copyright © 1953. Novartis. Reprinted with permission from the *Netter collection of medical illustrations*, illustrated by Frank H. Netter. All rights reserved.

Tears and saliva production is largely by reflex activation of the secretory glands, through sensory input via the trigeminal nerve into the brainstem. The efferent arms of these reflexes leave the brainstem through the facial and glossopharyngeal nerves. Blinking is important in the activation of tear production and chewing in the activation of saliva production. Both tears and saliva production respond to local chemical stimuli, especially acids. These reflexes are modulated by higher centres during the expression of emotions or in a conditioned reflex. It is well known that stress can dry up saliva in the mouth and fill the eyes with tears.

Gastric and intestinal secretions are largely activated through various local reflexes started by the arrival of food in the gut. Some of these reflexes involve afferent fibres in the vagus nerve from the gut to the brainstem, while other reflexes include the production of gut-hormones like gastrin, and cholecystokinin. Local stimuli include mechanical and chemical agents in the food. Vagal stimulation facilitates both gastric and intestinal secretions. The secretory reflexes of the vagus nerve are modulated by higher centres in the brain and can be conditioned to other unrelated sensory inputs like the sound of a bell. Rage is known to increase gastric secretion by increasing the secretive activity of the vagus nerve, known as the cephalic phase (Hightower 1966).

The local nervous network controls the baseline peristalsis in the gut. This is then modulated by both sympathetic and vagal activity. Vagal stimulation increases peristalsis and relaxes the tones of sphincters in the gut, while sympathetic stimulation reduces the motility of the gut and increases the tones of sphincters in the gut. The two nervous systems work in a balance as described above in the Reciprocal Innervation. Local stimuli that increase the activity of the vagus nerve include mechanical and chemical agents in the food. It is therefore true that peristalsis will be reduced and the tones of the sphincters will be high when the gut is empty, since vagal stimulation will be low while sympathetic tone is maintained by the pacemaker activity in the brainstem.

When there is an imbalance between sympathetic and parasympathetic tone in any organ, it is important to understand that sympathetic tone is maintained by pacemaker activity in the brainstem, while reflexes are responsible for the parasympathetic tone, some of these reflexes involving somatic nerves outside the autonomic network.

6.4.4 Medullary cardiorespiratory neurons

These are groups of neurons in the medulla oblongata that integrate the minute-volume of the respiratory system with the cardiac output. Richter and Spyer (1990) introduced the concept of cardiorespiratory neurons. Integration of the minute volume of the respiratory system and the cardiac output is done moment by moment through reflexes. The presympathetic neurons involved in cardiorespiratory integration are in the rostral VLM and their baseline discharges are maintained by pacemaker activity as described before. The respiratory neurons have a built-in inhibitory network to generate their baseline activity to be discussed later. However the parasympathetic neurons involved in cardiorespiratory integration appear to have no dedicated system for maintaining baseline tone but rely on reflex activity like other parasympathetic systems in the body. The parasympathetic reflexes for cardiorespiratory integration may have their afferent and efferent arms in different cranial nerves like others previously discussed.

The natural stimuli generating sensory inputs to the cardiorespiratory neurons are blood pO_2 and pCO_2, lung volume, blood pressure, blood volume and possibly force of contraction of the heart. The receptors are peripheral chemoreceptors in the carotid and aortic bodies, slowly adapting pulmonary stretch receptors (SAR), and baroreceptors in the carotid and aortic sinuses and coronary arteries and volume receptors in the walls of the heart and large blood vessels. A group of poorly defined neurons on the ventral surface of the medulla oblongata respond specifically to pCO_2 and are known collectively as the central chemoreceptor. It is possible that the mechanoreceptors in the wall of the heart can detect the force of ventricular contraction and this may set off certain reflexes in extreme situations. The sensory inputs from these receptors to the medulla oblongata come through two cranial nerves, glossopharyngeal and vagus.

The central relay station of the sensory input to the cardiorespiratory neurons is the nucleus of the tractus solitarius (NTS) (Spyer 1994). The NTS is derived from the common sensory pathway to the trigeminal, facial, glossopharyngeal and vagus nerve nuclei in early intrauterine development. This explains why the central relay station of the sensory inputs arriving through the glossopharyngeal and vagus nerves are located here, and also why sensory inputs from the trigeminal nerve can evoke cardiorespiratory responses. For example the diving reflex is initiated by pressure and temperature changes on the face and the oculocardiac reflex is initiated by exerting pressure on the eyeball; both reflexes increase cardiac vagal tone and alter the rate of breathing.

6.4.5 Viscerotopic organization of sensory input in the NTS

The cardiorespiratory sensory inputs are organized in the NTS according to their visceral origin. For example, sensory inputs from the respiratory tract receptors are grouped together in one central area of the NTS, surrounded by sensory inputs from the cardiovascular receptors. Sensory inputs from the gastrointestinal tract receptors are grouped together in a neuronal pool medial to the cardiovascular input, while the inputs from pulmonary receptors are grouped together in a different neuronal pool lateral to the cardiovascular inputs within the NTS (Loewy 1990). The viscerotopic arrangement of sensory neurons in the NTS makes it possible to have viscera-specific lesions or dysfunction at the level of the sensory integration within the NTS. There are inputs from different areas of the brain into the NTS. Inputs from the brainstem respiratory system and the neurons receiving these inputs are also grouped together in a discrete area of the NTS. There are projections from the supra-medullary autonomic areas such as the parabrachial nucleus in the pons, periaqueductal grey matter of the midbrain, the hypothalamic areas and the amygdala into the NTS. The different groups of sensory neurons in the NTS probably use different neurotransmitters and they are also connected with each other by interneurones using different neurotransmitters. The excitatory amino acid L-glutamate appears to be used by the baroreceptor sensory system and serotonergic, opioid and peptidergic neurons have all been demonstrated in the NTS, some as interneurones. Interconnections between secondary sensory neuronal groups within the NTS are both facilitatory and inhibitory. The NTS is therefore able to integrate cardiorespiratory sensory inputs for the varying needs of the rest of the body.

6.4.6 Cardiorespiratory motor neurons

The general arrangement of sensory and motor neurons in the lower brainstem can be loosely compared with that in the spinal cord, where sensory neurons are situated dorsally while motor neurons are found in the ventrolateral aspect of the grey matter. We should however appreciate that neuronal masses in the brainstem are arranged in elongated nuclei running caudo-cranially and do not form one confluent mass as in the spinal cord. The cardiorespiratory motor neurons are arranged from caudal to rostral ventrolateral medulla oblongata and consist of the nucleus ambiguus and the periambigual area (Fig 6.7). They comprise the cardiac parasympathetic motor neurons in the caudal VLM, presympathetic neurons of the rostral VLM and respiratory neurons including the caudal ventral respiratory group (cVRG), rostral ventral respiratory group (rVRG), pre-Bötzinger complex, Bötzinger complex and Kölliker-fuse nuclei in the parabrachial area of the pons (Fig. 6.7). There are some respiratory neurons situated dorsally in association with the NTS referred to as the dorsal respiratory group (DRG).

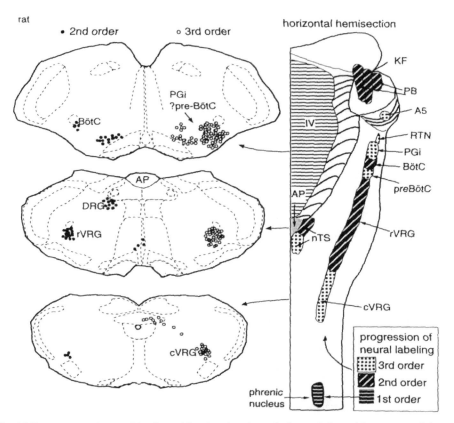

Fig. 6.7 Transverse sections and horizontal hemisection through the medulla and lower pons of the rat summarizing the successive distribution of virus-containing neurons after application of pseudorabies virus to one phrenic nerve. A5, group of nor-adrenergic neurons; AP, area postrema; BötC, Bötzinger complex; cVRG, caudal ventrolateral respiratory group; DRG, dorsal respiratory group; IV, fourth ventricle; KF, Kölliker-fuse nucleus; nTS, nucleus of tractus solitarius; PB, parabrachial nucleus; preBötC, pre-Bötzinger complex; rVRG, rostral ventrolateral respiratory group. Reprinted with kind permission from *The lower brainstem and bodily homeostasis*, W.W. Blessing, Oxford University Press, Copyright © 1997.

Cardiac parasympathetic neurons or cardiovagal motor neurons generate the cardiac vagal tone (CVT) and are found in the nucleus ambiguus in the caudal part of the ventrolateral medulla oblongata (Fig. 6.7). Cardiovagal motor neurons are parasympathetic preganglionic cholinergic neurons. The major source of excitatory input into the cardiovagal motor neurons generating CVT comes from the baroreflex through the nucleus of tractus solitarius and no other excitatory inputs have so far been clearly identified (Guyenet *et al.* 1996; Jordan 1995; Spyer 1993). However, the nucleus ambiguus receives inputs from many parts of the brain especially from the commissural part of the NTS. Also from the medullary reticular formation, the supra-medullary autonomic nuclei, most of the hypothalamic nuclei, the rostral VLM, Kölliker-fuse nucleus in the parabrachial area of the pons involved with respiratory activity and both the mesencephalic reticular formation and its central grey matter. There is some indication that cardiovagal motor neurons have serotonergic inputs of yet unknown origins. All other inputs into the nucleus ambiguus except those from baroreceptors appear to only modulate the CVT and none has been shown to participate in the generation of baseline tone. The cardiovagal motor neurons do not have pacemaker activity and their excitation depends on the baroreceptor input (McAllen and Spyer 1978). Baseline CVT is thus dependent on reflex activity, in this case originating from the baroreceptors and CVT like other parasympathetic activity in the body is maintained through reflexes. Baroreceptors are mainly found in the walls of the carotid and aortic sinuses and are stimulated maximally during the ejection period of each cardiac cycle (Rushmer 1972). The excitation of cardiovagal motor neurons therefore varies during the cardiac cycle and reaches peaks in synchrony with the arterial pulses (Katona *et al.* 1970). There is a group of neurons in the caudal VLM which use γ-aminobutyric acid (GABA) as their neurotransmitters and they project into the rostral VLM to inhibit the presympathetic neurons there. These GABAergic neurons receive excitation from the baroreceptors through the NTS and constitute the baroreceptor negative feedback control of sympathetic excitation at the level of the brainstem. Baroreceptor inputs also stimulate neurons in the lateral tegmental field, which inhibit sympathetic discharges in the spinal cord through the raphe nuclei, independent of the rostral VLM. This inhibition contributes to cardiorespiratory integration.

How is CVT regulated?
Spyer (1989) suggested a model for the regulation of the cardioinhibition originating from the cardiovagal motor neurons. The only excitatory input into the cardiovagal motor neurons in the Spyer model comes from baroreceptor afferents through the NTS. However, the cardiovagal motor neurons are inhibited both directly and indirectly by the inspiratory neurons via interneurones, while the hypothalamic defence area acts at several levels, either directly or through the NTS using GABAergic neurons or by activating the inspiratory neurons to reduce

cardioinhibition. Lung receptors excited by inflation are known to inhibit cardioinhibition and would therefore reduce CVT but their site of action in the brainstem is still uncertain, probably they act at the level of the interneurones between NTS and the cardiovagal motor neurons. A modification of the Spyer model was suggested by Jordan (1995) in which he included the anterior hypothalamus as another source of excitatory input to the cardiovagal motor neurons in addition to the baroreceptor afferents. The Jordan model suggested that chemoreceptor inputs may also contribute to baseline CVT, while other sources like the postinspiratory neurons, superior laryngeal nerve afferents and other yet unidentified sources of inputs augment CVT in various situations (Jordan 1995). There may be other excitatory afferent links to the cardiovagal motor neurons, including the trigeminal inputs in the oculo-cardiac reflex; however, there is very strong evidence that the baroreceptor afferents are the only major excitatory source of baseline CVT (Guyenet et al.1996). The CVT is the only common parasympathetic output of the cardiorespiratory neurons and forms the negative feedback arm for cardiorespiratory integration (Fig. 6.8).

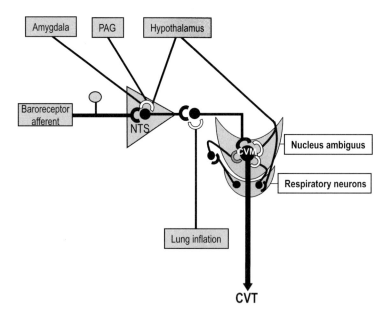

Fig. 6.8 A model of the regulatory processes involved in maintaining the baseline levels of cardiac vagal tone. Filled black crescents represent excitatory synapses, empty white crescents represent inhibitory synapses and the stippled white crescent represents cholinergic inhibitory synapses. The only proven excitatory input is from the baroreceptors. CVM, cardiovagal motor neurons; CVT, cardiac vagal tone; PAG, periaqueductal grey matter; NTS, nucleus of tractus solitarius.

6.4.7 Common autonomic pathways in cardiorespiratory integration

The fundamental aim of cardiorespiratory integration is to distribute optimally oxygenated blood to different tissues according to demand and to meet individual fluctuation of metabolic requirements in each organ. Tissues' demand for oxygen can change rapidly and the integrative responses must be equally rapid. To achieve optimal oxygenation of blood, it requires synchronization of air intake with the cardiac output into the lungs. This is achieved on a breath-by-breath basis, cardiac output increasing during inspiration when the lungs are inflated with air, and decreasing during expiration when air intake is minimal. This integrative process results in respiratory sinus arrhythmia (RSA) since the different cardiac outputs are achieved through changes in the heart rate (HR).

The body monitors blood oxygenation by continuously measuring the arterial pCO_2, pO_2 and pH through the arterial chemoreceptors and institutes the appropriate cardiorespiratory responses according to pre-set values. For example, ventilation will increase to expel excess CO_2 from the blood if pCO_2 exceeds a preset value, usually 45 mmHg. Distribution of oxygenated blood to tissues according to needs is achieved by first maintaining a pre-set level of mean arterial blood pressure (BP). Then by varying the vasomotor tone in individual organs according to the local metabolic or physiological requirements, the tissues requiring more oxygen will have low vasomotor tone and more blood flow, while those requiring less oxygen will have elevated vasomotor tone and less blood flow. The body measures the mean arterial BP continuously using the arterial baroreceptors and then institutes appropriate cardiorespiratory responses according to a pre-set level. A given value of mean arterial BP is maintained by a specific amount of cardiac output determined by the sum total of vasomotor tone in all tissues in the body, the total peripheral resistance (TPR). The fastest means of changing cardiac output is by altering the HR through changes in CVT, while the only means of changing TPR is through adjustment of vasomotor tone in various tissues. Cardiorespiratory adjustments usually require fast changes in cardiac output. It is therefore evident that all integrative processes to adjust the vasomotor tone must take place in the rostral VLM where that facility exists and the output will be through a common vasomotor pathway (Fig. 6.9). In the same way, all integrative processes for rapid change in the cardiac output must take place in the NTS and nucleus ambiguus and the output will be through a common parasympathetic pathway in the form of CVT (Fig. 6.8). Using the previous example of increased ventilation to expel CO_2, it will be coupled with increased cardiac output into the lungs and increased oxygen intake into the blood. The increased cardiac output will require adjustment of TPR in order to maintain the pre-set mean arterial BP. That will require changes in the vasomotor tone of various tissues. This one example illustrates how what is initially a respiratory response leads to changes in autonomic responses and readjustments in remote tissues in the body.

The concept of integrative inhibition

Here integration means the addition of signals from different sources, usually in the correct temporal sequences for a common output pathway (Fig. 6.9). The incoming signals inhibit or facilitate the common output pathway depending on

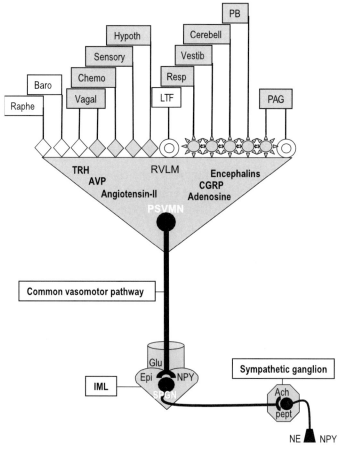

Fig. 6.9 A cocktailglass representation of the integrative function of the rostral ventrolateral medulla. Amino acid neurotransmitters are used for both excitation and inhibition during signal integration. Filled diamonds represent synapses using excitatory amino acids and empty diamonds represent synapses using the amino acid γ-aminobutyric acid (GABA) for inhibitions. There are other inhibitory and excitatory synapses that do not use amino acids, but their neurotransmitters are not known. White wheels represent inhibitory synapses and filled circles with spikes represent excitatory synapses. Known neurotransmitters that can influence the activity of the common vasomotor pathway if applied directly to rostral ventrolateral medulla are indicated. Ach, acetylcholine; AVP, arginine vasopressin; Baro, baroreceptor inputs; Cerebell, cerebellar inputs; CGRP, calcitonin gene related peptide; Chemo, chemoreceptor input; Epi, epinephrine; Glu, glutamate neurotransmitter; Hypoth, hypothalamic inputs; IML, intermediolateral cell column of spinal cord; LTF, lateral tegmental field inputs; NE, norepinephrine; NPY, neuropeptide Y neurotransmitter; PAG, periaqueductal grey matter inputs; PB, parabrachial nuclei inputs; pept, peptide neurotransmitters; PSVMN, presympathetic vasomotor neurons; Raphe, raphe nuclei inputs; Resp, respiratory neurons inputs; RVLM, rostral ventrolateral medulla; Sensory, somatic sensory inputs; SPGN, sympathetic preganglionic neurons in spinal cord; TRH, thyrotrophin-releasing hormone; Vagal, inputs from sensory nerves in the vagus nerve; Vestib, vestibular inputs.

the neurotransmitters used. There is clinical evidence to suggest that the inhibitory component of integration is lacking in the Rett disorder. It is evident that GABA is a prominent inhibitory neurotransmitter used by a number of integrative inputs in the rostral VLM (Fig. 6.9). This suggests that the neurotransmitter GABA could be important for integrative inhibition in the rostral VLM. Other sources of integrative inhibition in the rostral VLM may be serotonergic nerves from lateral tegmental field and periaqueductal grey matter and the peptidergic modulations discussed before. It is also apparent from Figure 6.8 that integrative inhibition for the common output transmitted as the CVT is achieved in the NTS and the nucleus ambiguus by cholinergic activity of the inspiratory neurons, GABAergic activity mainly from the hypothalamus and serotonergic activity from variable sources. It is worth noting that the excitatory input generating CVT also contributes to integrative inhibition in the rostral VLM through a GABAergic mechanism (Fig. 6.9). The CVT can be regarded as a form of integrative inhibition directed in this case towards the heart, the key peripheral target-organ in cardiorespiratory integration.

6.4.8 Generation of respiratory rhythm

This is reviewed at length by Richter (1996) and by Blessing (1997). There is evidence to suggest that respiratory rhythm is generated by pacemaker cells in the pre-Bötzinger complex (see Fig. 6.7) in neonatal rats and mice (Blessing 1997). There is however no such evidence in mature mammals (Richter 1996; St.-John et al. 1999). I will adopt the alternative model of the generation of respiratory rhythm suggested by Richter (1996). This model suggests a network of reciprocal inhibitions involving at least six groups of neurons which work together to generate a three-phased respiratory cycle, one inspiratory phase and two expiratory phases. The inspiratory phase facilitates a steady ramp increase in lung volume and ends abruptly followed immediately by a postinspiratory decrease in lung volume caused by relaxation of the inspiratory muscles and passive recoil of the lungs in phase-one expiration (postinspiration) (Fig. 6.10). In phase-two expiration (E2) there is further decrease in the lung volume but less steep than in phase-one expiration (Fig. 6.10). There is contraction of expiratory muscles during phase-two expiration as indicated by the activity of the internal intercostal nerve (Richter 1996). This pattern of breathing is achieved through accurate and precise firing sequence of the six groups of respiratory neurons in every breathing cycle. The breathing pattern is particularly sensitive to the behaviour of post-inspiratory neurons.

Respiratory neurons in the Richter model are classified according to their sequence of firing in a breathing cycle based on phrenic nerve activity. Neuronal groups are classified as early inspiratory, inspiratory or throughout inspiratory;

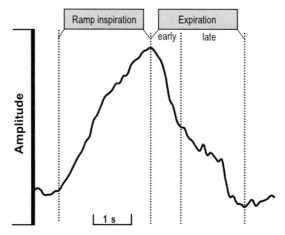

Fig. 6.10 Chest movements during a single normal breath, recorded using the MedullaLab™ (see Section 6.5.2) illustrating three phases of breathing representing the three-phased respiratory cycle. The two expiratory phases cannot be separated as clearly as shown here in forceful breathings such as tachypnoea and hyperventilation. 'Early' represents phase-one expiration and 'late' represents phase-two expiration. Obtained from Julu *et. al.* (manuscript submitted).

late inspiratory; postinspiratory; expiratory, and pre-inspiratory. The exact anatomical locations of these neurons in the brainstem are undetermined and this is a major criticism of the Richter model. Most of the neurons are thought to be in the ventral respiratory group (Fig. 6.7), and some neurons with postinspiratory activity are thought to be in the cVRG (Richter 1996). Rhythmogenesis in this model would require an extrinsic drive, possibly from the reticular activating system of the brainstem. Two primary oscillators, the early inspiratory and postinspiratory neurons, engage in reciprocal inhibitions largely using glycine and GABA as the neurotransmitters. Reciprocal inhibitions together with the neuronal membrane property of accommodation allow the primary oscillators to go into alternate bursts of neuronal activity which determine the main breathing rhythm like a see-saw. The other four groups of neurons modulate this basic rhythm using various mechanisms and a number of neurotransmitters are involved in the modulation process (Richter 1996).

The abrupt end of the inspiratory ramp is achieved at least in part in humans by the action of serotonergic neurons situated in the lower ventrolateral pons. Injury to the lower ventrolateral pons in a child caused apneustic breathing (failure to end the inspiratory ramp) which was treated successfully with serotonin-1_A receptor agonist (Wilken *et al.* 1997). These serotonergic neurons are not represented in the Richter model. GABAergic neurons in the Bötzinger complex are also thought to play a role in the transition between inspiration and expiration (Ezure 1990) and this is not represented in the Richter model. It is also difficult to explain hyperventilation and tachypnoea involving rapid and forceful breathing using this model, although rapid shallow breathing, hypoxic apnoea, and respiratory arrest following activation of laryngeal afferents can all be explained using the Richter model (Richter 1996).

6.4.9 Functional interactions between respiratory and autonomic neurons

The receptors supplying afferent inputs into the brainstem for the interactions of the respiratory and autonomic neurons include baroreceptors, arterial chemoreceptors, pulmonary SAR, pulmonary and airways irritant receptors (or rapidly adapting receptors), pulmonary J-afferents (or unmyelinated pulmonary C-fibre nerve ends), afferent nerves in the trigeminal and recurrent laryngeal nerves. The interaction of these neurons protects the airways during sneezing and coughing, and provides reflex cardiorespiratory regulation during asphyxia and breath holding in deep water diving. The overall responses to these afferent inputs are influenced by the respiratory phase at the arrival of the afferent nerve signals. The outcome of the interactions between the afferent nerve inputs and the autonomic neurons in the brainstem is detected as changing levels of the CVT, decreases or increases in the vasomotor tone and various changes in pulmonary ventilation.

The neuronal mechanisms of the interactions are not yet fully known, but the following responses have been reported; see Daly de Burgh (1995) for a review. The primary effect of arterial chemoreceptor stimulation, or activation of the afferents in the recurrent laryngeal and trigeminal nerves, is to facilitate baroreceptor input at the level of the NTS, thereby increasing the CVT and causing bradycardia (Fig. 6.11). However stimulation of the arterial chemoreceptors also increases the central inspiratory drive, which in turn inhibits CVT at the level of the nucleus ambiguus (Fig. 6.11). The overall effect of stimulating the arterial chemoreceptors on the CVT will depend on the respiratory phase when the input signals arrive in the brainstem. Chemoreceptor stimulation at full inspiration may have no effect on CVT or may reduce it causing tachycardia due to the combined inhibitory effects of the central inspiratory drive and lung inflation acting through the pulmonary SAR (Fig. 6.11). The overall effect of chemoreceptor stimulation at full inspiration is to increase the vasomotor tone due to increased central inspiratory drive and a direct excitation of the rostral VLM (see Fig. 6.9). This vasoconstrictor response is weakened by the inhibitory effect of lung inflation acting on vasomotor tone through the pulmonary SAR (Fig. 6.11). Chemoreceptor stimulation in full inspiration will augment the inspiratory phase of breathing (Daly de Burgh 1995). The maximum effect of chemoreceptor excitation of the CVT is achieved during end-expiratory apnoea with the risk of cardiac arrest. This is also the optimum condition for vasoconstrictor response to chemoreceptor stimulation because the inhibitory effect of lung inflation at that time is markedly reduced.

Activation of the afferents in the recurrent laryngeal and trigeminal nerves will abolish the central inspiratory drive in addition to facilitation of the baroreceptor input (Fig. 6.11), which can greatly increase CVT. Laryngeal afferents activate the postinspiratory neurons (Lawson *et al.* 1991; Remmers *et al.* 1986), upsetting the primary respiratory oscillator involved in the see-saw reciprocal inhibition and so causing reflex apnoea (Richter 1996). The vasomotor response to laryngeal afferents varies according to the balance between the central respiratory drive and lung inflation at the time of stimulus input. Excitation of the laryngeal afferents and the arterial chemoreceptors at the same time during apnoea will optimally increase CVT with the risk of cardiac arrest, for example during tracheal intubation in apnoea. Cardiac arrest caused by excessive CVT can be reversed by lung inflation, which acts through the pulmonary SAR stretch receptors to inhibit the excessive CVT (Angell-James and Daly 1978). Lung inflation can be achieved using mouth-to-mouth resuscitation. Combined activation of the arterial chemoreceptors and laryngeal afferents also produces optimal vasoconstrictor response.

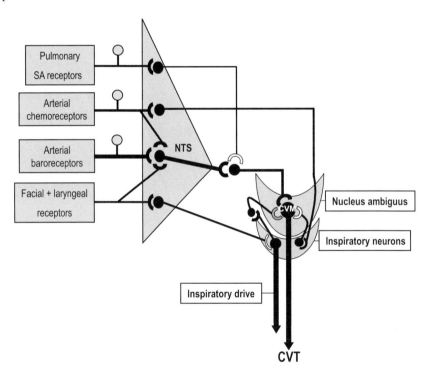

Fig. 6.11 A schematic model of the interactions between autonomic and respiratory afferent inputs at the level of the brainstem, showing the effects on the common autonomic pathway represented by cardiac vagal tone (CVT). Filled black crescents represent facilitatory synapses; empty white crescents represent inhibitory synapses; the stippled white crescent represents inhibitory cholinergic synapses. CVM, cardiovagal motor neurons; NTS, nucleus of tractus solitarius; SA, slowly adapting pulmonary stretch receptors.

Stimulation of the trigeminal afferents in the facial skin in the diving reflex is not sufficient to cause apnoea and it requires a central effort to stop breathing (Daly de Burgh 1995). Activation of the trigeminal afferents and arterial chemo-receptors simultaneously as in breath-hold deep water diving maximally increases CVT leading to extreme bradycardia. It also stimulates vasoconstriction maximally in all tissues except the coronary and cerebral circulation, turning the mammal into a heart-brain preparation with a slowly beating heart for maximum energy conservation. The diving reflex can be used in the treatment of supraventricular tachycardia resistant to other reflexes like the carotid massage (Wildenthal and Atkins 1979).

6.5 Clinical evaluation of brainstem function in the Rett disorder

6.5.1 Patient and carer preparation for autonomic examination session

Monitoring of the brainstem respiratory and autonomic functions in Rett syndrome requires at least one hour. A standard letter is sent to parents or carers to explain the procedures, indicating the non-invasive nature of the investigation. The subject may sit on her own, in a wheelchair or in a 'Tumble Form' chair with a seatbelt. Carers have free access during monitoring, and favourite music may be played during the autonomic monitoring to calm down the Rett person. The subject can eat and drink as she wishes. There is continuous video and sound recording and event markers are inserted in the computer records to facilitate matching of the record segments with the events.

6.5.2 Clinical measurement of breathing dysrhythmia

Breathing movements are monitored using a stretch sensitive plethysmograph placed around the chest at the level of the Xiphisternum. This is a strategic site for recording both thoracic and abdominal respiratory movements. Respiratory movements are recorded through an interface called the MedullaLab (MediFit Instruments Ltd, London, UK) into the microcomputer, time-locked with all other physiological markers. A typical record of a normal breathing movement captured by this method is shown in Figure 6.10. The shapes and rates of the breathing movements are important for characterizing the breathing rhythms. It is therefore important that accurate records of the chest movements contributing to breathing and not other aberrant movements of the body are kept. The video record and event markers of the computer data are used to achieve this aim. The plethysmograph is sensitive to gross body movements or external blows, for example from the arms or hands, and these are marked in the computer and are excluded from the final analysis of breathing rhythms.

6.5.3 Normal breathing movement

We need to define normal breathing movement in order to identify the abnormal ones. A ramp inspiratory expansion of the chest terminated abruptly and immediately followed by a double phased expiratory reduction in the chest volume (Fig. 6.10) is a normal breathing movement. This shape indicates that the rhythm generating respiratory neurons can sustain a ramp increase in the lung volume that is ended abruptly and is immediately followed by a two-phased reduction of the lung volume. This shape reflects the normal function of the brainstem respiratory neurons. The shape alone is not enough to define a breathing rhythm, therefore the rate and the relative depth of breathing are included. The normal breathing rate in Rett persons is below 35 breaths/min. Our system measures breathing movement and not the volume of air drawn by the lungs and the computer assigns arbitrary units to the amplitude of each breathing movement. We therefore measure the average depth of breathing for each Rett person in arbitrary computer units during normal breathing movements and this varies with each individual.

It is important to establish whether a given breathing effort is sufficient to ventilate the patient, so we measure the transcutaneous partial pressures of the respiratory gases, oxygen (pO_2) and carbon dioxide (pCO_2). Partial pressures of oxygen and carbon dioxide are monitored using a TCM3 membrane sensitive to both oxygen and carbon dioxide, placed on the skin in a warm fluid (Radiometer, Copenhagen, Denmark). The partial pressures of oxygen and carbon dioxide are recorded through the MedullaLab interface into the microcomputer time-locked with all other physiological markers. This arrangement ensures that not only the breathing rhythm, but its efficiency in the ventilation of the patient is being monitored throughout the clinical session.

6.6 Respiratory observations in the Rett disorder

Breathing has been noticed to be irregular in Rett syndrome since it was first described. Hyperventilation and prolonged breath holding are impressive respiratory anomalies and therefore are most often mentioned by families. In response to the British Isles questionnaire, families indicated hyperventilation (or deep breathing) in over 75% and breath holding in over 70% of the Rett persons (see Chapter 1). However, without accurate measurement, central apnoea and Valsalva's manoeuvre are readily mistaken for breath holds, and tachypnoea and rapid shallow breathing may be mistaken for hyperventilation. Subtler dysrhythmias may be missed altogether. In our experience of monitoring over 50 cases, although the range of abnormality was wide, we found breathing dysrhythmias in all cases of Rett syndrome, even in those whose families thought there was no breathing abnormality. The percentage of awake-time spent in each rhythm of breathing was calculated for each subject for the entire session (Julu *et al.* submitted).

6.6.1 Apneustic breathing rhythms which may cause inadequate ventilation

Breath hold A single full inspiration achieved fast with a very steep ramp, followed by a delayed expiration also achieved fast without the usual double-phase, the intervening period is variable and lacks respiratory movement (Fig. 6.12). The breath hold must not raise intrathoracic pressure enough to cause measurable blood pressure and heart rate changes characteristic of reduced venous return to the heart.

Regular breath holds Breath holds as described above but coming in successions, one on another for a variable duration (Fig. 6.12).

Protracted inspiration Is a prolonged and continuous inspiratory ramp ending abruptly in full expiration that is achieved fast, often forcefully without the usual double-phase (Fig. 6.12). This must not raise intrathoracic pressure enough to cause measurable blood pressure and heart rate changes characteristic of reduced venous return to the heart.

Apneustic breathing occupied over 35% of the monitoring period in those under 5 years old and fell to under 15% in those of 15 years of age. It is probably the earliest breathing dysrhythmia to appear in the Rett disorder. We observed protracted inspiration in a 2-year old girl in whom it was the only type of breathing dysrhythmia seen. This girl later developed the full classical characteristics of Rett syndrome with multiple breathing dysrhythmias.

6.6.2 Feeble breathing rhythms which may cause inadequate ventilation

Rapid shallow breathing Shallow inspirations are followed immediately by equally shallow expirations (Fig. 6.13). The rate of breathing is above 35 breaths/min and depth in arbitrary computer units is below 50% of the average normal amplitude for the individual.

Shallow breathing Shallow inspirations are followed immediately by equally shallow expirations. The rate is below 35 breaths/min and depth in arbitrary computer units is below 50% of the average normal breathing amplitude for the individual (Fig. 6.13).

Central apnoea Is the cessation of breathing movement at the end of expiration (Fig. 6.13).

Inadequate ventilation in our series occupied almost 20% of the monitoring time in the 10–15 year age group, but less in the older and younger age groups.

158 | Rett disorder and the developing brain

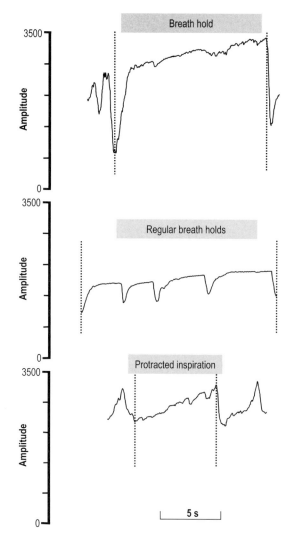

Fig. 6.12 Chest movements during apneustic breathings recorded using the MedullaLab™. See Section 6.6.1 for details. The amplitudes are measured in arbitrary computer display units. Obtained from Julu *et. al.* (manuscript submitted).

6.6.3 Forceful breathing rhythms which may cause excessive ventilation

Hyperventilation: Exaggerated inspirations are followed immediately by equally exaggerated expirations, usually without the double-phase, and contribute directly to a central apnoea as the end-point (Fig. 6.14).

Tachypnoea Rapid inspirations, usually with steep ramp that are followed immediately by expirations, usually without the double-phase, but without

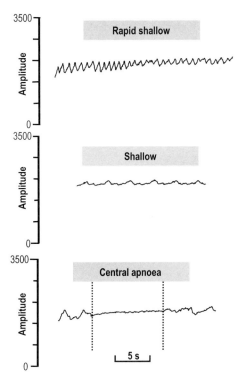

Fig. 6.13 Chest movements during feeble breathings recorded using the MedullaLab™. See Section 6.6.2 for details. The amplitudes are measured in arbitrary computer display units. Obtained from Julu *et. al.* (manuscript submitted).

causing central apnoea (Fig. 6.14). The rate of breathing is between 35–45 breaths/min but depth can be average or above for that individual.

Deep breathing Exaggerated inspirations, usually with steep ramps that are followed immediately by equally exaggerated expirations, usually with no double-phase but without causing a central apnoea (Fig. 6.14). The rate of breathing is below 35 breaths/min, but depth in arbitrary computer units is above average for that individual by 50% or more.

Forceful breathing was prominent in the young age group, occupying 25% of the monitoring time in those under 5 years old, falling to below 10% in adults. It is our impression that forceful breathing tends to occur in fit Rett persons and is associated with agitation.

6.6.4 Valsalva's manoeuvre

Is achieved by raising intrathoracic pressure using breathing movements resembling breath holds or protracted inspirations to create pressure sufficient to

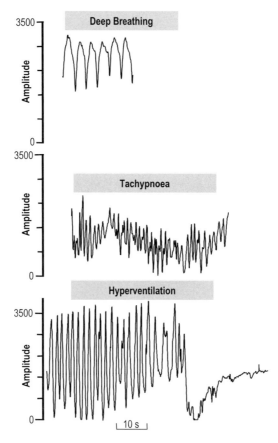

Fig. 6.14 Chest movements during forceful breathings recorded using the MedullaLab™. See Section 6.6.3 for details. The amplitudes are measured in arbitrary computer display units. Obtained from Julu *et. al.* (manuscript submitted).

obstruct venous return to the heart, causing a characteristic change in blood pressure and heart rate. Saw-tooth-shaped heart rate response with clear rebound bradycardia is characteristic of Valsalva's manoeuvre (Fig. 6.15).

Valsalva's breathing was mostly seen in teenagers and adults in our series, occupying about 10% of monitoring time in those over 25 years old.

6.6.5 Periodic breathing rhythms that can cause excessive ventilation

Biot's breathing Abrupt apnoea followed by equally abrupt regular and forceful breathing in which both the apnoea and regular breathing have variable lengths (Fig. 6.16). This is a very rare type of breathing dysrhythmia in the Rett disorder. It has been observed so far in only two girls with Rett syndrome in our series.

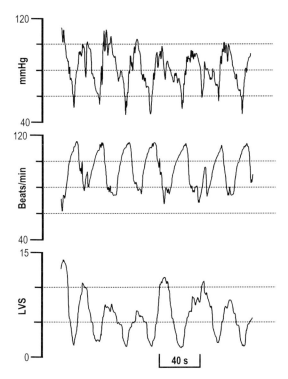

Fig. 6.15 The changes in the mean arterial blood pressure (MAP), measured in millimetres of mercury (mmHg, top trace); heart rate in beats per minute (beats/min, middle trace); cardiac vagal tone (CVT) measured in arbitrary units of a Linear Vagal Scale (LVS, bottom trace), in a 19-year old girl with Rett syndrome while she was having successive episodes of involuntary Valsalva's manoeuvres. The decrease in MAP during positive intrathoracic pressure is accompanied by vagal withdrawal and a sharp increase in heart rate. The drop in MAP is stopped and reversed, but vagal withdrawal continues while the increase in heart rate becomes less sharp in the middle of the positive intrathoracic pressure. The sharp increase in CVT at the end of the positive intrathoracic pressure is accompanied by a rebound bradycardia giving the characteristic saw-toothed appearance of the heart rate trace. Obtained from Julu *et. al.* (manuscript submitted).

Cheyne-Stokes breathing A periodic breathing interrupted by central apnoea during which the breathing movements gradually increase in amplitude and then decay again into apnoea (Fig. 6.16). This is sometimes associated with hyperventilation, but is often unprovoked in the Rett disorder. Unprovoked Cheyne–Stokes breathing is well known in premature neonates (Youmans 1966).

6.6.6 Breathing rhythms that cannot be classified

Atypical breathing Episodes of inspirations and expirations of variable patterns with rates below 35 breaths/min but with average depths for the individual. This forms a very small proportion of breathing abnormalities in the Rett disorder,

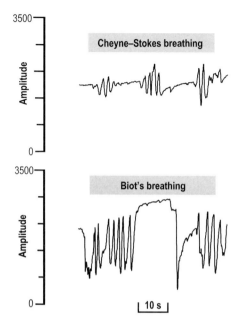

Fig. 6.16 Chest movements during periodic breathings recorded using the MedullaLab™. See Section 6.6.5 for details. The amplitudes are measured in arbitrary computer display units. Obtained from Julu *et. al.* (manuscript submitted).

often less than 1% of the monitoring time. Usually the breathing rhythms can be classified into episodes matching one of the above categories.

6.7 Clinical assessment of brainstem autonomic function in Rett syndrome

The methods are painless and non-invasive and were developed for diagnostic purposes in autonomic failure. A computerized, integrated monitoring machine called the NeuroScope™ (MediFit Instruments Ltd, London, UK) records beat-to-beat heart rate (HR) from ECG R-R intervals while beat-to-beat systolic, mean and diastolic blood pressures (BP) are recorded using the Finapres™ BP monitor (Ohmeda, Englewood, USA). A photoplethysmographic cuff applied on one finger obtains a continuous digital arterial BP waveform in the Finapres, which sends the waveform to a microcomputer for calculation of beat-to-beat BP (systolic, mean and diastolic). Since sympathetic activity is closely related to the mean arterial BP (Sun and Guyenet 1986), generalized sympathetic activity can be monitored indirectly and continuously from the readings of the mean BP. This provides a non-invasive means of monitoring the common autonomic pathway to the vasomotor system discussed above. Sympathetic stimulation to the heart can be deduced from the heart rate, in conjunction with cardiac vagal tone, which is measured independently as described below.

Cardiac vagal tone (CVT) is monitored continuously in real-time from the ECG signals using a modification of the principles described by Julu (1992) and now implemented in the NeuroScope™ (MediFit Instruments Ltd, London, UK). To understand how we quantify nerve impulses in the vagus nerve non-invasively, it must be appreciated that these impulses are integrated, or added up, in the sino-atrial node (SA node) and affect heart periods beat-by-beat. Work by Eckberg (1976) showed that baroreceptor stimulation using neck suction had maximal effect on the SA node when the stimulus was applied in synchrony with the ejection of blood into the great vessels indicated by a rise in arterial pressure. Most relevant to the measurement of CVT is that baroreceptor stimulation causes delays in the onset of the cardiac cycle immediately following the stimulus and this delay can be measured in the ECG P-P intervals. The delay in the onset of cardiac periods caused by baroreceptor stimulation is mediated through the cardiac vagal tone (Eckberg 1976). Baroreceptor signals are the main source of excitation for cardiovagal motor neurons in the medulla and to date are the only proven source of excitation of cardiovagal motor neurons as is discussed previously (see 'how is CVT regulated?' above). Since blood is ejected into the arteries in every cardiac cycle with enough strength to stimulate the baroreceptors (Rushmer 1972), there is a quantifiable pulse-synchronised fast alteration in R-R interval, which is measured continuously by the NeuroScope™ (Little et al. 1999). A scale of vagal tone known as the Linear Vagal Scale (LVS) has been derived using atropine (Julu 1992). The LVS will read 10 units in young adults in supine position and breathing normal tidal volumes quietly and zero units in every person at full atropinization (Julu 1992). This provides a non-invasive means of quantifying the only cardiovascular parasympathetic output from the brain and a very important common autonomic pathway as described above. The CVT is also an important indicator of the integrative inhibition in the brainstem as was discussed earlier.

If we define the cardiac sensitivity to baroreflex (CSB) as the increase in pulse intervals per unit change in systolic BP, we can measure CSB by quantifying cardiac responses to ejection pressures in each cardiac cycle as $\Delta RR/\Delta SBP$, where ΔRR is the difference between present and previous ECG R-R intervals and ΔSBP is the difference between systolic pressures in two preceding cycles to the current cardiac cycle. This method is based on the observation by Eckberg (1976) in which a brisk stimulation of baroreceptors affected the period of the cardiac cycle immediately following the stimulus. Beat-to-beat ΔBP is measured non-invasively using the Finapres, while beat-to-beat ΔRR is obtained from consecutive R-R intervals measured by the NeuroScope™. These two measurements are integrated into a single microcomputer, which calculates the CSB in real-time (Julu et al. 1996). The CSB is a measure of the integrative function of the NTS involving more than one neurotransmitter including L-glutamate and angiotensin-II (see Paton and Kasparov 1999*a*; *b* for more discussion). Monitoring the CSB therefore provides a non-invasive means of assessing the integrative function of the NTS in real-time. This is the major centre for cardiorespiratory integration as is discussed above (see Fig. 6.11) and therefore forms an important part of brainstem function.

Other neurophysiological functions measured
EEG is recorded simultaneously with the physiological markers of autonomic function in real-time, and epileptiform changes in the EEG and their timing are noted for later comparison with autonomic abnormalities and behavioural states observed in the video recording. The EEG records are time-locked with the video and autonomic data for accurate interpretation.

6.7.1 Baseline autonomic tone in the Rett disorder

We shall define baseline brainstem autonomic function as the autonomic activity recorded during the period when the subject is not agitated and has normal breathing rhythm as discussed above with blood gases within the normal range. We have fully analysed the brainstem autonomic functions in 45 girls with classical Rett syndrome (Julu *et al.*, in preparation) (age range 2–35 years, average 12.5) and 12 normal healthy girls (age range 5–28 years, average 9.8).

There was no significant difference between persons with the Rett disorder and their healthy age group, regarding the baseline vasomotor activity measured

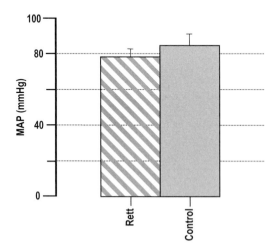

Fig. 6.17 Bar charts representing baseline mean arterial blood pressure (MAP) in a group of people with Rett syndrome and their healthy age group as control. Error bars are S.E.M. There was no statistically significant difference in the baseline MAP in the two groups. Obtained from Julu *et. al.* (manuscript submitted).

indirectly from the mean arterial blood pressure. This means that the baseline activity of the presympathetic neurons in the rostral VLM responsible for vasomotor tone is comparable in Rett syndrome with those in normal healthy girls (Fig. 6.17). Mean arterial blood pressure was about 76 mmHg in Rett girls and not significantly different from 84 mmHg in controls (Fig. 6.17). Pacemaker neurons maintain the baseline sympathetic vasomotor activity (see discussion under the relevant subheadings). It can therefore be inferred that the presympathetic pacemaker activity in the Rett disorder is comparable to that in the normal age group.

Integrative function of the NTS as measured by the CSB was significantly lower in people with Rett syndrome compared with healthy controls, by as much as 44% ($p<0.05$, Student's t-test). The average CSB was about 3.5 ms/mmHg in the Rett girls compared with about 6.2 ms/mmHg in control girls (Fig. 6.18). There is some evidence of a tonic regulation of the level of CSB in the NTS involving serotonergic nerves; at least the 5-HT_4 receptors are implicated (Edwards and Paton 1999). However the eventual response of the heart to the baroreflex is regulated by other neurotransmitters, including excitatory amino acids and peptidergic systems (Paton and Kasparov 1999a; Paton and Kasparov 1999b). The level of CSB indicates the overall gain of the negative feedback in the baroreflex system set up in the NTS by a complex integrative process in which several neurotransmitters are involved.

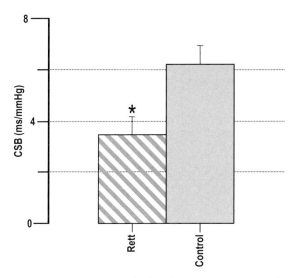

Fig. 6.18 Bar charts representing the baseline levels of cardiac sensitivity to baroreflex (CSB), a measure of the integrative function of the nucleus of tractus solitarius in the brainstem, in a group of people with Rett syndrome and their healthy age group as control. Error bars are S.E.M. There was a significant difference between the two groups; *$p<0.05$, unpaired Student's t-test. Obtained from Julu *et. al.* (manuscript submitted).

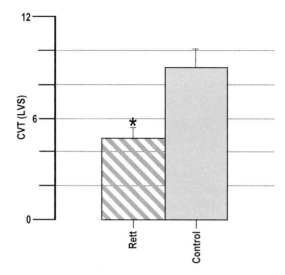

Fig. 6.19 Bar charts representing the baseline levels of cardiac vagal tone (CVT) measured in arbitrary units of a Linear Vagal Scale (LVS) in a group of people with Rett syndrome and their healthy age group as control. Error bars are S.E.M. There was a significant difference between the two groups; *$p<0.05$, unpaired student's t-test. Obtained from Julu *et. al.* (manuscript submitted).

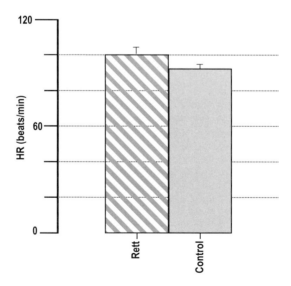

Fig. 6.20 Bar charts representing the baseline heart rates (HR) in a group of people with Rett syndrome and their healthy age group as control. The error bars are S.E.M. There was no significant statistical difference in baseline heart rate in the two groups. Obtained from Julu *et. al.* (manuscript submitted).

The low level of CSB in Rett syndrome should be interpreted as a reduction of the baseline inhibitory gain of the baroreflex system. This is part of the clinical evidence suggesting a lack of integrative inhibition in Rett syndrome mentioned earlier.

The level of CVT was very low in Rett girls compared with their age group controls. A reduction by as much as 47% was found ($p<0.05$). The CVT measured on average only 4.8 units in the LVS in Rett girls compared with the average 9 units in the same scale in control girls (Fig. 6.19). As discussed above, the level of CVT is regulated through complex integrative processes in the NTS, nucleus ambiguus and the bulbar reticular formation, involving several supra-medullary centres. The CVT being the only inhibitory output of the cardiorespiratory integrative system serves a very important function in situations requiring fast cardiovascular responses and is a major part of the integrative inhibition in the cardiorespiratory system.

The low level of CVT in Rett girls is an important clinical evidence of a lack of integrative inhibition in this syndrome.

The baseline heart rate averaged 101 beats/min in Rett, not significantly different from the 92 beats/min in control girls (Fig. 6.20). This illustrates the flexibility in the reciprocal innervation of the heart facilitated by the organotopic arrangement of the presympathetic neurons in the rostral VLM. The discrete tachycardia neuronal mass in the rostral VLM is independently readjusted to suit the low CVT (Jordan 1995) avoiding excessive tachycardia at rest. However, the heart rate response to other situations may be totally different due to the lack of integrative inhibitions.

The clinical evidence shows that the baseline brainstem functions maintained by complex integrative inhibitions of neurons are most affected in the Rett disorder, while the functions maintained by pacemaker activity of neurons are preserved.

Since breathing rhythm is invariably affected in Rett syndrome, there is a strong implication that rhythmogenesis of breathing movement is likely to be due to a complex network of neuronal inhibitions as suggested by Richter. Our observations in the Rett disorder therefore support the Richter model of breathing rhythmogenesis in humans.

6.8 Cardiorespiratory interactions

I will now discuss cardiorespiratory interactions during the generalized neuronal activation in hyperventilation, optimal stimulation of the pulmonary SAR in breath holding and increased brainstem excitability in the suppressed breathing of inadequate ventilation.

6.8.1 Autonomic tone during hyperventilation in the Rett disorder

Figure 6.21 shows the responses of HR, CVT, and mean arterial BP representing sympathetic activity, to hyperventilation in a healthy girl, and Fig. 6.22 shows the responses in a girl with the Rett disorder. The sharp increase in mean BP was immediately countered by a fall in HR in response to an increase in vagal tone; keeping blood pressure within the basal range, the HR was then restored back to normal in a V-shaped manner. Vagal tone remained elevated during the whole period of hyperventilation and was withdrawn to baseline level only when the girl stopped hyperventilating. This is the pattern in normal persons during voluntary hyperventilation. The heart and indeed the whole cardiovascular system are under increased parasympathetic regulation during hyperventilation compared to baseline levels. It illustrates a normal reciprocal innervation of the cardiovascular system, being a response to increased sympathetic tone during hyperventilation. The increase in sympathetic tone is indicated by the sharp rise in the mean BP.

In the girl with Rett syndrome whose hyperventilation was involuntary, CVT increased initially but was withdrawn in the middle of the hyperventilation and reinstated after the hyperventilation (Fig. 6.22). There was a sharp increase in the mean BP at the onset of hyperventilation which could not be countered by a sufficient fall in HR due to withdrawal of the CVT. Mean BP and the HR were

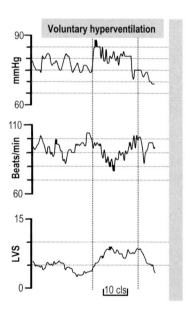

Fig. 6.21 Continuous and simultaneous records of the mean arterial blood pressure, measured in millimetres of mercury (mmHg, top trace); heart rate (middle trace); cardiac vagal tone, measured in arbitrary units of a Linear Vagal Scale (LVS, bottom trace) in a healthy 7-year old girl illustrating changes during 20 s of hyperventilation. See Section 6.8.1 for details. Obtained from Julu *et. al.* (manuscript submitted).

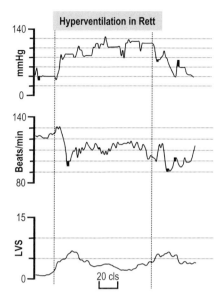

Fig. 6.22 Continuous and simultaneous records of the mean arterial blood pressure, measured in millimetres of mercury (mmHg, top trace); heart rate (middle trace); cardiac vagal tone, measured in arbitrary units of a Linear Vagal Scale (LVS, bottom trace) in an 8-year old girl with Rett syndrome illustrating changes during 50 s of hyperventilation. See Section 6.8.1 for details. Obtained from Julu et. al. (manuscript submitted).

therefore uncontrolled during hyperventilation and finally became unstable. This illustrates the effect of a lack of sufficient reciprocal innervation. Agitation, distress and sometimes vocalization were also present. This pattern was seen in most people with Rett syndrome who hyperventilated for more than 15 s continuously. Hyperventilation for less than 10 s was too brief to cause consistent cardiorespiratory interaction.

The sympatho-vagal balance during hyperventilation in healthy persons and in Rett syndrome is as follows. Cardiac vagal tone increases to counter increased sympathetic activity indicated by raised BP in normal healthy persons. This indicates the balanced reciprocal innervation of the cardiovascular system. The raised CVT is maintained throughout the hyperventilation and beyond in normal people. However, in Rett syndrome the CVT is withdrawn at the height of sympathetic activity creating severe imbalance between the two cardiac autonomic tones indicating faulty reciprocal innervation of the cardiovascular system during hyperventilation and failure of integrative inhibition by the cardiorespiratory neurons.

Pathological hyperventilation in Rett syndrome and voluntary hyperventilation in normal people are both associated with agitation and autonomic stimulation. Cold extremities and raised blood pressure and heart rate indicate activation of the sympathetic vasoconstrictors and cardioaccelerator in the rostral part of ventrolateral medulla both in Rett syndrome and normal people during the initiation of hyperventilation. At the same time there is parasympathetic activation in the caudal part of the ventrolateral medulla, shown by increase in CVT to check and control the increase in heart rate and blood pressure. The rise in CVT is adequate in normal people, achieving smooth regulation of heart rate and blood pressure whereas this damping effect of the parasympathetic system is lacking in Rett syndrome leading to excessive swings of blood pressure and heart rate during hyperventilation (Fig. 6.22).

The autonomic responses to hyperventilation suggest that rostral and caudal ventrolateral medulla are simultaneously activated during the initiation process and this is true for normal people as well as for Rett cases. It is not certain whether this medullary activation is achieved by neuronal excitation or by disinhibition (withdrawal of a tonic inhibition). Second and third order respiratory neurons including those suspected to be rhythm generators are arranged in a rostro-caudal chain in the ventrolateral medulla intermixed with the autonomic neurons (Fig. 6.7). We can therefore assume that there is generalized activation of the ventrolateral medulla during hyperventilation in all human beings although the origin of this activation is beyond the scope of our studies.

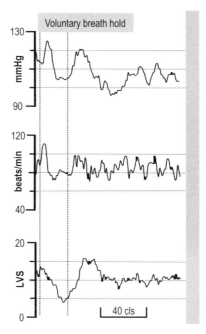

Fig. 6.23 Continuous and simultaneous records of the mean arterial blood pressure, measured in millimetres of mercury (mmHg, top trace); heart rate (middle trace); cardiac vagal tone, measured in arbitrary units of a Linear Vagal Scale (LVS, bottom trace) in a healthy 10-year old girl illustrating the changes during 20 s of end-of-inspiration breath hold. See Section 6.8.2 for details. Obtained from Julu *et. al.* (manuscript submitted).

6.8.2 Autonomic tone during breath holding in Rett

Figure 6.23 shows the responses of the HR, CVT, and mean arterial BP representing sympathetic activity in a normal girl (voluntary breath hold). Figure 6.24 shows similar responses in a girl with the Rett disorder during an involuntary end-of-inspiration breath hold. Parasympathetic control of the cardiovascular system indicated by CVT was promptly and appropriately withdrawn at the beginning of breath hold and restored immediately afterwards in the normal healthy girl (Fig. 6.23). The HR and BP had similar patterns of responses throughout breath holding, indicating the same regulatory influence by the sympathetic system with parasympathetic control withdrawn. This is the pattern of responses in all normal people demonstrating that the whole cardiovascular system comes under the dominant influence of the sympathetic nervous system during voluntary breath holding.

Breath holding in the girl with Rett syndrome also caused prompt withdrawal of the CVT regulation as in healthy girls (Fig. 6.24). However, the initial increase in sympathetic activity at the beginning of breath holding caused oscillation or 'ringing' in the BP, a sign of poor restraint of the sympathetic system by the negative feedback mechanism of the baroreflex known to control it (Spyer 1990).

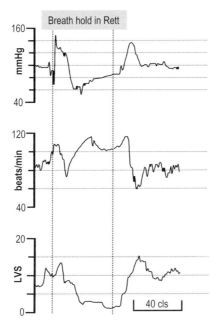

Fig. 6.24 Continuous and simultaneous records of the mean arterial blood pressure, measured in millimetres of mercury (mmHg, top trace); heart rate (middle trace); cardiac vagal tone, measured in arbitrary units of a Linear Vagal Scale (LVS, bottom trace) in a 10-year old girl with Rett syndrome illustrating the changes during 38 s of end-of-inspiration breath hold. See Section 6.8.2 for details. Obtained from Julu *et. al.* (manuscript submitted).

It is another sign of poor negative feedback control of the sympathetic system. The evidence from our series indicates that the whole cardiovascular system is left under the control of the sympathetic nervous system during the involuntary breath holding in Rett syndrome as in normal voluntary breath holding. But the negative feedback regulation of the sympathetic system during breath holding is poor in Rett syndrome. This provides a further sign that integrative inhibition in the cardiorespiratory neurons is deficient.

During normal initiation of end-of-inspiration breath hold, the lungs fill with air in a single inspiratory chest movement before holding the breath which stimulates pulmonary SAR, causing inhibition of both CVT and CSB (see Section 6.4.9 on cardiorespiratory interactions). This explains the reduction in CVT and CSB at onset of the normal breath hold. The central inspiratory drive at the beginning of the breath hold increases sympathetic tone and decreases CVT and CSB further. As long as the lungs are kept inflated, cardiovascular control is therefore left under the control of the sympathetic nervous system with little or no reciprocal parasympathetic activity. Our results show that normal healthy people can cope with the reduced negative feedback control during a breath hold, but this manoeuvre is precarious in Rett syndrome.

The cardiorespiratory interactions in various manoeuvres provide consistent clinical evidence of deficient integrative inhibition in Rett syndrome.

6.8.3 Abnormal brainstem function during inadequate ventilation in Rett syndrome

Brainstem shutdown
Feeble breathing was common in 10–15-years old girls with Rett syndrome in our series. Five girls developed a progressive drop in BP accompanied by a progressive fall in both CVT and CSB during inadequate ventilation (Fig. 6.25). Mean arterial BP approached 40 mmHg, the level of BP usually associated with spinal transection, both CSB and CVT came close to zero and HR approached the intrinsic rate of the sino-atrial node suggesting lower brainstem shutdown. I have therefore adopted the phrase 'brainstem shutdown' to describe this phenomenon. These girls looked vacant and staring. The electroencephalogram (EEG) changed to generalized very low voltage or flat during the episodes. Transcutaneous oxygen fell as the episode duration increased.

The cause of this brainstem shutdown is uncertain and requires further study in a larger series. One girl had brainstem shutdown after long successive episodes of Valsalva's manoeuvre, another following long episodes of hyperventilation, but in others there was no obvious provocation. If brainstem shutdown follows prolonged repetitive and exaggerated brainstem activation as in forceful breathing, or seizure, it might be argued that post-activation or post-ictal

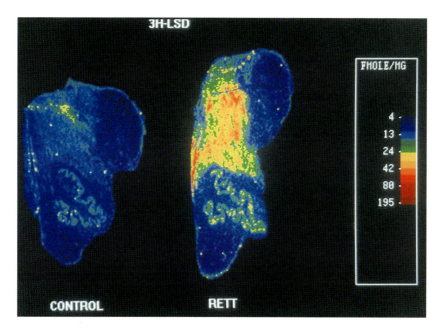

Fig. 3.4a Representative example of serotonin receptor binding in the medulla of a mature control brain (left) and a Rett brain (right). The photograph is colour-coded with a colour scale marking the specific binding activity levels in fmol/mg tissue. Note that there is a greater density of receptor binding in the regions of the nucleus of the solitary tract and the nucleus centralis in the Rett medulla.

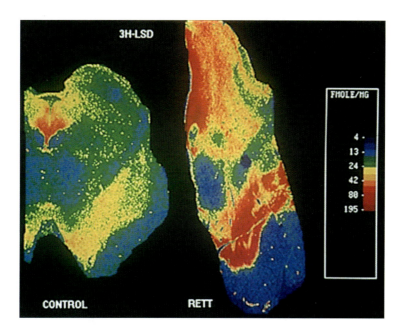

Fig. 3.4b Representative example of serotonin receptor binding in the midbrain of a mature control brain (left) and a Rett brain (right). The photograph is colour-coded with a colour scale marking the specific binding activity levels in fmol/mg tissue. Note that there is a greater density of receptor binding in the regions of the substantia nigra in the Rett midbrain.

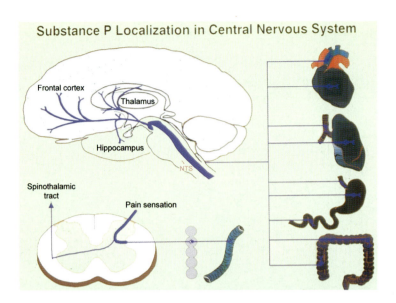

Fig. 3.5 Multiple sites of action of substance P. Note that in Rett syndrome there is a dysfunction of many of these sites, suggesting that the deficiency of substance P may be associated with the abnormality (illustrated by Kimiko Deguchi).

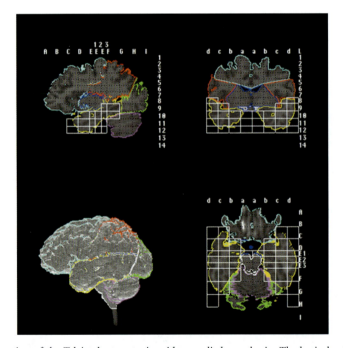

Fig. 4.1 Tri-planer view of the Talairach stereotaxic grid as applied on a brain. The brain has been positionally normalized and Talairach sectors designated as representing the temporal lobe are shown superimposed over manually derived sulcal-based, 'gold standard' regions. In this illustration, the gold standard temporal lobe, frontal lobe, parietal lobe and occipital lobe boundaries are designated in yellow, blue, red, and green, respectively. The Talairach sectors appear as white boxes in the three orthogonal views. The figure on the upper left corresponds to a midsagittal view. The coronal slice (upper right) corresponds to the level of the amygdala/third ventricle and includes anterior levels of the posterior insula. The figure on the lower right presents an axial view. Finally, a rendered three-dimensional display, without the grid, is illustrated on the lower left. Reproduced with permission from Kates *et al.* (1999).

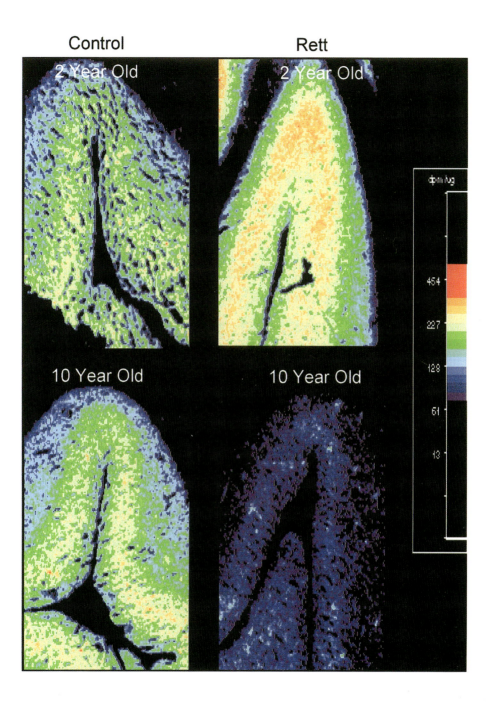

Fig. 5.2.1 Pseudocolor images of [3H] CGP39653 binding of N-methyl-D-aspartate (NMDA) receptors in 2-year-old (upper panel) and 10-year-old (lower panel) Rett syndrome (RS) patients and controls. The density of NMDA receptors appears markedly higher in the 2-year-old RS patient compared to her age-matched control. In contrast, the density of NMDA receptors is lower in the 10-year-old RS patient than in her age-matched control. Reprinted from Blue *et al.* (1999*b*), with permission of Lippincott Williams & Wilkins, Inc.

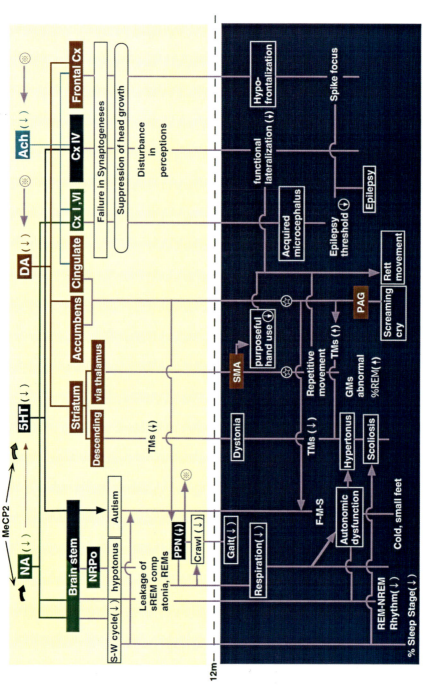

Fig. 8.2. Pathophysiology of Rett syndrom-hypothesis - ⊛ Receptor Supersensitivity; MeCP2, methyl-CpG-binding protein 2; NA, noradrenaline; 5HT, serotonin; DA, dopamine; Ach, acetylcholine; NRPo, nucleus reticularis pontis oralis; PPN, pedunculo-pontine nuclei; SMA, supplementary motor area; PAG, periaqueductal grey; Cx I,VI, cerebral cortex layer I and VI; Cx IV, cerebral cortex layer IV; Cx, cortex; FMS, friendliness-muricide-selfmutilation; S-W cycle, sleep-wake cycle; sREM, rapid eye movement sleep stage; REM(s), rapid eye movements; NREM, non-rapid eye movement; TMs, twitch movements; GMs, gross movements; 12m, age of 12 months. ⊛ indicates that decreased function of PPN leads to decreased DA and Arch.

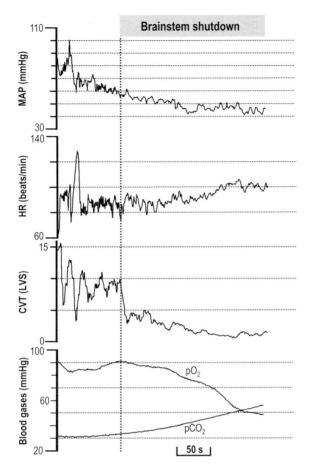

Fig. 6.25 Continuous and synchronized records of the mean arterial blood pressure (MAP), heart rate (HR), cardiac vagal tone (CVT) measured in arbitrary units of a Linear Vagal Scale (LVS), partial pressure of oxygen in the blood (pO_2), and partial pressure of carbon dioxide (pCO_2) in an 11-year old girl with Rett syndrome illustrating the changes during brainstem shutdown. The vertical dotted line marks the beginning of the shutdown. See Section 6.8.3 for details. Obtained from Julu *et. al.* (manuscript submitted).

neuronal quiescence is the cause of the shutdown. The longest duration of a shutdown in our series was three minutes. We do not know if prolonged shock caused by brainstem shutdown may occur in Rett syndrome.

Brainstem storm
Prolonged feeble breathing causes elevation of pCO_2 and a fall in pO_2. Weak central respiratory drive may be inferred, in which case respiratory inhibition of cardiovagal motor neurons will be reduced (see Section 6.4.9). A combination of hypercapnia and hypoxia will stimulate the chemoreceptors optimally and combined with weak central respiratory drive lead to maximal cardiovagal excitation

(see Section 6.4.9 and Fig. 6.11). An 11-year old girl illustrated this phenomenon very well during our monitoring session with abnormally large simultaneous increases in CSB, CVT and BP against a background of very low baseline levels in all these indices of brainstem function (a section of her record is shown in Figure 6.26). I have adopted the phrase 'brainstem storm' to describe this phenomenon because the functional indices of the whole brainstem, rostral, caudal and dorsal are simultaneously and momentarily increased to exaggerated levels much higher than the level immediately before the event. The reflex bradycardia and drop in the BP following increased level of the CVT was maintained throughout the brainstem storm (Fig. 6.26).

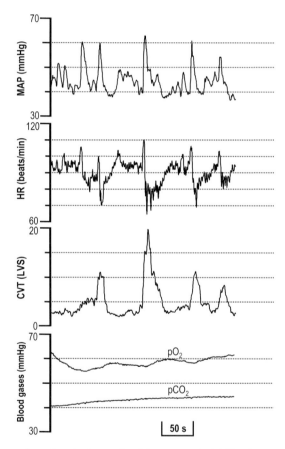

Fig. 6.26 Continuous and synchronized records of the mean arterial blood pressure (MAP), heart rate (HR), cardiac vagal tone (CVT) measured in arbitrary units of a Linear Vagal Scale (LVS), partial pressure of oxygen in the blood (pO_2), and partial pressure of carbon dioxide (pCO_2) in an 11-year old girl with Rett syndrome illustrating spontaneous and exaggerated excitation of the brainstem during feeble breathing. The pO_2 oscillated below 60 mmHg and at every trough there were spikes in MAP and HR. On four occasions, there were spikes in CVT too causing sharp and transient bradycardias. The exaggerated simultaneous spikes of MAP, HR and CVT constitute brainstem storm. See Section 6.8.3 for details. Obtained from Julu *et. al.* (manuscript submitted).

The clinical importance of brainstem storm is that it indicates the risk of large changes in the autonomic indices when inadequate ventilation is present for a long period. Sudden big increases in CVT and feeble breathing with high pCO_2 and low pO_2 are both conducive to cardiac arrest. It would be rational to direct therapy to alleviate hypoxia, and stimulate breathing.

Brainstem epilepsy
The brainstem autonomic neurons are activated either through reflexes or through pacemaker neurons, and the outputs are carefully integrated to fulfil physiological functions discussed above. We have observed outputs from the

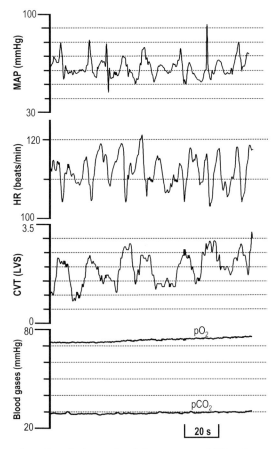

Fig. 6.27 Continuous and synchronized records of the mean arterial blood pressure (MAP), heart rate (HR), cardiac vagal tone (CVT) measured in arbitrary units of a Linear Vagal Scale (LVS), partial pressure of oxygen in the blood (pO_2), and partial pressure of carbon dioxide (pCO_2) in a 13-year old girl with Rett syndrome illustrating the changes during brainstem epilepsy. There was normal breathing rhythm and both pO_2 and pCO_2 were steady within the normal limits. The exaggerated and repeated simultaneous sharp increases in MAP, HR and CVT, best seen at the beginning and end of the traces, represent widespread aberrant excitation of the brainstem. See Section 6.8.3 for details. Obtained from Julu *et. al.* (manuscript submitted).

brainstem, which did not conform to known physiological activation of the neurons involved and the widespread nature of this aberrant, brief and often repetitive activation is consistent with epilepsy. I have therefore defined brainstem epilepsy as 'widespread brief aberrant activation of brainstem neurons (Fig. 6.27).

Brainstem epilepsy is different from brainstem storm in that the physiological conditions for brainstem storm such as feeble breathing, low pO_2 and high pCO_2 in the blood are absent. Extreme swings in levels of autonomic output are recorded without apparent cause. The clinical consequences of such wild autonomic output are unpredictable. Respiratory arrest can be possible if postinspiratory neurons are aberrantly activated. This is not unique to the Rett disorder and we have observed brainstem epilepsy in elderly patients presenting with syncope and in other known epileptic patients referred to us for autonomic examination (unpublished observations in our laboratory).

6.9 Clinical significance of the evidence of brain immaturity in the Rett disorder

In addition to our own studies, much physiological evidence points to immaturity of the brain in the Rett disorder. The EEG is immature and poorly responsive with slow background and poor development of α-rhythm. Functional imaging using Single positron emission computed tomography (SPECT) revealed a functional distribution of blood flow in the Rett brain similar to that of an infant of only a few months old (Nielsen *et al.* 1990). The CVT in Rett syndrome measured in our series is at the level of neonates. The maturity of the brainstem autonomic nuclei can be assessed at post-mortem using lysergic acid diethylamide (LSD) binding to serotonin receptors (Zec *et al.* 1996). The increased post-mortem LSD binding to brainstem nuclei in the Rett disorder discussed elsewhere (Chapter 3) suggests that the autonomic maturity is between mid-gestation and birth. Since it is evident that the consistent physiological description of the Rett brain is that of immaturity, a combination of maturity indices above including functional imaging may be of value for early diagnosis of the syndrome. A combination of an assessment of the brainstem autonomic function and functional imaging using a serotonin-binding ligand in positron emission tomography (PET) may be able to demonstrate the type of brainstem immaturity characteristic of Rett syndrome at an early age.

6.10 Clinical intervention in the abnormal brainstem function in Rett syndrome

There are risks, some of which are known to cause sudden deaths, which depend on the variable type and severity of the breathing dysrhythmia and level of autonomic incompetence in the Rett person. The type of sympatho-vagal imbalance seen during prolonged hyperventilation in the Rett disorder is known to cause sudden death in ischaemic heart disease *(Schwartz et al.* 1988) and in hypoglycaemia (Thomson *et al.* 1996). The physiological state of Rett persons during brainstem storm is conducive to cardiac arrest. Brainstem shutdown may carry a risk of sudden death if it is accompanied by extreme shock. Respiratory arrest or even cardiac arrest may occur during brainstem epilepsy. With such variation in clinical picture and risks, it is important to characterize the clinical features precisely for each individual in order to plan treatment specifically for that individual.

Clinical intervention in apneustic breathing
Serotonin (5-HT), acting through its 1_A receptors, is partly responsible for the transition from the ramp inspiration to expiration in the brainstem. We have used buspirone, a $5-HT1_A$ agonist, with some success to alleviate very severe apneusis (Kerr *et al.* 1998). This has been partially successful in four cases and is clearly justified only after detailed assessment and selection of cases with predominant severe apneusis. It was of no value in Valsalva's breathing nor in short breath holds (our observation and personal communication with Witt Engerström). Supervised by a physician, oral buspirone can be started at 5 mg daily, increasing gradually to 20 mg daily.

Clinical intervention in feeble breathing
An increased level of β-endorphin has been reported in the Rett brain (Budden *et al.* 1990). This might contribute to respiratory depression in the brainstem and if present would justify the use of an opioid antagonist. We gave intravenous naloxone, an opioid antagonist, to two persons with Rett syndrome who had very severe and long periods of central apnoea without useful effect. We have not yet found a useful intervention for feeble breathing in Rett syndrome.

Animal studies suggest that central apnoea may be caused by depletion of the second messengers participating in neuronal transmissions (Ballanyi *et al.* 1997; Richter *et al.* 1999). Second messengers are mostly essential fatty acids, arachidonic acid being an important one. Theoretically, a clinical means of replenishing neuronal essential fatty acids in the central nervous system would be expected to ameliorate feeble breathing. However, the route followed by essential fatty acids from the gut to the central nervous system is complex and a simple oral administration of free arachidonic acid is futile.

Clinical presentation of classical Rett syndrome is heterogeneous in association with a broad spectrum of central autonomic competence and variable risk factors in different individuals, while all physiological indices so far show that the brain is immature.

6.11 Appraisal of the non-invasive methods of examination of the brainstem

The brainstem has been inaccessible to neurophysiological assessment except for the auditory evoked potential that examines a restricted pathway. The non-invasive methods of monitoring brainstem autonomic function described here provide a new neurophysiological approach to the evaluation of brainstem function. The method covers both sensory and efferent systems in the brainstem as well as dorsal and ventral aspects of most of the lower brainstem. The respiratory system is also covered in our methods and its disturbance in Rett syndrome provides a means to explore the physiological abnormalities that underlie the disorder.

Earlier autonomic indices do indicate the disturbances in the Rett disorder, but they are indirect measures thus limiting their value. Heart rate variability caused by respiratory modulation of the CVT is measured using mathematical manipulation of heart periods and is commonly interpreted to represent the level of CVT. However, the extent of respiratory modulation of CVT is affected by the depth and rate of breathing (Hirsch and Bishop 1981) and other factors not usually taken into account by the procedure (see cardiorespiratory interactions in Section 6.4.9). These early measurements are usually discontinuous and not performed in real-time; however autonomic tone may change very rapidly and this will be missed. More invasive methods are unacceptable to patients and liable to interfere with the phenomena to be measured.

Our non-invasive methods for monitoring brainstem autonomic function have the advantage of ready acceptability by disabled subjects and they provide direct continuous measures of central autonomic competence throughout a prolonged recording period. By displaying all the results continuously throughout the recording, it is possible to match the behaviour of the subject with the full range of physiological variables on the screen, immediately and accurately. Continuous video recording time-locked with the autonomic data allows replay and a detailed study of the time sequence of individual event, and facilitates interpretation since noise created by body movements and other unwanted events can be excluded. We have found it a convenient way to explore the otherwise elusive physiological abnormalities that underlie the Rett disorder.

Acknowledgements

I am very grateful to many colleagues who participated in the studies described in this chapter. Alison M. Kerr from the Monitoring Centre, University Department of Psychological Medicine, Gartnavel Royal Hospital Glasgow; Stig Hansen and Flora Apatopolous from the Institute of Neurological Sciences, Southern General

Hospital Glasgow; Lars Engerström and Witt Engerström from Swedish Rett Centre, Frösön; all do deserve special mention. I am also grateful to families of all the girls and women with Rett syndrome who participated and gave their consents in the many studies I have carried out. I acknowledge with heartfelt thanks the unfunded supports and partnerships given by Pavel Belichenko from Brain Research Institute (INTAS), Russian Academy of Medical Sciences Moscow and by Dawnna Armstrong from Department of Neuropathology, Texas Children Hospital, Houston. Most of all, I acknowledge the patience of my wife Helen who tolerated the long hours of work and absence during all of the studies.

References

Angell-James, J.E. and Daly, M.D. (1978). The effects of artificial lung inflation on reflexly induced bradycardia associated with apnoea in the dog. *J. Physiol. (London)*, **274**, 349–66.

Ballanyi, K., Lalley, P.M., Hoch, B., and Richter, D.W. (1997). cAMP-dependent reversal of opioid- and prostaglandin-mediated depression of the isolated respiratory network in new-born rats. *J. Physiol. (London)*, **504**(Pt. 1), 127–34.

Blessing, W.W. (1997). *The lower brainstem and bodily homeostasis*. Oxford University Press, Oxford.

Budden, S.S., Myer, E.C., and Butler, I.J. (1990). Cerebrospinal fluid studies in the Rett syndrome: biogenic amines and beta-endorphins. *Brain Dev*, **12**, 81–4.

Cechetto, D.F. and Chen, S.J. (1992). Hypothalamic and cortical sympathetic responses relay in the medulla of the rat. *Am J Physiol*, **263**, R544–52.

Daly de Burgh, M. (1995). Aspects of the integration of the respiratory and cardiovascular systems. In *Cardiovascular regulation* (ed. D.Jordan and J.M. Marshall), pp. 15–35. Portland Press, London.

Damsey, R.A.L. and McAllen, R.M. (1988). Differential control of sympathetic fibres supplying hindlimb skin and muscle by subretrofacial neurons in the cat. *J.Physiol. (London)*, **395**, 41–56.

Eckberg, D.L. (1976). Temporal response patterns of the human sinus node to brief carotid baroreceptor stimuli. *J. Physiol. (London)*, **258**, 769–82.

Edwards, E. and Paton, J.F.R. (1999). Modulatory effect of 5-HT$_4$ receptor stimulation at the level of the nucleus tractus solitarii on cardiorespiratory reflexes in a working heart-brainstem preparation. *J.Physiol. (London)*, **518.P**, 174P–5P.

Ezure, K. (1990). Synaptic connections between medullary respiratory neurons and considerations on the genesis of respiratory rhythm. *Prog. Neurobiol.*, **35**, 429–50.

Gootman, N.G. and Gootman, P.M. (1983). *Perinatal cardiovascular function*, Marcel Dekker, New York.

Guyenet, P.G., Koshiya, N., Huangfu, D., Baraban, S.C., Stornetta, R.L., and Li, Y.W. (1996). Role of medulla oblongata in generation of sympathetic and vagal outflows. In *The emotional motor system* (ed. G. Holstege, R. Bandler, and C.B. Saper), pp. 127–44. Elsevier, Amsterdam Lausanne.

Hightower, N.C. (1966). Gastric secretion. In *The physiological basis of medical practice* (ed. C.H. Best and N.B.Taylor), (8 edn), pp. 1081–121. E. & S. Livingstone Limited, Edinburgh, London.

Hirsch, J.A. and Bishop, B. (1981). Respiratory sinus arrhythmia in humans: how breathing pattern modulates heart rate. *Am J Physiol.*, **241**, H620–29.

Jordan, D. (1995). CNS integration of cardiovascular regulation. In *Cardiovascular regulation* (eds. D. Jordan and J. Marshall), pp. 1–14. Portland Press, London.

Julu, P.O.O. (1992). A linear scale for measuring vagal tone in man. *J. Auton. Pharmacol.*, **12**, 109–15.

Julu, P.O.O., Hansen, S., Barnes, A. and Jamal, G.A. (1996). Continuous measurement of the cardiac component of arterial baroreflex (ccbr) in real-time during isometric-exercise in human volunteers. *J. Physiol. (London)*, **497P**, P7–8.

Julu, P.O., Kerr, A.M., Hansen, S., Apartopoulos, F., and Jamal, G.A. (1997). Functional evidence of brainstem immaturity in Rett syndrome. *Eur. Child Adolesc. Psychiatry*, **6** (**Suppl. 1**), 47–54.

Julu, P.O., Kerr, A.M., Hansen, S., Apartopoulos, F., Witt Engerström, I., and Engerstrom, L. Characterisation of the breathing abnormality and associated central autonomic dysfunction in the Rett disorder, in press 2001.

Katona, P.G., Poitras, J.W., Barnett, G.O., and Terry, B.S. (1970). Cardiac vagal efferent activity and heart period in the carotid sinus reflex. *Am. J. Physiol.*, **218**(4), 1030–7.

Kerr, A., Julu, P., Hansen, S., and Apartopoulos, F. (1998). Serotonin and breathing dysrhythmia in Rett syndrome. In *New developments in child neurology* (ed. M.V.Perat), pp. 191–5. Monduzzi Editore Bologna.

Kissel, P., Andre, J.M., and Jacquier, A. (1981). *The Neurocristopathies*, Year Book Medical Publishers, Chicago.

Lawson, E.E., Richter, D.W., Czyzyk-Krzeska, M.F., Bischoff, A., and Rudesill, R.C. (1991). Respiratory neuronal activity during apnea and other breathing patterns induced by laryngeal stimulation. *J Appl Physiol.*, **70**, 2742–9.

Little, C.J., Julu, P.O., Hansen, S., and Reid, S.W. (1999). Real-time measurement of cardiac vagal tone in conscious dogs. Am. J. Physiol, **276**, H758–65.

Loewy, A.D. (1990). Central autonomic pathways. In *Central regulation of autonomic functions* (ed. A.D. Loewy and K.M.), pp. 88–103. Oxford University Press' New York.

McAllen, R.M. and Spyer, K.M. (1978). The baroreceptor input to cardiac vagal motorneurones. *J. Physiol. (London)*, **282**, 365–74.

Nielsen, J.B., Friberg, L., Lou, H., Lassen, N.A., and Sam, I.L. (1990). Immature pattern of brain activity in Rett syndrome. *Arch Neurol*, **47**, 982–6.

O'Rahilly, R., Muller, F. and Meyer, D.B. (1990). The human vertebral column at the end of the embryonic period proper. 3. The thoracicolumbar region. *J. Anat.*, **168**, 81–93.

Papp, J.G. (1988). Autonomic responses and neurohumoral control in the human early antenatal heart. *Basic Res. Cardiol.*, **83**, 2–9.

Paton, J.F.R. and Kasparov, S. (1999a). Differential effects of angiotensin II on cardiorespiratory reflexes mediated by nucleus tractus solitarii—a microinjection study in the rat. *J.Physiol. (London)*, **521.1**, 213–25.

Paton, J.F.R. and Kasparov, S. (1999b). Differential effects of angiontensin II in the nucleus tractus solitarii of the rat—plausible neuronal mechanisms. *J.Physiol. (London)*, **521.1**, 227–38.

Remmers, J.E., Richter, D.W., Ballantyne, D., Bainton, C.R., and Klein, J.P. (1986). Reflex prolongation of stage I of expiration. *Pflugers Arch.*, **407**, 190–8.

Richter, D.W. (1996). Neural regulation of respiration: rhythmogenesis and afferent control. In *Comprehensive human physiology* (ed. R.Greger and U.Windhorst), pp. 2079–95. Springer, Berlin.

Richter, D.W. and Spyer, K.M. (1990). Cardiorespiratory control. In *Central regulation of autonomic functions* (ed. A.D. Loewy and K.M. Spyer), pp. 186–207. Oxford University Press, Oxford.

Richter, D.W., Schmidt-Garcon, P., Pierrefiche, O., Bischoff, A.M., and Lalley, P.M. (1999). Neurotransmitters and neuromodulators controlling the hypoxic respiratory response in anaesthetized cats (see comments). *J. Physiol. (London)*, **514**(**Pt. 2**), 567–78.

Rushmer, R.F. (1972). Systemic arterial pressure. In *Structure and function of the cardiovascular system* (ed. R.F. Rushmer), pp. 148–91. W.B. Saunders, Philadelphia.

Schwartz, P.J., Vanoli, E., Stramba Badiale, M., De Ferrari, G.M., Billman, G.E., and Foreman, R.D. (1988). Autonomic mechanisms and sudden death. New insights from analysis of baroreceptor reflexes in conscious dogs with and without a myocardial infarction. *Circulation*, **78**, 969–79.

Spyer, K.M. (1989). Neural mechanisms involved in cardiovascular control during affective behaviour. *Trends. Neurosci.*, **12**, 506–13.

Spyer, K.M. (1990). The central nervous organisation of reflex circulatory control. In *Central regulation of autonomic functions* (ed. A.D.Loewy and K.M.Spyer), pp. 168–88. Oxford University Press, Oxford.

Spyer, K.M. (1993). Central nervous control of the cardiovascular system. In *Autonomic failure: a textbook of clinical disorders of the autonomic nervous system* (ed. R. Bannister and C. Mathias) (3 edn), pp. 54–77. Oxford University Press, Oxford.

Spyer, K.M. (1994). Central nervous mechanisms contributing to cardiovascular control. *J. Physiol. (London)*, **474.1**, 1–19.

St.-John, W.M., St. Jacques, R., Li, A., and Darnall, R.A. (1999). Modulation of hypoxic depressions of ventilatory activity in the newborn piglet by mesencephalic mechanisms. *Brain Res.*, **819**, 147–9.

Sun, M.-K. and Guyenet, P.G. (1986). Medulospinal sympathoexcitatory neurons in normotensive and spontaneously hypertensive rats. *Am.J.Physiol.*, **250**, R910–7.

Thomson, G.A., Galloway, P., Julu, P.O.O., Hansen, S., Burns, L., Fisher, B.M., and Semple, C.G. (1996). Reduced cardiac parasympathetic tone during acute hypoglycemia. *Diabetologia*, **39**, 241.

Walker, D. (1974). Functional development of the autonomic innervation of the human fetal heart. *Biol. Neonate.*, **25**, 31–43.

Wildenthal, K. and Atkins, J.M. (1979). Use of the diving reflex for the treatment of paroxysmal supraventricular tachycardia. *Am Heart J.*, **98**, 536–7.

Wilken, B., Lalley, P., Bischoff, A.M., Christen, H.J., Behnke, J., Hanefeld, F., and Richter, D.W. (1997). Treatment of apneustic respiratory disturbance with a serotonin-receptor agonist. *J. Pediatr.*, **130**, 89–94.

Youmans, W.B. (1966). The control of breathing. In *The physiological basis of medical practice* (ed. C.H.Best and N.B.Taylor) (8 edn), pp. 1007–29. E. & S. Livingstone Limited, Edinburgh.

Zec, N., Filiano, J.J., Panigrahy, A., White, W.F., and Kinney, H.C. (1996). Developmental changes in [3H]lysergic acid diethylamide ([3H]LSD) binding to serotonin receptors in the human brainstem. *J Neuropathol Exp Neurol.*, **55**, 114–26.

7 The role of genetic and environmental factors in brain development: development of the central monoaminergic nervous system

Masaya Segawa

Summary

The monoaminergic (MA) neurons have important roles in the morphological and functional maturation of the brain in man as they do in rodents and these are specific for each type of MA neuron. Furthermore, the modulating influence of each type of MA neuron on the development of the brain changes during its maturational course and lesions in MA neurons which mature in the foetal and early infancy periods lead to later brain dysfunction. The effects of these lesions can be studied in rodents; however the lesions occurring in late infancy or early childhood in man lead to specific symptoms observed only in humans.

In considering human disease it is therefore necessary to study the MA neurons which mature after late infancy as well as those maturing before early infancy. For this, studies on the neurons which modulate the development of the biphasic circadian day–night cycle and human type locomotion are particularly important because they are specific for humans and may throw light on the processes of development of the much higher functions of the human being as compared to other primates.

7.1 Introduction

The MA neurons in the brainstem, namely the noradrenalin (NA), serotonin (5HT) and dopamine (DA) neurons, project their axons to various areas of the brain including the neocortex. There is regional specialization of innervation and the pattern for each of the three systems is distinctly different. The anatomical characteristics relate to the specific patterns of modulation which these systems exert on the functions of the brain. During the development of the brain, these neurons have roles in the morphogenesis or synaptogenesis and in the functional maturation of the brain. Early lesions of each of these neurons are known to cause specific and varied functional abnormalities of the brain which become evident after maturation. These processes have been studied mainly in rodents. Although recently there has been increased investigation of primates, studies on humans are still very few. In particular, the relationship between the development of these neurons and the functional maturation of the human brain is still unclear.

In this chapter, I will briefly review the basic science research and try to relate the existing evidence to the development of sleep parameters and locomotion in the human being because these biological phenomena directly reflect the activities of MA neurons and are specific for each type. Furthermore, I will try to illustrate the roles of the MA neuron during development with reference to idiopathic or inherited disorders of MA neurons in which particular symptoms occur in an age-dependent fashion.

7.2 Monoaminergic neurons in mature and immature brains

The MA neurons, particularly 5HT and NA systems, are phylogenetically old and have several features in common. The rate limiting pterin-dependent aromatic amino acid hydroxylases, tryptophen hydroxylase for 5 HT and tyrosine hydroxylase (TH) for NA, are homologous. The molecule in the nerve-cell membrane which transports NA in the reuptake process is similar to the molecule which transports 5HT (Baker and Halliday 1995). The MA neurons, located in the midbrain and the brainstem, modulate the activities of the central nervous system (CNS) through their axons which are widely distributed throughout the brain but are specific to each.

The NA innervation of the neocortex arises solely from the nucleus locus coeruleus (LC) which is located in the pontine brainstem. Individual LC neurons innervate widely separated brain regions. The NA innervation of primate cortex exhibits a high degree of regional specialization with regard both to the density and the laminar pattern of innervation (Morrison and Magistretti 1983) (Fig. 7.1). Thus the primary somatosensory and motor regions are densely innervated in all six laminae while the temporal cortical regions are very sparsely innervated. In the primary visual cortex the density of innervation is intermediate but there is a striking absence of fibres in lamina IV (Fig. 7.1).

The 5HT innervation of adult monkey neocortex is very dense and exhibits variations in density and laminar distribution of axons (Takeuchi and Sano 1983). This pattern of innervation is characteristically shown in the primary visual cortex

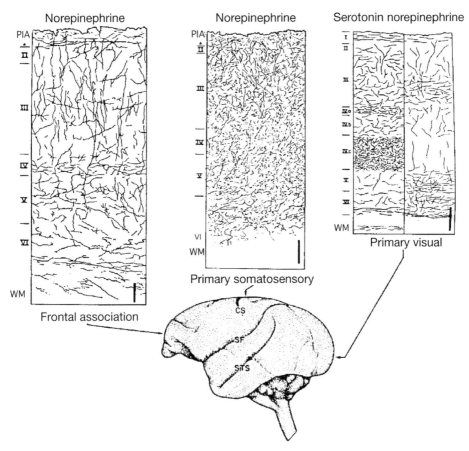

Fig. 7.1 NA innervation of three different regions of primate neocortex. WM, white matter; CS, central sulcus; SF, sylvian fissure; STS, superior temporal sulcus; PIA, pial surface. Calibration bars=200#mm. From Morrison and Magistretti (1983), with permission.

(area 17) where, in contrast to the NA neurons, the 5HT fibres are distributed densely in laminated fashion in layer IV (Fig. 7.1). It is noteworthy that lamina IV is the primary recipient of thalamo-cortical afferents and contains the highest density of 5HT fibres and the lowest density of NA fibres (Foote and Morrison 1984).

Biochemical data from monkey studies showed high DA levels throughout the frontal lobe, although there is a clear decrease of its concentration in more posterior areas (Goldman-Rakic *et al.* 1982). By means of histochemical examination, Lewis *et al.* (1986) showed that DA axons are widespread in the frontal, temporal and parietal lobes in monkeys and exhibit a high degree of regional and laminar specificity. The highest densities were observed in the dorsolateral prefrontal areas, anterior cingulate, motor cortices and inferior

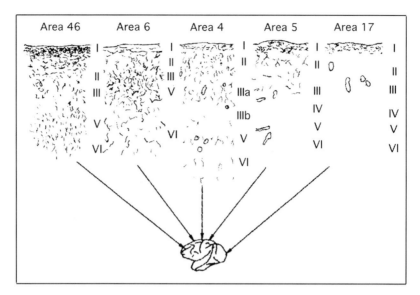

Fig. 7.2 Area difference of the density and bilaminar pattern of DA innervation. Camera Lucida drawings of DA-IR fibres observed on coronal sections in the prefrontal (area 46), frontal (area 4), parietal (are 5) and occipital (area 17) cortices of the macaque. Note that the bilaminar distribution pattern is conspicuous in agranular cortices (areas 46, 6 and 4) and also note the rostrocaudal gradient of decrease in density (Meada and Ikemoto 1995).

parietal lobes (Lewis et al. 1986). That is, the fibres were most dense in the anterior cingulate cortex and least dense in the visual cortex. The central sulcus formed a rough boundary between densely innervated and lightly innervated regions of the cortex. A bilaminar pattern of DA innervation was also bounded by the central sulcus (Maeda et al. 1995) (Fig 7.2).

The DA afferents were very dense in the medial wall of the hemisphere in monkey cortex, including the medial part of the supplementary motor area and cingulate cortex (areas 24 and 23) (Maeda et al. 1995) (Fig. 7.3).

The projections of each MA neuron are specific to the neurons within the nuclei from which they project, and each neuron targets one or more specific areas of the brain and subserves specific functions in each area (Baker and Halliday 1995). This has been studied extensively in DA neurons.

In humans, as in rodents, the DA neurons are located in three cell groups, A8, A9 and A10. Each group is further divisible into a number of regions: A8 includes the retrorubral field and the midbrain reticular fields; A9 includes the substantia nigra consisting of the pigmented pars compacta and the more ventrally positioned, non-pigmented pars reticulata; A10 includes the paranigral, parabrachial pigmented nuclei, the small interfascicular pigmented nucleus in the interpeduncular nucleus, the parapeduncular, caudal and rostral linear nuclei and the ventral tegmental area (VTA) (McRitchie and Halliday 1995). The range of

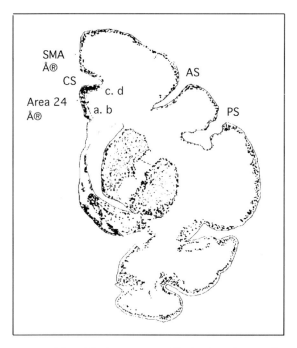

Fig. 7.3 Target of DA neurons of the midbrain Camera Lucida drawing of DA-IR fibres in a coronal section through the striatum. Dense innervation is present in the medial wall of the cerebral hemisphere including the supplementary motor cortex (SMA) and cingulate cortex (area 24). AS arcuate sulcus; CS, cingulate sulcus; PS, principal sulcus (Maeda and Ikemoto 1995).

morphological types of neurons throughout these regions correlates with the differential distribution of calcium binding proteins. That is, calbindin was found in medium sized bipolar, non-pigmented neurons, while calretinin was found in medium sized bipolar non-pigmented neurons and parvalbumin in small, non-pigmented multipolar neurons (Baker and Halliday 1995). In the macaca fuscata, the DA neurons in the midbrain are subdivided into two groups, one group located in the ventral and the other in the dorsal area (Maeda *et al.*, unpublished data). Those in the ventral area project to the cortex. In the dorsal tier of the monkey mesencephalon there are two kinds of DA neurons, calbindin positive (63%) and calbindin negative (37%) (Fig. 7.4). They are highly developed in primates and project to whole cortical areas. The DA projection to the cortex has a predominance of calbindin-D28. However in the cingulate cortex motor associated areas (4 and 24c,d) show lower percentage of calbindin-D28 (69%) as compared with the limbic area (area 24a,b, 91%). In the substantia nigra of macaca fuscata, parvalbumin positive neurons were located exclusively in the non-DA containing area (pars reticulata), the ventral area, while calbindin and calretinin positive neurons were distributed in both the dorsal (pars compacta) and ventral area of DA positive neurons (Fig. 7.4).

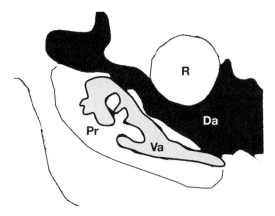

Fig. 7.4 Schematic illustration of the distribution of two types of DA neurons in the midbrain: calbindin positive and negative neurons (courtesy of Prof. Toshihiro Maeda). ■ DA containing area with calbindin D28 positive neurons; ☐ DA containing area with calbindin D28 negative neurons; Da dorsal area; Va ventral area; Pr pars reticulata; R red nucleus.

The MA neurons appear early in the developmental course of the brain.

In the human foetus cells destined for the future LC appear early around 32 days post-fertilization and those for the raphe nucleus appear in the septum medulla around 36–38 post fertilization days (Müller and O'Rahilly 1997).

Among DA containing cells, the ventricular zone (containing future cells of the interpeduncular nucleus) and the VTA have been shown by immunological methods to be the first regions to display TH-immunoreactivity in human embryos at about 6.5 (Freeman et al. 1991) or 7 weeks post-fertilization (Verney et al. 1991). The nigrostriatal fibres develop at about 7 post-fertilization weeks (Verney et al. 1991).

Using immunocytochemical techniques Zecevic and Verney (1995) examined the catecholaminergic (CA) cell groups and fibres in the human CNS from 6 to 13 gestational weeks. According to these authors, at 6 gestational weeks, TH-like immunoreactive (TH-IR) cell groups were widespread throughout the caudorostral extension of the CNS, corresponding to the different dopaminergic mesencephalic and hypothalamic groups. Noradrenergic groups also were labelled in the medulla oblongata and in the LC as well as in other areas in the pons. Additional TH-IR cell groups may represent a transient developmental expression of TH. Dopamine beta hydroxylase (DBH) immunoreactivity was found chiefly to label the noradrenergic pontine cell groups and to a lesser extent the groups of neurons located in the medulla oblongata. Rare phenylethanolamine-N–methyltransferase-IR neurons were detected in the medulla oblongata at 13 gestational weeks.

The main CA bundles described in the adult were also observed in human embryos and foetuses (Zecevic and Verney 1995).

At 6 gestational weeks, TH-IR pathways extended caudorostrally with the central tegmental tract and the dorsal tegmental bundle. At 7–8 gestational weeks the TH-IR fibres extended to the basal ganglia and the telencephalic wall. The first TH-IR and to a lesser extent DBH-IR fibres penetrated the frontal lateral cortical anlage through the intermediate zone and a few crossed through the marginal zone but did not pass through the thin cortical plate. The second stream entered the telencephalic anlage frontomedially, ventral to the septal area. At 11 gestational weeks, numerous TH-IR fibres invaded the subplate layer, but they penetrated the cortical plate only at 13 gestational weeks. At that time, TH-IR and DBH-IR fibres had reached the occipital cortex in a rostrocaudal gradient.

These studies showed a well-organized CA system already at the embryonic stages in man (Zecevic and Verney 1995). During the development of the brain these catecholaminergic neurons regulate the functional maturation of the cortex through their involvement in synaptogenesis and their regulatory or trophic roles affecting target neurons (Levitt *et al.* 1997: Müller *et al.* 1999).

In primates the MA ergic neurons have important roles among the afferents which are waiting for migrating neurons during the processes of columnar organization of the neocortex (Rakic 1995). In animals synaptogenesis in the cerebral cortex, modified by the 5HT neurons, occurs after birth (Mazer *et al.* 1997). This is seen in the 'barrel formation' of the fourth layer of the visual cortex. At this time a large number of axons project to the cortex and they disappear following the critical neonatal period (Koh *et al.* 1991). In humans this critical period corresponds to the 18 or 24 months after birth. Studies on autopsied brain show that the number of 5HT1A receptors in the frontal cortex is high in the foetal period and decreases in adulthood (Bar-Peled *et al.* 1991). These processes involving 5HT and NA neurons, particularly those occurring after birth, are regulated by environmental factors at critical ages, while in DA neurons the processes follow a timetable which is determined genetically.

MA neurons, particularly 5HT and NA neurons, have roles in stage setting. This is seen in the regulation of the sleep–wake (S-W) cycle. In this cycle both 5HT and NA neurons are active during wakefulness. During NREM sleep they reduce their activities but in sREM they become silent (Hobson *et al.* 1975). These cyclic activities provide the REM–NREM cycle (Hobson *et al.* 1975). However 5HT and NA act as opposing central neurochemical systems (Baker and Halliday 1995). NA neurons habituate to sensory stimuli, while 5HT neurons do not. NA neurons become active when an organism is active or stressed, while 5HT neurons do not. 5HT neurons are active during vegetative activities, whereas NA neurons are not (Jacobs and Azmitia 1992). In a mature brain, both 5HT and NA neurons are implicated in affective disorders and the DA neurons are involved in movement disorders and psychiatric illnesses, particularly disorders of thought. Early lesions of the MA neurons are known to cause behavioural disorders and to affect cognitive function after maturation (Levitt *et al.* 1997; Mazer *et al.* 1997; Müller *et al.* 1997).

7.3 Clinical and neurophysiological correlates reflecting the development of the activities of the MA neurons

Since most of the parameters of sleep are modulated by the MA neurons, functional development of the MA neurons in *man* can be studied through observation of the development of sleep parameters (Segawa 1999).

Examination of the foetus with ultrasound and of premature babies with polysomnography (PSG) revealed that the development of rapid eye movement sleep (sREM) starts with the periodic occurrence of twitch movements in the 20th gestational week and that almost all components of sREM and REM–non-REM (NREM) rhythm appear by the 36th week of gestation (Parmelee and Stern 1972; Segawa 1999), while the parameters of slow wave sleep (SWS) begin to develop in the later weeks of gestation. Although most components of sREM are modulated by cholinergic neurons, twitch movements are modulated by the nigrostriatal (NS)-DA neurons through the basal ganglia and its descending efferents (Segawa *et al.* 1987). This evidence suggests that the NS-DA neurons and related neuronal pathways modulating twitch movements in sREM begin to function around the 20th gestational week and the NA neurons of the LC which produce cyclic inhibition of the cholinergic neurons of the pons are almost mature by the end of the foetal period (Hobson *et al.* 1975). All the components of sREM mature completely by 3–4 months of post-natal age when atonia begins to appear restricted to this sleep stage (Segawa 1999). However the foetal period when the cyclic occurrence develops differs with regard to the components of sREM (Segawa 1999). This suggests that specific NA neurons prevent the occurrence of particular components of sREM in NREM and each has a distinct developmental course: that for twitch movements matures earliest and that for atonia the latest. The 5HT neurons are also thought to have an important role in prevention of the leakage of atonia into NREM (Segawa 1999).

In the period from around 38 gestational weeks until early infancy (3–4 months) there is developmental modulation in the components of sREM and also of the relationships between the parameters of sREM. This is observed in the development of burst occurrence of REMs and phasic inhibition of muscle activity by REMs bursts (Kohyama and Iwakawa 1991). The latter is considered to reflect the development of the NA neurons (Segawa 1999). This period is also the critical age for development of the S-W cycle, which is mainly modulated by 5HT neurons. From this period until early childhood modulation of phasic movements of the mentalis muscle is observed. Activities lasting >0.5 s decrease, while those lasting <0.5 s increase (Kohyama and Iwakawa 1991). The cholinergic neurons of the brainstem are thought to be involved in these processes (Kohyama and Iwakawa 1991). Development of the components of sleep, particularly those of SWS, continues into childhood and in this development all three MA neurons have important roles. It is possible however that these neurons involved in the development of sleep parameters in childhood may be different from those modulating developments of the parameters in the foetus and infant.

It should be noted that the process of development of the components of sREM and the REM–NREM cycle is genetically determined, while that of SWS, as well as that of the S-W cycle, is influenced by the epigenetic factors. For normal development of these parameters, specific and adequate environmental factors, including day–night light–dark cycle, are required at critical ages.

The neural pathway for atonia in sREM (Satai 1984) is considered to be the same pathway as for postural suppression or suppression of the antigravity muscles (Mori *et al.* 1992). Thus restriction of the atonia in sREM implies development of the neuronal pathway for postural augmentation that is, activation of the antigravity muscles. The 5HT and NA neurons, particularly the former, activate postural augmentation, and suppress the postural suppression pathways (Mori *et al.* 1992). Postural augmentation is necessary in order to execute locomotion and this is modulated by a neuronal system originating from the midbrain locomotor region (MLR) (Mori *et al.* 1992). In executing locomotion both 5HT and NA neurons also have important roles (Mori *et al.* 1992). Thus attainment of head control at 4 months and of crawling, a locomotor activity, around 8 months reflect the development of the brainstem MA neurons which modulate these antigravity activities, head control and locomotion, each at critical stage.

Autopsy studies have revealed high activity of TH at the terminals of the NS-DA neurons in early childhood which show exponential age-dependent decrement in the first three decades of life, whereas the activity of TH in the substantia nigra shows no apparent age variation (McGeer *et al.* 1973). The former can be observed in decremental change with age in the numbers of twitch movements during sREM, the sleep parameter which reflects the levels of the activities of the NS-DA neurons (Segawa and Nomura 1995). PET studies revealed the existence of an enormous number of DA-D_2 receptors in the third decade which decreased to base levels around the end of the decade (Antonini *et al.* 1993).

In man however, it is not exactly known how the specific development of these MA neurons is involved in the development of particular areas of the brain or how this modifies the particular functions of the brain at these critical periods. However since lesion studies in animal experiments indicate that a particular disorder of the CNS follows lesion of MA neuron at a particular point in its developmental course, I will try to illustrate this principle with illustrations from clinical observations of inherited or idiopathic disorders with early but non-progressive lesions of the MA neurons.

7.4 Involvement of the monoaminergic neurons in inherited or idiopathic neuropsychological disorders with onset in infancy and childhood

Since the involvement of MA neurons in Rett syndrome is discussed in Chapter 8, I will concentrate here upon some other disorders of the first three decades of life in which inherited or idiopathic lesions of the MA neurons are involved. These include infantile autism, Down's syndrome, Tourette's syndrome and dopa-responsive basal ganglia disorders. In these disorders there are no progressive degenerative changes in the CNS. Thus the explanation for the clinical features of these disorders appears to be specifically early lesion of the MA neurons.

Infantile autism shows delay in development of the circadian S-W cycle, hypotonia and abnormalities in locomotion from infancy (Segawa 1989). The abnormal S-W cycle is improved by strengthening of the day time environmental factor but more markedly by administration of 5-hydroxy-tryptophan (5HTP), the precursor of 5HT (Segawa 1989). PSGs and biochemical studies have shown hypofunction of the 5HT and the DA neurons occurring in early infancy (Segawa 1989) and brain PET (positron emission tomography) studies revealed upward regulation of the DA-D_2 receptors (Watanabe, personal communication). These imply early disturbance of 5HT and DA neurons in infantile autism (Segawa *et al.* 1992*b*). Abnormalities in the distribution of the axons of the inferior olivary nucleus in autopsied brain of infantile autism suggest that the abnormalities in the CNS develop before the 30th gestational week (Kemper and Bauman 1992).

In Down's syndrome 5HT neurons and 5HT1A receptors are decreased both in the cortex (Bar-Peled *et al.* 1991) and the brainstem (Fukumizu, personal communication). Coleman (1973) showed increased muscle tone in a patient with Down's syndrome after administration of 5HTP. Failure in locomotion observed in infancy, as well as reduced postural tone, suggests hypofunction of the 5HT neuron in Down's syndrome which develops early in development. (Segawa 1993: Segawa *et al.* 1998).

Leakage of the atonia from sREM into NREM sleep, that is the presence of atonic NREM in infants with Down's syndrome and in infantile autism, also suggests dysfunction of 5HT neurons in early infancy, before 3–4 months.

Tourette's syndrome is diagnosed when two or more motor tics and one or more phonic or vocal tics have continued for more than one year. In this syndrome co-morbidity with obsessive compulsive disorders is common. Most symptoms start in childhood around 6 years of age with motor tics and soon phonic or vocal tics appear. Obsessive compulsive disorders appear later, around the end of childhood. PSGs in Tourette's syndrome revealed reduction of twitch movements with amplitude of more than $20\,\mu V$ in sREM to around 30% of normal values (Fukuda *et al.* 1995). But the number of twitch movements with amplitude less than 20 µV is significantly increased (Nomura 1985). PSGs also showed a decrease in the number of gross movements in sREM but an increase during sleep stage I (Fukuda et al. 1995: Nomura 1985). These findings of PSGs imply DA receptor supersensitivity following hypofunction of the NS-DA neurons. Neuroimaging studies also revealed up-regulation of DA-D_2 receptors (Wolf et al. 1996). In Tourette's syndrome both the limbic system and the cortico-striato-thalamo-cortical circuit seem to be involved (Peterson et al. 1999). This implies involvement of the DA neurons projecting to the limbic striatum and the cingulate cortex. PSG studies also suggested reduced function of the 5HT neurons. There are leakages of atonia into NREM sleep and abnormalities of sleep structure with disturbance of slow wave sleep (SWS) (Nomura 1985). Disturbance of SWS induces disturbance of the circadian S-W cycle in late childhood including a delayed sleep stage syndrome (DSPS), disturbed 24 h S-W cycle with a free-running pattern, typically with a 25 h S-W cycle, or frequent disruption of night sleep with profound daytime sleep. As patients with Tourette's syndrome show normal development in the S-W cycle and of locomotion in infancy and early childhood, the 5HT neurons involved in this syndrome may be those with critical ages for development later in childhood.

Early lesions of the NS-DA neurons cause specific dopa-responsive basal ganglia disorders in the first three decades (Segawa 2000). These are hereditary progressive dystonia with marked diurnal fluctuation or strictly defined dopa-responsive dystonia (HPD/DRD) (Segawa's disease), dystonic type juvenile parkinsonism (dJP) (Yokochi) and autosomal recessive early onset parkinsonism with diurnal fluctuation (AR-EPDF) (Yamamura). Typical ages of onset in these disorders are in the first decade, early in the second decade and early in the third decade, respectively. All are inherited disorders. Segawa's disease is a dominantly inherited GTP-cyclohydrolase I (GCH-I) deficiency, caused by heterozygotic abnormalities of the gene of the enzyme located on 14q22.1-q22.2 (Ichinose et al. 1994). AR-EPDF is caused by a fault in parkin gene located on 6q25.2-q27 (Kitada et al. 1998: Matsumine et al. 1997). Segawa's disease with partial deficiency of GCH-I causes partial deficiency of tetrahydrobiopterin (BH_4), the cofactor of hydroxylases, among which TH, with the lowest affinity to BH_4 is affected rather selectively (Nomura et al. 1998). Neurohistochemical examination of Segawa's disease in an 18 year old female who died in a *traffic* accident revealed decrease of TH in the striatum but not in the substantia nigra and in the striatum DA was decreased predominantly in the ventral area of the caudate nucleus (Hornykiewicz 1995). In dJP TH and DA are reduced only at the terminal of the NS-DA neuron (Yokochi et al. 1984), but in AR-EPDF both TH and DA are decreased in the substantia nigra as well as in the striatum, whereas in these diseases pteridine metabolism is preserved. Moreover in AR-EPDF the DA decreases in the dorsal as well as in the ventral area of the striatum (Kondo et al. 1997). Neuropathologically there are no degenerative changes in Segawa's disease. Glial infiltration is observed in the substantia nigra in dJP and AR-EPDF, and Lewy bodies in that of dJP: however there are no degenerative changes in either disorder.

Although there is postural tremor, typically from around the fourth decade in Segawa's disease, postural dystonia is the main feature throughout its course. The dystonia starting in childhood, progresses markedly in the first one and one half decades but later progression slows with age and from the fourth decade it is stationary. Dystonic juvenile parkinsonism and AR-EPDF may show postural dystonia if they have onset in childhood but from around the middle of the second decade the features of parkinsonism predominate (Segawa and Nomura 1998).

7.5 Clinical correlates of the early disturbances in the monoaminergic neurons

In infantile autism and Down's syndrome, the behavioural and mental disabilities and the neurological and neurophysiological findings reflect the early involvement of brainstem MA neurons. Abnormalities in the S-W cycle, the presence of atonic NREM in the PSGs and abnormalities of inter-limb coordination or locomotion observed in these diseases are considered to be due to abnormalities of the 5HT neurons which develop in early infancy before 4 months and also in late infancy around 8 months and suggest involvement of these neurons in these disorders (Segawa et al. 1992a,b).

In typical infantile autism there is failure in communication during infancy. In early childhood there is insistence on sameness with extreme rote memory, specific language disturbance with echolalia which is soon followed by pronominal reversals, hyperkinesia, stereotypy and aggressive behaviour with or without self-mutilation. Apart from the last three, these behavioural abnormalities improved after normalization of the circadian S-W cycle by strengthening the daytime environmental stimulus for awakening (Segawa et al. 1992b). All these behavioural abnormalities also responded to 5HTP administered before 5 years (Segawa et al. 1992b). This seems to confirm the impression that they are due to hypofunction of the 5HT neuron and can be influenced by environmental factors. On the other hand, hyperkinesia, stereotypy and aggressive behaviour responded to a low dose of l-Dopa with 0.5 mg per kilogram per day without decarboxylase inhibitor (Segawa 1989: Segawa et al. 1992b). This is the dose which alleviates supersensitivity of DA receptors (Tanaka et al. 1983). These three behaviours were not improved by adjustment of the environment. This suggests involvement of the DA neuron with receptor supersensitivity in these three features.

In middle or late childhood, infantile autism shows delay in the determination of hand dominance with increase in left-handedness or an ambidextrous state. This suggests a delay in development of the functional lateralization of the cortex. Failure to close the eyes on command and to pronate and supinate are also observed. These are signs of developmental oro-facial apraxia and limb-kinetic apraxia, respectively and imply a delay in the development of functional specialization of the cortex.

Age at determination of hand dominance correlated with normalization of the circadian S-W cycle (Segawa *et al.* 1992b). The age when normal stepping emerged correlated with the disappearance of the signs suggesting developmental oro-facial and limb kinetic apraxia and these ages were significantly inversely correlated with intelligence quotients (IQ) (Segawa *et al.* 1998).

In Down's syndrome the IQ and developmental quotients also correlated inversely with ages at crawling and walking unsupported (Segawa *et al.* 1998). These levels were significantly and inversely correlated with the ages when atonic NREM disappeared (Segawa 1993: Segawa *et al.* 1998).

Patients with Tourette's syndrome were slow and clumsy in pronation and supination which induce rigidity on the contralateral arm. Stepping with closed eyes most patients rotated towards the clumsy side. These signs suggest reduction in DA neuron activity with consequent receptor supersensitivity (Nomura, in preparation). Patients, particularly those older than 10 years, with abnormalities in the circadian S-W cycles showed obsessive compulsive disorders. In particular, patients with DSPS were associated with failure in adaptation, such as school refusal. Tic symptoms, particularly simple motor and vocal tics, improved on a low dose of l-Dopa or DA receptor antagonists (Nomura, in preparation). This pharmacological evidence indicates that in Tourette's syndrome tics are caused by DA receptor supersensitivity. Obsessive compulsive disorders or behaviours were alleviated when the abnormal S-W cycle was improved by strengthening daytime awakening (Nomura, in preparation). These effects were age dependent and more marked in childhood. Hypofunction of the 5HT neurons is considered to be one of the causes of obsessive compulsive disorders in Tourette's syndrome (Anderson *et al.* 1999) as well as the disturbance of SWS with some S-W cycle abnormalities which occurs after late childhood.

The postural dystonia and other signs of Segawa's disease are reversed by a relatively low dose of l-Dopa (20 mg per kilogram daily with plain L-Dopa) unrelated to duration of the clinical course and sustained without side effects. The dose can be decreased after the 4th decade. *Postural* dystonia *and* parkinsonian symptoms in *dJP* and *AR-EPDF* also respond well to levodopa but 'on and off' phenomena and levodopa induced dyskinesia appear *soon but from around the middle of the second decade*. In these dopa-responsive disorders, neither the favourable effects nor the side effects of l-Dopa are influenced by environmental factors and are entirely dependent on the doses and the ages of administration (Segawa and Nomura 1998). This clinical evidence indicates that functional abnormalities of the NS-DA neurons and their response to L-dopa depend on the age of onset and relate to timing relative to the developmental programme of the NS-DA neurons.

7.6 Animal correlates of age-related human behaviour and specific behavioural abnormalities

In animals, early lesions of 5HT neurons lead to abnormal behaviour similar to early social isolation with impairment of instinctive behaviours (Valzelle 1978). These are comparable to the failure in development of social relatedness and accommodation to a novel environment in infantile autism, which are considered to be caused by early lesions of the 5HT neurons (see above).

Early lesions of the NA neurons impair developmental growth of the brain after birth (Brenner *et al.* 1983) and this is reminiscent of the stagnation of head growth in Rett syndrome. Early lesions of the dorsal bundle of LC-NA neurons cause failure in extinction of acquired memory while preserving memory function normally (Tanaka *et al.* 1987). This is reminiscent of the extreme rote memory with insistence on sameness observed in infantile autism. Animal experiment showed that in rat early DA neuron dysfunction in association with dysfunction of 5HT and NA neurons causes 'friendliness' (groom mice) in comfortable situations and 'muricide' (kill mice without the purpose of eating) in isolation (Valzelle and Garattini 1972). These could account for the particular selfishness with aggressive behaviour and self-mutilation observed in infantile autism in early childhood.

In animals early lesions of 5HT neurons induce abnormal cognitive function in adults (Levitt *et al.* 1997: Müller *et al.* 1997). Studies of infantile autism suggest that in man early lesion or hypofunction of the 5HT neurons causes delay in development of the S-W cycle in early infancy which leads to delay in the development of hand dominancy, that is in the functional lateralization of the cortex in early childhood (Segawa *et al.* 1992b). This shows that development of the circadian S-W cycle in early infancy has an important role for development of functional lateralization of the cortex (Segawa *et al.* 1992b).

In animals a 5HT lesion causes failure in the development of locomotion (Nakajima *et al.* 1998). In humans it may cause failure in the development of crawling or inter-limb coordination in late infancy and also leads to developmental oro-facial and limb-kinetic apraxia, that is to say abnormalities or delay in the development of the functional specialisation of the cortex. This also relates to lowering of IQ levels.

Then how do locomotor movements relate to the functional development of the brain? The neurons of the pedunculopontine nuclei (PPN) are considered key neurons in this process. The PPN executes locomotion with its descending projection and is known to have ascending projections. Kojima *et al.* (1997) showed that a unilateral excitotoxic lesion in the PPN of a monkey led to damage in the ipsilateral substantia nigra, decrease in TH activity and development of parkinsonian symptoms in the contralateral extremities. The PPN has been shown to have projections to the Meynert nucleus. The PPN is functionally activated by the 5HT and NA neurons. Early lesions in these MA neurons might cause dysfunction of the PPN and so of the Meynert nucleus leading to developmental abnormalities of the neocortex through disturbance in the processes of synaptogenesis.

These examples indicate that the 5HT neurons which modulate development of the circadian S-W cycle in early infancy and those involved in the execution of normal crawling in late infancy have specific roles in the development of neocortical function. These abnormalities become apparent in early childhood but not in infancy or before the age of 2 years. These two functions, biphasic circadian S-W cycle and locomotion with inter-limb coordination, are particularly important because they are observed only in humans. Furthermore, as observed in Tourette's syndrome, there seem to be other 5HT neurons which modulate SWS leads to disorders and various abnormalities the of S-W cycle or obsessive compulsive behaviors which become apparent in the second decade.

Studies of HPD revealed that depletion of BH_4 due to the reduction in GCH-I early in the developmental course leads to a decrease in the TH content in the terminals of NS-DA neurons and so to a decrease in the levels of DA chiefly in the ventral area of the striatum (Horneykiewicz 1993) where *striosome/patches* (Graybiel and Ragsdale 1978), that is D_1 receptors and the striatal direct pathways are prominent (Gibb. 1996). So in Segawa's disease the D_1 receptors of the striatal direct projection are rather selectively involved (Segawa and Nomura 1998). Early BH_4 deficiency in Segawa's disease may also reduce DA contents in the tubulo-infundibular DA neurons which connect to D_4 receptors (Segawa and Nomura 1998). D_4 receptors belong to the D_2 family but mature earlier than D_2 receptors (Nair and Mishra 1995). Through the DA-D_4 receptors, stagnation in linear growth appears in children with Segawa's disease. In AR-EPDF pteridine metabolism is not affected and the content of DA is decreased in the dorsal area of the striatum as well as in the ventral area (Kondo *et al.* 1997). Kondo *et al.* (1997) showed selective decrease in TH in the dorsal area of the striatum in an isolated case of JP who showed no clinical signs of dystonia and had no neurohistochemical abnormalities in pteridin metabolism. The dorsal area of the striatum is rich in the matrix compartment (Graybiel and Ragsdale 1978) of the indirect pathways (Gibb 1996). In AR-EPDF involvement of the D_2 receptors and the indirect pathways in addition to the direct pathways leads to parkinsonian symptoms and levodopa induced dyskinesia in addition to dystonia (Segawa and Nomura 1995).

These studies of dopa-responsive disorders suggest that decrease in TH due to the reduction of its cofactor BH_4 causes decrease of DA in the ventral striatum and chiefly affects D_1 receptors and the direct striatal pathway, while primary decrease of TH or that not due to deficiency of BH_4 affects the D_2 receptors and the indirect striatal pathway.

In animal experiments the projection of the patches/striosome to the substantia nigra matures earlier (Van der Kooy *et al.* 1987) and studies of voluntary saccades suggest that the functional maturation of the indirect pathways is attained around the middle of the second decade while that of the direct pathways occurs the early first decade (Fukuda 1996). With reduced TH activity restricted to the terminals of the NS-DA neurons, Segawa's disease and dJP develop symptoms in childhood and early in the first two decades as TH activity at the terminal undergoes age-related reduction. Segawa's disease develops in childhood through the D_1-direct pathways which have already matured whereas dJP develops its full manifestations in the second decade after functional maturation of the indirect pathways. With its main lesion in the substantia nigra and with involvement of the indirect pathways, AR-EPDF shows its characteristic features in the third decade, along with age-related decrease in D_2 receptors.

This suggests that there are at least two NS-DA neurons with different biochemical characteristics and different distribution of the axons in the striatum each with a distinct developmental course.

The level of neopterin is high in the brain in the early period of development (Yoshida *et al.* 2000). Excretion of neopterin in the urine is high in infancy and decreases to base levels around 5 years of age (Shintaku 1994). This suggests increased pteridine metabolism early in the development of the brain. Inherited disorders of pteridine metabolism other than Segawa's disease show L-Dopa-responsive postural dystonia but do not develop parkinsonism (Nomura *et al.* 1998). Thus for the NS-DA neurons, early increase of TH or DA activity due to increased pteridine metabolism may regulate D_1 and D_4 receptors in early childhood, whereas the primary increase of TH activity in late childhood and adolescence may be involved in regulation of D_2 receptors (Segawa and Nomura 1998). Each of these processes may be modulated by particular DA neurons which are regulated by specific genes.

Hypofunction of the DA neuron and related dopamine D_2 receptor supersensitivity may be involved in the pathogenesis of Tourette's syndrome and in infantile autism (Nomura, in preparation). However, the increased D_2 receptors in these disorders may not be those of the NS-DA neurons projecting to the striatal indirect pathways since, as mentioned above, these pathways are too immature to express specific clinical manifestations before 15 years. The limbic DA system with its high content of DA in childhood may be involved in the development of partially instinctive behaviours which are programmed by routine stresses imposed on children in daily life. In Tourette's syndrome, with reduced levels of DA, exposure to these stresses may lead to the limbic DA system executing the programmed behaviour with up-regulation of the D_2 receptors compensating for the decreased DA levels, so inducing the tic movements. Vocal tics are considered to be due to dysfunction of the limbic DA neurons which project to the cingulate cortex. It is known that tics sometimes develop in infantile autism but, interestingly, such patients tend to be relatively able.

Among DA neurons projecting to non-motor areas are some which project to the frontal cortex. Early dysfunction of these neurons should be expected to become apparent at later ages as seen in the hypofrontalization of Rett syndrome and the frontal spike discharges in EEGs of infantile autism, both of which are observed in later childhood. The NS-DA neuron modulates the supplementary motor area via the basal ganglia and thalamus and may also control purposeful hand use. By such a mechanism, early lesion of the supplementary motor area may lead to the loss of purposeful hand use in early childhood as observed in Rett syndrome (Segawa 1997).

This clinical evidence suggests that in man there are more than two types of DA neuron projecting to the non-motor area, each with a particular course of development.

Although it will require further investigation, evaluation of the clinical disorders with early MA disturbance has shown that in the human as well as in animals each MA neuron has a particular developmental course and specific roles in the functional maturation of particular parts of the brain. Moreover, for the development of the higher cortical function of the human being, the two age periods, early and late infancy, are both important. Development of the S-W cycle and crawling or locomotion at these periods provide important biological markers which reflect the development of the MA neurons involved in the development of the higher cortical functions.

References

Anderson, G.M., Leckman, J.F., and Cohen, D.J. (1999). Neurochemical and neuropeptide systems. In *Tourette's syndrome. Tics, obsessions, compulsions. developmental psychopathology and clinical care* (ed. J.F. Leckman and D.J. Cohen), pp. 261–81, John Wiley & Sons, New York.

Antonini, A., Leenders, K.L., Reist, H., Thomann, R., Beer, H.F., and Locher, J. (1993). Effect of age on D_2 dopamine receptors in normal human brain measured by positron emission tomography and ^{11}C-raclopride. *Archives of Neurology*, **50**, 474–80.

Baker, K.G. and Halliday, G.M. (1995). Ascending noradrenergic and serotonergic systems in the human brainstem. In *Neurotransmitters in the human brain* (ed. D.J. Tracey, G. Paxinos, and Jc. Stone), pp. 155–71. Plenum Press, New York.

Bar-Peled, O., Gross-Isseroff, R., Ben-Hur, H., Hoskins, I., Groner, Y., and Biegon, A. (1991). Fetal human brain exhibits a prenatal peak in the density of serotonin 5-HT1A receptors. *Neuroscience Letters*, **127**, 173–76.

Brenner, E., Mirmiran, M., Uylings, H.B.M., and Van Der Gugten, J. (1983). Impaired growth of the cerebral cortex of rats treated neonatally with 6-hydroxydopamine under different environmental conditions. *Neuroscience Letters*, **42**, 13–17.

Coleman, M. (1973). *Serotonin in Down syndrome*. Elsevier, Amsterdam.

Cooper, J.R., Bloom F.E., and Roth, R.H. (1991). *The Biochemical basis of neuropharmacology*. Oxford University Press, New York.

Freeman, T.B., Spence, M.S., and Boss, B.D. (1991). Development of dopaminergic neurons in the human substantia nigra. *Experimental Neurology*, **113**, 344–53.

Foote, S.L. and Morrison, J.H. (1984). Postnatal development of laminar innervation patterns by monoaminergic fibres in monkey (Macaca fascicularis) primary visual cortex. *Journal of Neurosicence*, **4**, 2667–80.

Fukuda, H. (1996). Changes of saccade in development and aging. *Advances in the neurological science (Tokyo)*, **40**, 462–70. (In Japanese).

Fukuda, H., Segawa, M., Nomura, Y., Nishihara, K., and Ono, Y. (1995). Phasic activity during REM sleep in movement disorders. In *Age-related dopamine-dependent disorders*, Monographs in Neural Science, Vol. 14 (ed. M. Segawa and Y. Nomura), pp. 69–76. Karger, Basel.

Gibb, W.R.G. (1996). Selective pathology, disease pathogenesis and function in the basa ganglia. In *Recent advances in clinical neurophysiology* (ed. J. Kimura and H. Shibasaki), pp. 1009–15. Elsevier, Amsterdam.

Goldman-Rakic, P.S. and Brown, R.M. (1982). Postnatal development of monoamine content and synthesis in the cerebral cortex of rhesus monkeys. *Brain Research*, **256**, 339–49.

Graybiel, A.M. and Ragsdale, C.W., Jr (1978). Histochemically distinct compartments in the striatum of human, monkey and cat demonstrated by acetylthiocholinesterase staining. *Proceedings of the National Academy of Sciences*, **75**, 5723–6.

Hobson, J.A., McCarley, R.W. and Wyzinzki, R.W. (1975). Sleep cycle oscillation: reciprocal discharge by two brainstem neuronal groups. *Science*, **189**, 55–8.

Hornykiewicz, O. (1995). Striatal dopamine in dopa-responsive dystonia. Comparison, with idiopathic Parkinson's disease and other dopamine-dependent disorders. In *Age-related dopamine-dependent disorders*, Monographs in Neural Science, Vol. 14 (ed. M. Segawa and Y. Nomura), pp. 101–8. Karger, Basel.

Ichinose, H., Ohye, T., Takahashi, E., Seki, N., Hori, T., Segawa, M., et al. (1994). Hereditary progressive dystonia with marked diurnal fluctuation caused by mutations in the GTP cyclohydrolase I gene. *Nature Genetics*, **8**, 236–42.

Jacobs, B.L. and Azmitia, E.C. (1992). Structure and function of the brain serotonin system. *Physiol. Review*, **72**, 165–229.

Kemper, T.L. and Bauman, M. (1992). Neuropathology of infantile autism. In *Neurobiology of infantile autism*, International Congress Series No. 965 (ed. H. Naruse and E.M. Ovnitz), pp. 43–57. Excerpta Medica, Elsevier, Amsterdam.

Kitada, T., Asakawa, S., Hattori, N., Matsumine, H., Yamamura, Y., Minoshima, S., et al. (1998). Mutations in the parkin gene cause autosomal recessive juvenile parkinsonism. *Nature*, **392**, 605–8.

Koh, T., Nakazawa, M., Kani, K., and Maeda, T. (1991). Investigation of origin of serotonergic projection to developing rat visual cortex: a combined retrograde tracing and immunohistochemical study, *Brain Research Bulletin*, **27**, 675–84.

Kohyama, J. and Iwakawa, Y. (1991). Interrelationships between rapid eye and body movements during sleep: polysomnographic examinations of infants including premature neonates. *Electroencephalography and Clinical Neurophysiology*, **79**, 277–80.

Kojima, J., Yamaji, Y., Matsumura, M., Nambu, A., Inase, M., Tokuno, H., et al. (1997). Excitotoxic lesions of the pedunculopontine tegmental nucleus produce contralateral hemiparkinsonism in the monkey. *Neuroscience Letters*, **226**, 111–14.

Kondo, T., Mori, H., Sugita, Y., Mizuno, Y., Mizutani, Y., and Yokochi, M. (1997). Juvenile Parkinsonian—clinical, neuropathological and biochemical study. *Movement Disorder*, **12**, S1 32.

Levitt, P., Harvey, J.A., Friedman, E., Simansky, K. and Murphy, H. (1997). New evidence for neurotransmitter influences on brain development, *Trends in Neuroscience*, **20**, 269–74.

Lewis, D.A., Campbell, M.J., Foote, S.L. and Morrison, J.H. (1986). The monoaminergic innervation of primate neocortex. *Human Neurobiology*, **5**, 181–8.

Maeda, T., Ikemoto, K., Satoh, K., Kitahama, K., and Geffard. M., (1995). Dopaminergic innervation of primate cerebral cortex—an immunohistochemical study in the Japanese macaque. In *Age related dopamine-dependent disorders*, Monographs in Neural Sciences, Vol. 14 (ed. M. Segawa and Y. Nomura), pp. 147–159. Karger, Basel.

Matsumine, M., Saito, M., Shimoda-Matsubayashi, S., Tanaka, H., Ishikawa, A., Nakagawa-Hattori, Y., *et al*. (1997). Localization of a gene for an autosomal recessive form of juvenile parkinsonism to chromosome 6q25.2–27. *American Journal of Human Genetics*, **60**, 588–96.

Mazer, C., Muneyyirci, J., Taheny, K., Raio, N., Borella, A., and Whitaker-Azmitia, P. (1997). Serotonin depletion during synaptogenesis leads to decreased synaptic density and learning deficits in the adult rat: a possible model of neurodevelopment disorders with cognitive deficits. *Brain Research*, **760**, 68–73.

McGeer, E.G., and McGeer, P.L. (1973). Some characteristics of brain tyrosine hydroxylase. In *New concepts in neurotransmitter regulation* (ed. J. Mandel) pp. 53–68. Plenum Press, New York.

McRitchie, D.A. and Halliday, G.M. (1995). Cytoarchitecture and chemistry of midbrain dopamine cell groups. In *Neurotransmitters in the human brain* (ed. D.J. Tracey, G. Paxinos, and Jc. Stone), pp. 115–27. Plenum Press, New York.

Müller, F. and O'Rahilly, R. (1997). Development of the human central neurons system. *Principles of neural aging* (ed. S.V. Dani, A. Hori, and G.F. Walter), pp. 175–91. Elsevier, Amsterdam.

Mori, S., Matsuyama, K., Kohyama, J., Kobayashi, Y., and Takakusaki, K. (1992). Neuronal constituents of postural and locomotor control systems and their interactions in cats. *Brain and Development*, **14**, S109–20.

Morrison, J.M. and Magistretti, J.P. (1983). Monoamines and peptides in cerebral cortex—contrasting principles of cortical organization. *Trends in Neuroscience*, **6**, 146–51.

Nair, V.D. and Mishra, R.K. (1995). Ontogenic development of dopamine D4 receptor in rat brain. *Development Brain Research*, **90**, 180–183.

Nakajima, K., Matsuyama, K. and Mori, S. (1998). Prenatal administration of para chlorophenylalanine results in suppression of serotonergic system and disturbance of swimming movements in newborn rats. *Neuroscience Research*, **31**, 155–69.

Nomura, Y. (1985). Tics–including Gilles de la Tourette syndrome. *Advances in neurological sciences (Tokyo)*, **29**, 265–75.

Nomura, Y., Uetake, K., Yukishita, S., Hagiwara, H., Tanaka, T., Tanaka, R., *et al*. (1998). Dystonias responding to levodopa and failure in biopterin metabolism. In *Advances in neurology*, Dystonia 3, Vol. 78 (ed. S. Fahn, D.C. Marsden, and M.R. DeLong), pp. 253–66. Lippincott-Raven Publishers, Philadelphia.

Parent, A., Poctras, D., and Dube, L. (1984). Comparative anatomy of central monoaminergic systems. In *Handbook of chemical neuroanatomy* (ed. A. Björklund and T. Hökfelt) Elsevier, Amsterdam.

Parmelee, A.H. Jr and Stern, E. (1972). Development of states in infants. In *Sleep and the maturing nervous system* (ed. C.D. Clement, D.P. Purpura, and F.E. Mayer), pp.199–228 Academic Press, New York.

Peterson, B.S., Leckman, J.F., Arnsten, A., Anderson, G.M., Staib, L.M., Core, J.C., *et al*. (1999). Neuroanatomical circuitry. In *TouretteÕs syndrome. Tics, obsessions, compulsions. developmental psychopathology and clinical care* (ed. J.F. Leckman and D.J. Cohen). pp. 230–60. John Wiley & Sons, New York.

Rakic, P. (1995). A small step for the cell, a giant leap for mankind: a hypothesis of neocortical expansion during evolution. *Trends in Neuroscience*, **18**, 383–88.

Sakai, K. (1984). Central mechanisms of paradoxical sleep. In *Sleep mechanism* (ed. A. Borbely and J.L. Valax), pp. 3–18. Springer-Verlag, Berlin.

Segawa, M. (1989). A neurological model of early infantile autism, *No-To-Hattatsu, (in Japanese)*, **21**, 170–80.

Segawa, M. (1993). Pathophysiology of Down Syndrome: Consideration from Clinical Neurology. *Neuropathology*, **13**, 301–3.

Segawa, M. (1997). The pathophysiology of Rett syndrome from the standpoint of early catecholamine disturbance. *European Child and Adolescent Psychiatry.* **6**, 56–60.

Segawa, M. (1999). Ontogeny of REM sleep. In *Rapid eye movement sleep.* (ed. B.N. Mallick and S. Inoue), pp. 39–50. Narosa Publishing House, New Delhi.

Segawa, M. (2000). Development of the nigrostriatal dopamine neuron and the pathways in the basal ganglia. *Brain and Development*, 22, supplement No. 1, S1–S4.

Segawa, M., Katoh, J., and Nomura, Y. (1992a). Neurology: as a window to brainstem dysfunction. In *Neurobiology of infantile autism* (ed. H. Naruse and E.M. Ovnitz), pp. 187–200. International Congress Service 965 Excepta, Amsterdam.

Segawa, M., Katoh, M., and Katoh, J., and Nomura Y. (1992b). Early modulation of sleep parameters and its importance in later behavior. *Brain Dysfunction*, 5, 211–223.

Segawa, M. and Nomura, Y. (1995). Hereditary progressive dystonia with marked diurnal fluctuation and dopa-responsive dystonia: pathognomonic clinical features. In *Age-related dopamine-dependent disorders*, Monographs in Neural Sciences, Vol. 14 (ed. M. Segawa and Y. Nomura), pp. 10–24. Karger, Basel.

Segawa, M. and Nomura, Y. (1998). Pathophysiology of hereditary progressive dystonia with marked diurnal fluctuation—its characteristics in contrast to other dopa-responsive disorders. In *Progress in Alzheimer's and Parkinson's diseases*, (ed. A. Fisher, *et al.*), pp. 363–9. Plenum Press, New York.

Segawa, M., Nomura, Y., Hikosaka, O., Soda, M., Usui, S., and Kase, M. (1987). Roles of the basal ganglia and related structures in symptoms of dystonia. In *The basal ganglia II* (ed. M.B. Carpenter and A. Jayaraman), pp. 489–504. Plenum Press, New York.

Segawa, M., Takano, M., Shimohira, M., Tanaka, R., Hachimori, K., and Nomura, Y. (1998). Locomotion in late infancy and development of higher cortical function at later ages. In *New development in child neurology* (ed. M.V. Perat), pp. 27–30. Monduzzi Editore, Bologna.

Takeuchi, Y. and Sano, Y. (1983). Immunohistochemical demonstration of serotonin nerve fibers in the neocortex of the monkey (Macaca fuscata). *Anatomical Embryology*, **166**, 155–68.

Shintaku, H. (1994). Early diagnosis of 6-pyruvoyl-tetrahydroptern synthase deficiency. *Pteridine* 5, 18–27.

Tanaka, S., Igawa, C., Ogiso, M., Nomura, Y. and Segawa, M. (1983). Epileptic seizure with rotational behavior in tuberous sclerosis—pathophysiological consideration. *Folia Psychiatrica Neurologica Japonica*, 37, 331–32.

Tanaka, S., Miyagawa, F., and Imai, T., and Hidano, T. (1987). Effects on learning of the lesion on the dorsal noradrenergic bundle. *Juntendo Medical Journal (Tokyo)*, 33, 271–72.

Valzelle, L. (1978). Affective behavior and serotonin. In *Serotonin in health and disease*, (The central nervous system), Vol. 3 (ed. W.B. Essman), pp. 145–201. Spectrum, New York.

Valzelle, L., and Garattini, S. (1972). Biochemical and behavioral changes induced by isolation in rats. *Neuropharmacology*, **11**, 17–22.

van der Kooy, D., Fishell, G., Krushel, L.A., and Jhonston, J.G. (1987). The development of striatal compartments: from proliferation to patches. In *The basal ganglia II* (ed. M.B. Carpenter and A. Jayaraman), pp. 81–98. Plenum, New York.

Verney, C., Zecevic, N., Nikolic, B., Alvarez, C., and Berger, B. (1991). Early evidence of catecholaminergic cell groups in 5- and 6 weeks old human embryos using tyrosine hydroxylase and dopamine-3-hydorozylase immunocytochemistry. *Neuroscience Letters*, 131, 121–24.

Wolf, S.S., Jone, D.W., Knable, M.B., Gorey, J.G., Lee, K.S., Hyde, T.M., *et al.* (1996). Tourette syndrome: prediction of phenotypic variation in monozygotic twins by caudate nucleus D2 receptor binding. *Science*, 273, 1225–7.

Yokochi, M., Narabayashi, H., Izuka, R., and Nagatsu, T. (1984). Juvenile parkinsonism—some clinical, pharmacological and neuropathological aspects. In *Advances in neurology*, Vol. 40 (ed. R.G. Hassler and J.F. Christ), pp. 407–13. Lippincott-Raven, Publishers, Philadelphia.

Yoshida, Y., Eda, S. and Masada, M. (2000). Alterations of Tetrahydrobiopterin Biosynthesis and Pteridine Levels in Mouse Tissues during Growth and Aging. *Brain and Development*, 22, supplement No. 1, S45–S49.

Zecevic, N., and Verney, C. (1995). Development of catecholamine neurons in human embryos and foetuses, with special emphasis on with innervation of cerebral cortex. *Journal of comparative neurology*, 351, 509–35.

8 The monoamine hypothesis in Rett syndrome

Yoshiko Nomura and Masaya Segawa

Since the brainstem neural systems which develop before the 36th gestational week seem to be normal in Rett syndrome but those which mature between that gestational week and the end of the 2–3 postnatal months seem to be abnormal, we must assume that the onset of Rett syndrome lies within this period.

Summary

It is proposed that Rett syndrome (RS), a neurodevelopmental disorder, is due to early lesion of the monoamine neurons. The sleep-wake rhythm and sleep components indicate hypofunction of the noradrenergic and serotonergic neurons which develop between the 36th gestational week and 2–3 postnatal months. Deficiency of dopamine neurons follows with subsequent receptor supersensitivity. The early monoaminergic abnormalities cause later failure in cortical synaptogenesis. Cholinergic neurons seem to be preserved initially.

Mutations in the gene encoding methyl-CpG-binding protein 2 (MeCP2) were found to cause RS. The mutated gene abnormally regulates the expression of target genes, probably involving monoamine systems, initially from the 36th gestational week to 2–3 postnatal months, then with spatial and temporal specificity.

8.1 Introduction

Rett syndrome (RS) is a unique neurodevelopmental condition predominantly affecting females and presenting with characteristic symptoms and signs. It is caused by mutation in the gene encoding X-linked methyl-CpG-binding protein 2 (MeCP2) (Amir *et al.* 1999) but its pathophysiology still remains to be clarified.

Because of the presence of the regressive period in the course of the disorder it had been thought of as a degenerative disorder (Rett 1977). Based on the analysis of the clinical symptoms and signs from early infancy to the later stage of the clinical course, we emphasized that it is rather a peculiar disorder in the development of the central nervous system (Nomura *et al.* 1984, 1985, 1987; Nomura and Segawa 1986).

Evaluation of the clinical features and application of polysomnography (PSG) examinations led us to speculate that the disorder is due to deficiency of the monoaminergic (MA) neurons occurring at an early stage in the development of the brain (Nomura *et al.* 1984, 1985, 1987; Nomura and Segawa 1986; Segawa and Nomura 1990, 1992). In this chapter we will review the publications on MA neurons in RS, summarize our own original clinical and neurophysiological observations and finally discuss the pathophysiology of RS from the standpoint of the MA hypothesis.

8.2 Studies of monoamines and Rett syndrome

Almost all the characteristic features of RS were described in the original articles by Andreas Rett (Rett 1966, 1977). There he stressed that its clinical characteristics start after a certain period of apparently normal development and later take a progressive course. He initially considered hyperammonaemia to be a prominent feature (Rett 1966, 1977). In fact with later evaluation hyperammonaemia was not confirmed as a cardinal laboratory finding in general (Riederer *et al.* 1985; Percy *et al.* 1985).

From the initial neuropathological examinations, Rett described delay in the development of melanin pigmentation in the brainstem neurons (Rett 1977). This was the very first description implicating the involvement of the MA system in this disorder. The MA hypothesis for the pathophysiology of RS, as first proposed by us, was based on analyses of the clinical features and the sleep parameters obtained from PSG (Nomura *et al.* 1984, 1985, 1987; Nomura and Segawa 1986; Segawa and Nomura 1990, 1992). The data are summarized in a later section of this chapter.

In the first workshop organized by Andreas Rett in Vienna in April 1983, Walther Birkmayer pointed out the importance of the role of the basal ganglia for understanding the very characteristic motor signs of RS. He described a case with akinesia who showed paradoxical movement and discussed the similarity with aspects of the motor signs of RS (Birkmayer, unpublished thesis, 1983). At that conference Nomura showed the data on biopterin metabolism, serum levels of biopterin and neopterin of 9 cases of RS and 10 age matched disease controls. There were no differences between levels but the ratio of biopterin against neopterin was higher in RS. This suggested the possibility of involvement of

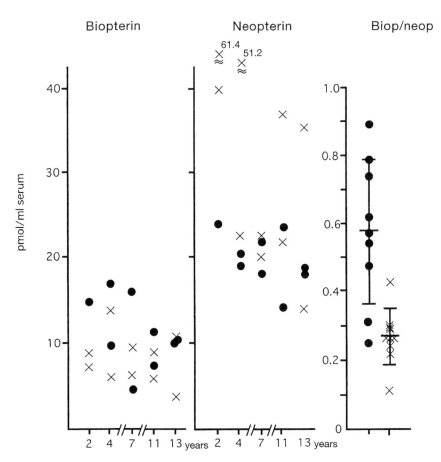

Fig. 8.1 Levels of serum biopterin (pmol/ml serum) and neopterin (pmol/ml serum) in Rett syndrome and pathological controls. ● Rett syndrome (*N*=9); × Disease control (*N*=10).

catecholamine metabolism but needed more study particularly in reference to the normal controls (Fig. 8.1) (Nomura *et al.*, unpublished thesis, 1983, Chapter 5.4).

In a second workshop organized again by Andreas Rett in 1984, we further extended our clinical analyses and PSG studies and suggested that the deficiency of MA in the brainstem and midbrain in the early period of development accompanied by dopamine (DA) receptor supersensitivity formed the pathophysiological basis of RS (Nomura *et al.* 1985). At this meeting biochemical data were presented by Riederer *et al.* (1985) revealing no severe changes in peripheral neurotransmitter synthesis and turnover; however autopsy of the brain in an advanced case showed severe reduction of biogenic amine synthesis with enhanced turnover and reduced DA-D2 receptor activity in the putamen. This early work encouraged research on the possible role of the biogenic amines in the pathogenesis of RS and gave direction to the MA hypothesis.

Evaluation of MA metabolites in the cerebrospinal fluid (CSF) showed reduced homovanillic acid (HVA) (Percy et al. 1985, 1987; Zoghbi et al. 1985, 1989), 3-methoxy-4-hydroxyphenylethylglycol (MHPG) (Zoghbi et al. 1989) and 5-hydroxyindoleacetic acid (5-HIAA) (Zoghbi et al. 1989; Nielsen et al. 1992). Reduced MA metabolites were reported only in the oldest patient aged of 15 years 2 months (Budden et al. 1990) and reduced HVA in the younger patients (Nielsen et al. 1992). There were also reports however showing normal MA metabolites in the CSF (Harris et al. 1986; Perry et al. 1988; Lekman et al. 1990; Budden et al. 1990; Nielsen et al. 1992). CSF tetrahydrobiopterin (BH4) was reported to be elevated (Zoghbi et al. 1989).

A study of MA metabolism by positron emission tomography (PET) was performed in a case aged 25 years. This revealed low normal range of DA-D2 receptor binding activity in the caudate measured by $[^{11}C]$-N-methylspiperone (Harris et al. 1986; Wagner 1986). Single photon emission computer tomography (SPECT) was used to measure the binding potential of 1231-iodolisuride, a specific D2 ligand. This study demonstrated significantly increased binding in RS and suggested increased density of D2 receptors due to reduced DA neurotransmission (Chiron et al. 1993).

Detailed neuropathological examination revealed reduced pigmentation of the substantia nigra (SN) as the most conspicuous finding. There were fewer well-pigmented neurons and fewer pigmented granules per neuron for age, while the total number of nigral neurons and the triphasic substructure of neuromelanin were normal for age. Furthermore the report indicated that no pathological changes were seen in the locus ceruleus, basal nucleus of Meynert (BNM) or nucleus dorsalis raphe (Jellinger and Seitelberger 1986; Jellinger et al. 1988).

Another postmortem examination showed that the concentration of kynurenine, the first stable compound in the tryptophan-nicotinamide pathway, showed increased concentration in the putamen, caudate nucleus, globus pallidus, raphe and amygdaloid nuclei. In contrast, 5-hydroxytryptamine (5HT, serotonin) and its metabolite, 5-HIAA, were below normal levels and DA-D2 receptor numbers were decreased in the putamen while their affinity was marginally increased as measured by $[^{3}H]$-spiroperidol (Riederer et al. 1986).

Further postmortem biochemical evaluation showed severe reduction of DA, noradrenaline (NA) and 5HT in most brain regions, and increase in the ratios of 3,4-dihydroxyphenyl acetic acid (DOPAC)/DA, HVA/DA and 5-HIAA/5HT, indicating increased metabolism of DA and 5HT and decreased $[^{3}H]$-spiroperidol binding in putamen (Brucke et al. 1987). Another examination showed differences in the biogenic amines, DA, 5HT and NA, according to age. The metabolites HVA and 5-HIAA measured in autopsied brains showed a decrease in the SN of the older patients but those in younger patients were normal (Lekman et al. 1989).

The number of DA-D2 receptors was decreased in the putamen (Riederer et al.

1986; Wenk 1995) but the number of D1 receptors in the caudate was unchanged (Wenk 1995). The DA uptake site was decreased in the caudate and putamen but unchanged in the cingulate and midfrontal gyri (Wenk 1995). Another report, however, suggested normal DA transporter in the caudate and putamen in RS (Wong et al. 1996).

These biochemical data on autopsied brains were compatible with the consistent neuropathological findings of decreased melanin content in SN neurons (Jellinger and Seitelberger 1986; Lekman et al. 1989; Kitt et al. 1990; Kitt and Wilcox 1995) and in agreement with the idea that a defect in the maturational process of the central monoaminergic system underlies the pathophysiology of RS.

The clinical features and results of CSF, biochemical, neuroimaging and neuropathological studies of MA metabolism stimulated further research. Histopathological studies of the cerebral cortex showed selective changes suggesting arrest of brain development in the early postnatal period (Armstrong 1992, 1995; Armstrong et al. 1995; Chapter 3). The neurons in the cerebral cortex showed normal layer specific arrangement but they were small with increased cell packing density throughout the brain and no active degeneration, suggesting curtailment of diffuse brain development from before birth (Bauman et al. 1995). The pathological findings in the basal ganglia are characterized by greater severity in the intermediate part of pallidum which is thought to represent the upper extremities (Belichenko et al. 1997). Endogenous levels of DA were decreased in superior frontal and superior temporal gyri, occipital cortex and putamen (Wenk et al. 1991, 1993; Wenk 1995).

The unchanged DA uptake in the midfrontal and cingulate cortex in spite of the decreased DA activity in the basal ganglia suggested that DA activity in the cortex may increase to compensate for fewer terminals with less DA (Wenk 1995). In 1996 the same author presented evidence conflicting with his earlier findings and suggested altered cholinergic function (Wenk 1996). In several cortical and subcortical regions, choline acetyltransferase (ChAT) activity was decreased, associated with decreased numbers of basal forebrain cholinergic cells (Wenk et al. 1993; Wenk 1996, 1997), and it was further speculated that the cholinergic cells fail to produce the ChAT enzyme due to failure to respond to a nerve growth factor (Wenk et al. 1999).

In 1995 Kaufmann et al. reported immunohistochemical investigations indicating decreased expression of microtubule-associated protein 2 (MAP-2) immunoreactivity throughout the neocortex. MAP-2 immunoreactivity was virtually undetectable in the white matter. These findings together with normal γ-aminobutyric acid (GABA) and peptidergic profiles were interpreted as indicating a marked disruption of a major cytoskeletal component in the neocortex. Since MAP-2 expression appears early in the neuronal maturation of the neocortex, these reported abnormalities in RS suggest a developmental disturbance involving several neurotransmitter systems particularly DA and cholinergic afferents regulating expression of MAP-2 (Kaufmann *et al.* 1995). The possible cholinergic deficit in RS was emphasized since a similar reduction of MAP-2 in the cortex was observed later in life in mice which had received neonatal lesions to the basal forebrain (Kaufmann *et al.* 1997).

8.3 Our own observations

8.3.1 Clinical characteristics (see Chapter 1)

(a) *Onset and early symptoms and signs of Rett syndrome*
The onset of RS is in the early part of infancy (Nomura *et al.* 1984, 1985, 1987). The deviation from normal in early infancy is very subtle except in severe cases who are obviously abnormal from birth, and our retrospective questionnaire to mothers of RS patients revealed autistic features among the earliest characteristics of the behaviour (Nomura *et al.* 1984, 1985, 1987; Nomura and Segawa 1990). The most frequent of these early autistic behaviours was pervasive lack of social relatedness and delay in development of sleep-wake rhythm (SWR) being characterized by profound daytime sleep. Decreased postural muscle tone with normal deep tendon reflex was found to be another sign characteristic of RS in early infancy (Nomura *et al.* 1984, 1985, 1987; Nomura and Segawa 1990). These behavioural and motor signs are shared by RS and early infantile autism (EIA) (Segawa 1982) and we suggest the existence of the common pathophysiological mechanism with autism in the initial stages of RS.

The developmental milestones show delay in gaining head control in the most severely affected cases but in the majority the delay is seen only after rolling over. The difficulty in crawling is most distinctive (Nomura *et al.* 1984, 1985, 1987; Nomura and Segawa 1990) indicating involvement of the locomotor system in RS (Nomura *et al.* 1984, 1985, 1987; Nomura and Segawa 1990).

(b) *The Characteristic features of RS*
These appear within specific age ranges and include behavioural, mental, cognitive, motor and autonomic signs. The autistic behaviours observed in the early period become less noticeable as the child grows (Nomura *et al.* 1984, 1985, 1987) and tests for developmental quotient (DQ) reveal rather severe retardation. The motor signs are most striking and stand out as the hallmark of RS (Nomura *et al.* 1984; Nomura and Segawa 1990, 1992). Among these the stereotyped hand movements are the core signs of RS. Their appearance is often preceded by the loss of purposeful hand use.

In RS the development of hand function is delayed after mid-infancy, that is, most patients have the ability to reach out and to grasp an object but often are unable to perform the pincer grasp. Hand to hand transfer is also difficult. Handedness is often undetermined and girls are commonly ambidextrous (Nomura and Segawa 1990, 1992, Chapter 1).

Long before the onset of the hand stereotypy, patients with RS show excessive or abnormal behaviour of the hands and mouth, such as patting the hands or licking. Hypersalivation and bruxism are also common features. The pathognomonic hand wringing movements appear between late infancy and early toddler age. Initially, they are rather simple patterns and they often change into complicated movement. They frequently occur in front of the chest or near the mouth in the midline. The hand stereotypy of RS is characterized by a fixed position of each hand and later accompanied by dystonic posture (Nomura *et al.* 1984, 1985; Nomura and Segawa 1990, 1992).

The gait abnormality initially described as gait apraxia by Rett (Rett 1977) is another characteristic symptom and we believe it to be a part of the abnormality of locomotion (Nomura *et al.* 1984, 1985; Nomura and Segawa 1990, 1992).

In later childhood scoliosis develops and dystonic postures of the extremities become more noticeable (Nomura and Segawa 1990, 1992). Epilepsy usually starts from late infancy to early childhood. Infantile spasm is rare. The growth of the head is also characteristic; it develops normally in the earlier half of infancy but stagnation begins in most patients in the later half of infancy.

8.3.2 Neurophysiological evaluation: abnormalities of sleep-wake rhythm and sleep components (refer also to Chapter 7)

Analyses of the neurological symptoms and signs suggest that abnormality of the monoaminergic system is involved in the pathophysiolgy of RS (Nomura *et al.* 1984, 1985, 1987; Nomura and Segawa 1986; Segawa 1997). To study this we analysed sleep-wake rhythm (SWR) using a day by day plot method recorded by mothers and performed PSG. SWR and each sleep parameter are known to be controlled by and to reflect function of the brainstem MA neurons and midbrain DA neurons (McCarley and Hobson 1971; Sakai 1984; Hobson *et al.* 1974, 1975; Segawa *et al.* 1986). The outline of the physiological background of these phenomena and the results of our studies in RS are shown below (Nomura *et al.* 1984, 1985, 1987; Nomura and Segawa 1986; Segawa and Nomura 1990, 1992).

(a) *Sleep-wake rhythm*
The generator of the endogenous circadian oscillation in man and rodent is in the suprachiasmatic nuclei at the base of the hypothalamus (Swaab *et al.* 1985). In normal infants the circadian SWR develops by 16 weeks of age synchronizing to a 24 h day-night cycle (Parmelee and Stern 1972). A lesion of the dorsal raphe nucleus in animals during early development led to persistent disturbances in the adjustment of endogenous circadian rhythms to a 24 hour light and dark cycle

(Takahashi *et al.* 1986). This indicates that the dorsal raphe 5HT neurons have an important role as synchronizer in early development of the SWR. It is also known that hypofunction of the NA neurons can disturb SWR with reduction in waking levels.

The SWR in RS showed irregularity in the time of waking up and of falling asleep at night and also profound daytime sleep by comparison with normal children of that age. This abnormal SWR continued into later childhood even after 10 years of age. The free running pattern was not observed in RS. Environmental stimulation or strengthening time cues for waking in daytime was not effective in correcting the abnormal SWR in RS. In contrast, in early infantile autism (EIA) a free running pattern is often found and environmental stimulation was effective to some extent in improving the abnormal SWR (Segawa 1982).

The abnormal SWR in RS was not corrected by the administration of l-threo 3,4-dihydroxyphenylserine (l-threo-DOPS) (a chemical precursor of NA) (Nomura *et al.* 1985, 1987), 5-hydroxytryptophan (5HTP) (Nomura *et al.*1985) or levodopa (Nomura *et al.* 1985, 1987). This indicates that in RS the dysfunction of either 5HT or NA neurons had been present before 16 weeks of age or that RS people lack sensitivity of response to environmental stimulation due to damage in early development. In contrast administration of melatonin was found to result in improved night-time sleep and increased arousal in daytime (McArthur and Budden 1998; Nomura and Segawa, unpublished theses, 1999; Chapter 5.3).

(b) *Polysomnography*

The rapid eye movement (REM)-non-rapid eye movement (NREM) cycle reflects the reciprocal activation of two cell groups in the brainstem: paradoxical sleep (PS) 'on-cells' which are cholinergic neurons of the giant cellular area of the pontine reticular formation and PS 'off-cells' which are NA neurons of the locus ceruleus (McCarley and Hobson 1971; Hobson *et al.* 1974, 1975; Sakai 1984).

These cholinergic neurons, PS on-cells, produce stage REM (sREM) by executing most components of sREM. In animal experiments, ponto-geniculo-occipital (PGO) spikes, discharges which are coordinated with rapid eye movements (REMs) in sREM, are triggered by PGO executive nuclei located in the caudal mesencephalic and rostral pontine tegmental structures and are cholinergic neurons. These are part of the mesencephalic reticular formation area in and around the brachium conjunctivum. The activating discharges project to the occipital cortex via the lateral geniculate nucleus, the pulvinar and the central lateral nucleus of thalamus. The atonia associated with sREM is also executed by the cholinergic neurons located in the dorsal tegmentum. Excitation of these cholinergic neurons is directed to the nucleus reticularis magnocellularis via the lateral tegmentoreticular tract, from which they project to the inhibitory interneurons of the spinal cord via the ventrolateral reticulospinal tract. This inhibition decreases the activity of anterior horn cell outflow and leads to axial atonia. On the other hand the NA neurons of locus ceruleus, with the 5HT neurons of the dorsal raphe nucleus, PS off-cells, show periodic activation by feed forward mechanism.

The ascending and descending excitatory cholinergic systems are under inhibitory regulation at multiple levels by projection from NA and 5HT systems. The NA and 5HT systems by increasing the discharges in NREM sleep inhibit cholinergic activity and prevent the occurrence of the components of sREM in NREM stages (McCarley and Hobson 1971; Hobson 1983; Sakai 1984).

During development almost all the components of sREM are restricted to sREM by 36 gestational weeks with the exception of axial atonia which becomes restricted to sREM by 2–3 months postnatally (Parmelee and Stern 1972; Segawa 1999). This suggests that the cholinergic system controlling the parameters associated with sREM, and 5HT and NA systems which prevent the REM associated components leaking into the NREM stage becomes mature by those ages.

In RS the components of sREM are present normally from the early stage but they tend to leak out to NREM stages, as shown by the appearance of axial atonia and REMs in NREM stages. This suggests that in RS the sREM executing cholinergic neurons of the pons are not affected, whereas activity is reduced in the neurons of the locus ceruleus and the dorsal raphe nuclei, failing to prevent the leakage of the components of sREM into the NREM stage.

Normally the ratio of sREM to slow wave sleep (SWS) in total night sleep decreases with age. In RS no abnormalities were observed in percentage of sleep stage (% sleep stage) in the younger cases, but in the older cases percentage of sREM (% sREM) was higher and percentage of SWS stage (% SWS) was lower than in normal subjects and showed irregularity of rhythm indicating the reverse of the normal developmental pattern.

Normal sleep structure in one night's sleep is characterized by prominent SWS in the earlier half of the sleep and sREM in the later half of the sleep. In younger girls with RS the sleep structure showed the normal nocturnal alteration and distribution of each sleep stage. In older RS patients this normal sleep structure was lost with decrease of nocturnal variation of SWS and the abnormally prominent % sREM with age.

The abnormal REM-NREM cycle observed in older people with RS suggests either the dysfunction of cholinergic or of noradrenergic neurons. The abnormal increase of REM sleep with age and the abnormal phasic components of sREM which also develop in older RS as described below can cause an abnormal REM-NREM cycle. These findings suggest that the abnormal REM-NREM cycle in RS may be caused by DA dysfunction.

Body movements during sleep reflect the function of specific neuronal systems. Two types of body movements were evaluated during sleep: gross movements (GMs), involving the axial muscle and muscles of extremities lasting more than 2 s, and twitch movements (TMs), localized in one muscle and lasting less than 0.5 s.

GMs are controlled by the ascending efferents and TMs by the descending efferents of the basal ganglia (Segawa et al. 1986). The numbers of TMs in sREM reflect the activities of nigrostriatal (NS)-DA neurons (Segawa et al. 1986, 1987) while the NS-DA neurons decrease the number of REMs (Segawa et al. 1987; Segawa and Nomura 1991) and regulate the sleep stage dependent occurrence of GMs by projection to the thalamus (Segawa et al. 1986, 1987; Uchiyama et al. 1987). The modulation of TMs reaches maturity around 3 months of age and of GMs around 8–10 months of age (Fukumoto et al. 1981).

Early DA lesions during the fetal period in animals lead to later exaggeration of TMs during sleep and increase of % sREM, which are the opposite of normal development (Mirmiran 1986; Segawa 1999; Fukuda et al. 1995). These altered phasic and tonic components of sleep are due to the occurrence of DA receptor supersensitivity due to the early lesion of the DA neurons. These components, regulated by the DA neurons, are not influenced by environmental factors but are thought to be determined by innate or genetic factors.

In younger cases with RS the sleep stage dependent modulation of GMs showed a normal pattern, that is the numbers per hour in each sleep stage was highest in stage 1, next in sREM and lowest in SWS stages. In older people with RS the pattern became abnormal with a decrease in the rate of occurrence in sREM (Nomura and Segawa 1986).

TMs of the mentalis muscle were normal in number and pattern against the sleep stages in younger RS groups, showing the highest rate of occurrence in sREM, next in stage 1 and lowest in SWS stages, while at older ages a marked increase was observed in the number of occurrences in each sleep stage although the pattern remained normal. On the other hand the number of TMs of the extremities was significantly greater in the younger cases and fewer in the older cases although still above the normal range (Nomura and Segawa 1986).

Markedly increased TMs in the mentalis muscles with age together with the development of abnormal sleep stage dependent modulation of GMs in girls with RS who are older than 5 years suggest the development of DA receptor supersensitivity (Nomura and Segawa 1986; Segawa and Nomura 1990, 1992), affecting the particular DA neurons involving axial muscles. In one case aged 3 years 11 months, administration of l-threo-DOPS led to a reduction in the number of TMs to within the normal range and also normalized the pattern but did not alleviate the abnormalities of GMs (Nomura et al. 1985, 1987).

Normally, except in early infancy, TMs do not appear during the period of REMs burst, that is REMs occurring at intervals of less than 1 s. The ratio of TMs during the period of REMs burst against total number of TMs in sREM, calculated as phasic inhibition index (PII), decreases markedly in the first 4 months and becomes almost zero by 1 year of age (Kohyama and Iwakawa 1991; Kohyama et al. 1995). In cases with lesion of NA neurons TMs are abnormally observed in REMs burst period (Segawa and Nomura 1990).

In RS an increase of PII was observed in younger cases and this further increased abnormally in older cases, suggesting dysfunction of the NA neurons in RS. A precursor of NA, l-threo-DOPS was effective in reducing this ratio in one case and supports this notion (Nomura *et al.* 1987).

Taking these observations into account, the findings of the SWR and PSG studies in RS indicate the presence of hypofunction of 5HT, NA and DA neurons followed by DA receptor supersensitivity; however the cholinergic neurons in the brainstem were thought to be preserved initially, at least until early infancy. Since the brainstem neural systems which develop before the 36th gestational week seem to be normal in RS but those which mature between that gestational week and the end of the 2–3 postnatal months seem to be abnormal, we must assume that the onset of RS lies within this period. The sequential age related abnormalities documented by PSG in RS reflect manifestation of the lesions from specific caudal to rostral neuronal systems (Nomura *et al.* 1984, 1985).

8.4 Discussion

8.4.1 Pathophysiology of Rett syndrome (Fig. 8.2)

The studies of sleep components indicate the onset of RS between 36 gestational weeks and 2–3 postnatal months and suggest that the initial disturbances of RS are hypofunction of the locus ceruleus and raphe nucleus leading to decreased NA and 5HT, delaying development of SWR and causing lack of interest in the environment. In EIA similar features are observed in the early stages. The delay in the development of SWR leads to delay in the development of functional lateralization and the delay in development of locomotion leads to delay in the development of specialization of the cortex in early childhood (Segawa 1997).

The descending pathways of NA and 5HT are known to give off collaterals to both the cervical and the lumbar spinal cord (Hayes and Rustioni 1981; Martin *et al.* 1981; Huisman *et al.* 1980, 1982). The function of these pathways is to exert a facilitatory action and determine the overall responsiveness of the motoneurons and the interneurons in the intermediate zone of the spinal cord (Kuypers 1985).

In animals normal locomotion is executed by activation of the midbrain locomotion region or pedunculo-pontine nuclei (PPN) in the rostral pons through the descending reticulospinal tracts and is suppressed by the postural suppression pathway which begins in the nucleus reticularis pontis oralis (NRPo) in the rostral pons (Mori *et al.* 1992). Locomotion is also known to be under chemical control; for example, in a decerebrated cat injection of carbachol, a cholinomimetic agent, into the NRPo suppresses induced locomotion, and injection of 5HT or NA into the NRPo restores it with increase in postural tone (Mori *et al.* 1992). This pathway which is involved in postural suppression is the same as that mediating axial

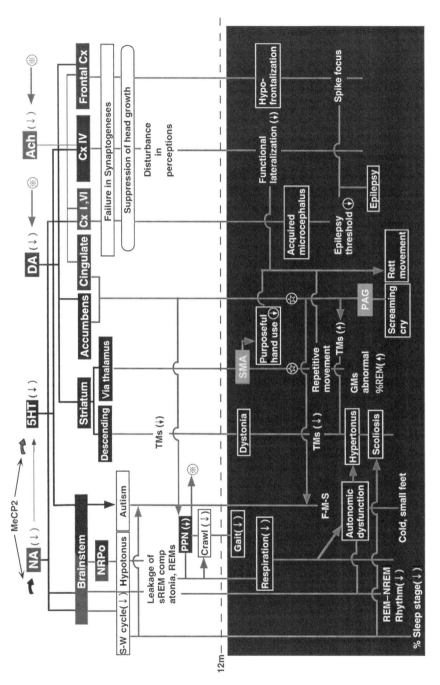

Fig. 8.2 Pathophysiology of Rett syndrome-hypothesis - ⊛ Receptor Supersensitivity; MeCP2, methyl-CpG-binding protein 2; NA, noradrenaline; 5HT, serotonin; DA, dopamine; Ach, acetylcholine; NRPo, nucleus reticularis pontis oralis; PPN, pedunculo-pontine nuclei; SMA, supplementary motor area; PAG, periaqueductal grey; Cx I, VI, cerebral cortex layer I and VI; Cx IV, cerebral cortex layer IV; Cx, cortex; FMS, friendliness-muricide-selfmutilation; S-W cycle, sleepwake cycle; sREM, rapid eye movement sleep stage; REM(s), rapid eye movements; NREM, non-rapid eye movements; TMs, twitch movements; GMs, gross movements; 12 m, age of 12 months. ⊛ indicates that decreased function of PPN leads to decreased DA and Ach. (See also colour plate section.)

atonia in sREM (Sakai 1984). Thus the hypofunction of NA and 5HT neurons in RS may cause hypotonia, a decrease in postural muscle tone and suppression of locomotion which manifests as difficulty with crawling and abnormal gait.

The characteristic stereotyped hand movements associated with involuntary movements of the mouth and tongue, such as licking and teeth grinding, are the hallmark of RS and we suggest that these stereotypies are fragments of the normal, immature, motor behaviour which occur in the presence of defective inhibitory or excitatory control (Nomura and Segawa 1990).

A young monkey injected with 1-methyl-4-phenyl-1,2,3,6-tetrahydropyridine (MPTP) into unilateral putamen developed rhythmic stereotyped movements of both hands similar to the stereotypy observed in RS (Hikosaka, 1992, personal communication). DA was depleted in the putamen and DA receptor super-sensitivity was found (Imai, 1992, personal communication). This animal model suggests that decreased DA in the striatum with receptor supersensitivity may underlie the stereotypy of RS.

Purposeful hand use is often lost when hand stereotypy begins in RS.

The supplementary motor area (SMA) is involved in purposeful hand use. In primates unilateral lesion of the SMA results in a deficit in bimanual coordination (Brinkman 1984). The opposite hand to the lesioned SMA performs movements against the purposeful movement of the normal hand.

NS-DA neurons modulate the SMA through the basal ganglia and their ascending pathway to the thalamus. Therefore the reduced function of NS-DA neurons in RS could induce disturbance of the SMA and cause the loss of purposeful hand use and stereotyped hand movements as a sign of defective bimanual coordination.

In RS postural dystonia and scoliosis are observed after childhood. In Segawa disease the decreased DA in the ventral striatum causes postural dystonia through descending efferents of the basal ganglia via the striatal direct pathway (Segawa and Nomura 1995, Chapter 7).

In RS hypofunction of the NS-DA neurons has been shown in the substantia nigra pars compacta (SNc) (Jellinger and Seitelberger 1986; Kitt *et al.* 1990), and within the basal ganglia the ventral portion seems to be most involved (Belichenko *et al.* 1997). This area of the striatum contains the striatal direct pathway and projections to and from the limbic system. Thus the hypofunction of the NS-DA neurons in RS is responsible for the postural dystonia and some behavioural disturbance through these pathways. The DA neuron has innate asymmetry in content and function. Its primary hypofunction leads to asymmetry in postural tone of the trunk muscles and may cause scoliosis with concavity to the more affected side (Duvoisin 1976). The scoliosis of RS can be explained by the asymmetrical involvement of the DA neurons. However the dystonia and scoliosis of RS are not relieved by levodopa; therefore mechanisms other than hypofunction of the NS-DA system are thought to be involved. NA lesion is known to be also involved in postural dystonia (Hornykiewicz *et al.* 1986) and the remedial effects of sympathectomy on postural dystonia of leg and foot in RS (Naidu *et al.* 1987) may suggest the possible involvement of NA neuron in dystonia and scoliosis in RS.

Furthermore, depletion of melatonin in the early developmental stage in chicken causes scoliosis by involving antigravity muscles (Machida *et al.* 1995) and since the sympathetic nerves are involved in the secretion of melatonin, disturbances of melatonin or the sympathetic nerves may also be related to the pathophysiology of scoliosis in RS (Nomura *et al.* 1997).

Suppression of the postural suppression pathway is also necessary for regular respiration (Schloon *et al.* 1976). Postural atonia in sREM blocks all reflex systems including those of the autonomic nervous system (ANS). In contrast with the presence of postural tone, the reflexes appear in NREM sleep. In RS however postural atonia is present not only in NREM sleep but also in awake periods. The abnormal respiratory pattern in RS with spontaneous occurrence of Valsalva manoeuvre (Kerr *et al.* 1998) may be due to the disturbance of regular respiration and the failure of autonomic reflexes caused by the lack of postural tone. Abnormalities in the ANS observed in RS (Nomura *et al.* 1997) could be explained by the disturbance of its reflex systems.

The early depletion of NA in animal experiments leads to poor development of head size (Brenner *et al.* 1983). In RS early lesion of the locus ceruleus NA neurons around 36–40 weeks of gestation may cause the stagnation of head growth in the latter half of the first year due to disturbance in synaptogenesis of the cortex. Bauman *et al.* (1995) reported histological changes of the cerebral cortex which may implicate the early hypofunction of the NA neurons.

The DA neurons in the midbrain send axons to the cerebral cortex and these are broadly distributed, particularly to the frontal and limbic cortex and cingulate gyrus (Rosenberg and Lewis 1995). These are involved in synaptogenesis in the early period of development (refer also Chapter 3). Marked reduction in the size of the frontal cortex (Armstrong 1995) and the abnormal MAP-2 staining in the cortex in RS (Kaufmann *et al.* 1995) suggest early involvement of the DA neurons which project to the frontal cortex.

The periaqueductal grey matter (PAG) is a key station for species specific vocalization and produces emotional vocalization by receiving signals from the cingulate gyrus (Jürgens and Pratt 1979; Jürgens 1986). PAG has afferents from substantia nigra pars reticulata (SNr) (Harting *et al.* 1991; Jayaraman *et al.* 1977). We suggest the involvement of PAG and the cingulate cortex in the characteristic screaming or vocalization of RS, and dysfunction of the DA neurons of the ventral tegmental area (VTA) as well as those of SNc play roles in the pathophysiology of RS.

Disturbed cognition is a major problem in RS. Of great interest in this regard is the failure of synaptogenesis and poor dendritic development without degenerative changes, as demonstrated by neuropathological investigations (Armstrong

1995; Armstrong *et al.* 1995). From the stage of neuronal migration in the early fetal period to the postnatal period the brainstem MA neurons play a part in cortical synaptogenesis (Levitt *et al.* 1997).

The neuropathological findings in RS suggest that the abnormality of the brainstem MA neurons occurs after the stage of migration and results in the deficient cortical synaptogenesis leading to defective cognitive function while preserving visual and auditory perception (Nomura *et al.* 1985; Nomura and Segawa 1986; Segawa 1997). As the synaptogenesis of the occipital lobe occurs latest in the cerebral cortex, visual involvement may be expected to be mild in RS. During the development of the primary visual cortex in monkeys, 5HT fibres are present in the highest density (Takeuchi *et al.* 1992), while the NA fibres are lowest. Thus the failure of synaptogenesis may be milder in the occipital cortex.

The somatosensory pathways which mature after birth are affected in RS as shown by somatosensory evoked potential measures (Kimura *et al.* 1992). Sleep stage REM in the fetal period has an important role in the development of neural pathways, particularly those involved in perception through activity dependent neural development (Mirmiran 1995). The pathway for visual perception from the retina to the visual cortex is established by the neural activity in sREM during the fetal period (Marks *et al.* 1995). Thus the normal development of the parameters of sREM sleep in the fetal period may also relate to the relative preservation of visual and auditory perception in RS.

In the rat 5HT neurons give rise to dense projections to the cortex during a certain period of development but after that period most of the 5HT neurons lose their cortical projections without cell death in the brainstem (Koh *et al.* 1991). This neonatal period corresponds to the first year in humans.

Lack of reports of pathology in the brainstem MA neurons at autopsy in RS may be due to the fact that the cases had passed the critical age for MA neurons. Alternatively in RS the axons of the MA neurons involved in synaptogenesis may disappear earlier or may be maldeveloped.

Involvement of cholinergic neurons in the pathogenesis of RS is conceivable based on the recent substantial evidence of abnormalities in the basal nucleus of Meynert (BNM) (Johnston *et al.* 1995; Wenk *et al.* 1999), reduction of MAP-2 immunoreactivity in the RS brain (Kaufmann *et al.* 1995) and an animal model with early lesion in the BNM which showed reduction of MAP-2 similar to RS (Kaufmann *et al.* 1997). The early signs of RS however cannot be explained by a primary lesion of cholinergic neurons (Segawa 1997). The study of sleep components shows that the cholinergic neurons, which are the executive neurons for sREM, are preserved normally in the early stages of RS (Segawa and Nomura 1990, 1992; Segawa 1997).

Therefore it remains to be clarified whether this involvement of the cholinergic neurons restricted to the BNM in RS is primary or secondary to the dysfunction of the brainstem MA neurons.

The pedunculo-pontine nucleus (PPN) is known to have ascending projections to SN and it also projects to the BNM.

An excitotoxic lesion of the unilateral PPN in monkey causes functional disturbance of the ipsilateral SN and leads to parkinsonism in the contralateral extremities (Kojima *et al.* 1997). In this experiment, tyrosine hydroxylase (TH) in the SN was decreased but there was no degenerative change (Kojima *et al.* 1997). In an autopsied case of RS, Saito and colleagues (unpublished thesis) found similar findings, that is decrease of TH in the SN and locus ceruleus without any degenerative change.

In RS we consider the PPN to be affected from the early period because of the marked failure in postural tone and locomotion. Lesion of PPN might cause functional disturbance in the BNM as well as the SN. The disturbances of these nuclei become apparent from late infancy and lead to the development of particular symptoms and signs in RS without any degenerative changes in these neurons.

In conclusion, the symptoms and signs of RS are explained by an early lesion of the MA neurons in the brainstem and midbrain (Nomura *et al.* 1984, 1985 1987; Nomura and Segawa 1986; Segawa 1997). These lesions may cause maturational arrest or insufficient synaptogenesis at each level of the brain (Levitt *et al.* 1997), which do not show progression except for the appearance of receptor supersensitivity. The maturational arrest is manifested in a caudal to rostral sequence, leading to the age dependent clinical features.

8.4.2. Etiology

Mutations in the gene encoding MeCP2 have been found to be causative in RS (Amir *et al.* 1999). How does the MA hypothesis for the pathophysiology of RS relate to these mutations? MECP2 is a regulatory gene for many genes which have methylated CpG and it is known to suppress the transcription of target genes and also to play an important role in maturation of the neuronal system from early development (Tate *et al.* 1996). The genes which are involved in the development of the MA systems in the CNS and express particularly between 36 gestational weeks and the second and third postnatal months and thereafter with temporal and spatial specificity, will be the important candidate genes in regard to the etiology and pathophysiology of RS.

References

Amir, R.E., Van den Veyver, I.B., Wan, M., Tran, C.Q., Francke, U., and Zoghbi, H.Y. (1999). Rett syndrome is caused by mutations in X-linked MECP2, encoding methyl-CpG-binding protein 2. *Nature Genetics*, **23**, 185–8.

Armstrong, D.D. (1992). The neuropathology of the Rett syndrome. *Brain and Development*, **14**(**Suppl.**), S89–98.

Armstrong, D.D. (1995). The neuropathology of Rett syndrome—overview 1994. *Neuropediatrics*, **26**, 100–4.

Armstrong, D., Dunn, J.K., Antalffy, B., and Trivedi, R. (1995). Selective dendritic alterations in the cortex of Rett syndrome. *Journal of Neuropathology Experimental Neurology*, **54**, 195–201.

Bauman, M.L., Kemper, T.L., and Arin, D.M. (1995). Microscopic observations of the brain in Rett syndrome. *Neuropediatrics*, **26**, 105–8.

Belichenko, P.V., Leontovich, T., Mukhina, J., Hagberg, B., and Dahlstrom, A. (1997). Morphological studies of neocortical areas and basal ganglia in Rett syndrome. *European Child and Adolescent Psychiatry*, **6**, 78.

Brenner, E., Mirmiran, M., Uylings, H.B.M., and Van Der Gugten, J. (1983). Impaired growth of the cerebral cortex of rats treated neonatally with 6-hydroxydopamine under different environmental conditions. *Neuroscience Letters*, **42**, 13–7.

Brinkman, C. (1984). Supplementary motor area of the monkey's cerebral cortex: short- and long-term deficits after unilateral ablation and the effects of subsequent callosal section. *Journal of Neuroscience*, **4**, 918–29.

Brucke, T., Sofic, E., Killian, W., Rett, A., and Riederer, P. (1987). Reduced concentrations and increased metabolism of biogenic amines in a single case of Rett-syndrome: a postmortem brain study. *Journal of Neural Transmission*, **68**, 315–24.

Budden, S.S., Myer, E.C., and Butler, I.J. (1990). Cerebrospinal fluid studies in the Rett syndrome: biogenic amines and beta-endorphins. *Brain and Development*, **12**, 81–4.

Chiron, C., Bulteau, C., Loc'h, C., Raynaud, C., Garreau, B., Syrota, A., and Maziere, B. (1993). Dopaminergic D2 receptor SPECT imaging in Rett syndrome: increase of specific binding in striatum. *Journal of Nucleus Medicine*, **34**, 1717–21.

Duvoisin, R.C. (1976). Parkinsonism: Animal analogues of the human disorder. In *The basal ganglia* (ed. M.D. Yahr), pp. 293–303. Raven Press, New York.

Fukuda, H., Segawa, M., Nomura, Y., Nishihara, K., and Ono, Y. (1995). Phasic activity during REM sleep in movement disorders. In *Age-related dopamine-dependent disorders*, Monographs in Neural Sciences (ed. M. Segawa and Y. Nomura), pp. 69–76. Karger, Basel.

Fukumoto, M., Mochizuki, N., Takeishi, M., Nomura, Y., and Segawa, M. (1981). Studies of body movements during night sleep in infancy. *Brain and Development*, **3**, 37–43.

Harris, J.C., Wong, D.F., Wagner, H.N., Jr, Rett, A., Naidu, S., Dannals, R.F., Links, J.M., *et al.* (1986). Positron emission tomographic study of D2 dopamine receptor binding and CSF biogenic amine metabolites in Rett syndrome. *American Journal of Medical Genetics* (**Suppl.** 1), 201–10.

Harting, J.K., Van Lieshout, P.V., and Feig, S. (1991). Connectional studies of the primate lateral geniculate nucleus: distribution of axons arising from the thalamic reticular nucleus of Galago crassicaudatus. *Journal of Comparative Neurology*, **310**, 411–27.

Hayes, N.L. and Rustioni, A. (1981). Descending projections from brainstem and sensorimotor cortex to spinal enlargements in the cat. Single and double retrograde tracer studies. *Experimental Brain Research*, **41**, 89–107.

Hobson, J.A. (1983). Sleep: order and disorder. *Behavioral biology in medicine*, A Monograph Series, Vol. 1, pp. 1–36.

Hobson, J.A., McCarley, R.W., Pivic, R.T., and Freedman, R. (1974). Selective firing by cat pontine brain stem neurons in desynchronized sleep. *Journal of Neurophysiology*, **37**, 497–511.

Hobson, J.A., McCarley, R.W., and Wyzinzki, R.W. (1975). Sleep cycle oscillation: reciprocal discharge by two brainstem neuronal groups. *Science*, **189**, 55–8.

Hornykiewicz, O., Stephen, J., Becker, L.E., Farley, I., and Shannak, K. (1986). Brain neurotransmitters in dystonia musculorum deformans. *New England Journal of Medicine*, **315**, 347–53.

Huisman, A.M., Kuypers, H.G.J.M., and Verburgh, C.A. (1980). Quantitative differences in collateralization of the descending spinal pathways from red nucleus and other brainstem cell groups in rat as demonstrated with the multiple fluorescent retrograde tracer technique. *Brain Research*, **209**, 271–86.

Huisman, A.M., Kuypers, H.G.J.M., and Verburgh, C.A. (1982). Differences in collateralization of the descending spinal pathways from red nucleus and other brainstem cell groups in cat and monkey. In *Descending pathways to the spinal cord, Progress in Brain Research*, Vol. 57 (ed. H.G.J.M. Kuypers and G.F. Martin), pp. 185–217. Elsevier, Amsterdam.

Jayaraman, A., Batton, R.R., and Carpenter, M.B. (1977). Nigrotectal projections in the monkey: an autoradiographic study. *Brain Research*, **135**, 147–52.

Jellinger, K. and Seitelberger, F. (1986). Neuropathology of Rett syndrome. *American Journal of Medical Genetics* (**Suppl.**1), 259–88.

Jellinger, K., Armstrong, D., Zoghbi, H.Y., and Percy, A.K. (1988). Neuropathology of Rett syndrome. *Acta Neuropathologica* (Berlin), **76**, 142–58.

Johnston, M.V., Hohmann, C., and Blue, M.E. (1995). Neurobiology of Rett syndrome. *Neuropediatrics*, **26**, 119–22.

Julu, P.O.O., Kerr, A.M., Hansen, S., Apartopoulos, F., and Jamal, G.A. (1998). Cardio-respiratory instability in Rett syndrome suggests medullary serotonergic dysfunction. *Brain and Development*, **20**, 324.

Jürgens, U. (1986). The squirrel monkey as an experimental model in the study of cerebral organization of emotional vocal utterances. *European Archives of Psychiatry and Neurological Sciences*, **236**, 40–3.

Jürgens, U. and Pratt, R. (1979). Role of the periaqueductal grey in vocal expression of emotion. *Brain Research*, **167**, 367–78.

Kaufmann, W.E., Naidu, S., and Budden, S. (1995). Abnormal expression of microtubule-associated protein 2 (MAP-2) in neocortex in Rett syndrome. *Neuropediatrics*, **26**, 109–13.

Kaufmann, W.E., Taylor, C.V., Hohmann, C.F., Sanwal, I.B., and Naidu, S. (1997). Abnormalities in neuronal maturation in Rett syndrome neocortex: preliminary molecular correlates. *European Child and Adolescent Psychiatry*, **6**, 75–7.

Kerr, A.M., Julu, P.O.O., Hansen, S., and Apartopoulos, F. (1998). Results from Rett autonomic assessments during the workshop in Meeting report: Workshop on Autonomic Function in Rett Syndrome, Swedish Rett Centre, Frösön, Sweden, May 1998. Witt Engerström, I. and Kerr, A.M. *Brain and Development*, **20**, 323–6.

Kimura, K., Nomura, Y., and Segawa, M. (1992). Middle and short latency somatosensory evoked potentials (SEPm, SEPs) in the Rett syndrome: chronological changes of cortical and subcortical involvements. *Brain and Development*, **14**(**Suppl.**), S37–42.

Kitt, C.A. and Wilcox, B.J. (1995). Preliminary evidence for neurodegenerative changes in the substantia nigra of Rett syndrome. *Neuropediatrics*, **26**, 114–8.

Kitt, C.A., Tronoso, J.C., Price, D.C., Naidu, S., and Moser, M.W. (1990). Pathological changes in substantia nigra and basal forebrain neurons in Rett syndrome. *Annals of Neurology*, **28**, 416–7.

Koh, T., Kakazawa, M., Kani, K., and Maeda, T. (1991). Investigation of origin of serotonergic projection to developing rat visual cortex: a combined retrograde tracing and immunohistochemical study. *Brain Research Bulletin*, **27**, 675–84.

Kohyama, J. and Iwakawa, Y. (1991). Interrelationships between rapid eye and body movements during sleep: polysomnographic examinations of infants including premature neonates. *Electroencephalography and Clinical Neurophysiology*, **79**, 277–80.

Kohyama, J., Shinohira, M., Hasegawa, T., Kouji, T., and Iwakawa, Y. (1995). Phasic motor activity reduction occurring with horizontal rapid eye movements during sleep in humans. *Experimental Brain Research*, **107**, 137–44.

Kojima, J., Yamaji, Y., Matsumura, M., Nambu, A., Inase, M., Takubo, H., Takada, M., and Imai, H. (1997). Excitotoxic lesions of the pedunculopontine tegmental nucleus produce contralateral hemiparkinsonism in the monkey. *Neuroscience Letters*, 226, 111–4.

Kuypers, H.G.J.M. (1985). The anatomical and functional organization of the motor system. In *Scientific basis of clinical neurology* (ed. M. Swash and C. Kennard), pp. 3–18. Churchill Livingstone, Edinburgh.

Lekman, A., Witt Engerström, I., Gottfries, J., Hagberg, B.A., Percy, A.K., and Svennerholm, L. (1989). Rett syndrome: biogenic amines and metabolites in postmortem brain. *Pediatric Neurology*, 5, 357–62.

Lekman, A., Witt Engerström, I., Holmberg, B., Percy, A., Svennerholm, L., and Hagberg, B. (1990). CSF and urine biogenic amine metabolites in Rett syndrome. *Clinical Genetics*, 37, 173–8.

Levitt, P., Harvey, J.A., Friedam, E., Simansky, K., and Murphy, E.H. (1997). Monoamines in neural differentiation (P. Levitt *et al.*). New evidence for neurotransmitter influences on brain development. *Trends in Neurosciences*, 20, 269–74.

Machida, M., Dubousset, J., Imamura, Y., Iwaya, T., Yamada, T., and Kimura, J. (1995). Role of melatonin deficiency in the development of scoliosis in pinealectomised chickens. *The Journal of Bone and Joint Surgery*, 77-**B**, 134–8.

Marks, G.A., Shaffery, J.P., Oksenberg, A., Speciale, S.G., and Roffwarg, H.P. (1995). A functional role for REM sleep in brain maturation. *Behavioural Brain Research*, 69, 1–11.

Martin, G.F., Cabana, T., and Humbertson, A.O. (1981). Evidence for collateral innervation of the cervical and lumbar enlargement of the spinal cord by single reticular and raphe neurons. Studies using fluorescent markers in double-labeling experiments on the North American opossum. *Neuroscience Letters*, 24, 1–6.

McArthur, A. and Budden, S.S. (1998). Sleep dysfunction in Rett syndrome: a trial of exogenous melatonin treatment. *Developmental Medicine and Child Neurology*, 40, 186–92.

McCarley, R.W. and Hobson, J.A. (1971). Single unit activity in cat gigantocellular tegmental field: selectivity of discharge in desynchronized sleep. *Science*, 174, 1250–2.

Mirmiran, M. (1986). The role of the central monoaminergic system and rapid eye movement sleep in development. *Brain and Development*, 8, 382–89.

Mirmiran, M. (1995). The function of fetal/neonatal rapid eye movement sleep. *Behavioural Brain Research*, 69, 13–22.

Mori, S., Matsuyama, K., Kohyama, J., Kobayashi, Y., and Takakusaki, K. (1992). Neuronal constituents of postural and locomotor control systems and their interactions in cats. *Brain and Development*, 14(**Suppl.**), S109–20.

Naidu, S., Chatterjee, S., Murphy, M., Uematsu, S., Phillipart, M., and Moser, H. (1987). Rett syndrome: new observations. *Brain and Development*, 9, 525–8.

Nielsen, J.B., Bertelsen, A., and Lou, H.C. (1992). Low CSF HVA levels in the Rett syndrome: a reflection of restricted synapse formation? *Brain and Development*, 14(**Suppl.**), S63–5.

Nomura, Y. and Segawa, M. (1986). Anatomy of Rett syndrome. *American Journal of Medical Genetics* (**Suppl.** 1), 289–303.

Nomura, Y. and Segawa, M. (1990). Characteristics of motor disturbances of the Rett syndrome. *Brain and Development*, 12, 27–30.

Nomura, Y. and Segawa, M. (1992). Motor symptoms of the Rett syndrome: abnormal muscle tone, posture, locomotion and stereotyped movement. *Brain and Development*, 14(**Suppl.**), S21–8.

Nomura, Y., Honda, K., and Segawa, M. (1987). Pathophysiology of Rett syndrome. *Brain and Development*, 9, 506–13.

Nomura, Y., Kimura, K., Arai, H., and Segawa, M. (1997). Involvement of the autonomic nervous system in the pathophysiology of Rett syndrome. *European Child and Adolescent Psychiatry*, 6, 42–6.

Nomura, Y., Segawa, M., and Hasegawa, M. (1984). Rett syndrome—clinical studies and pathophysiological consideration. *Brain and Development*, 6, 475–86.

Nomura, Y., Segawa, M., and Higurashi, M. (1985). Rett syndrome—an early catecholamine and indolamine deficient disorder? *Brain and Development*, 7, 334–41.

Parmelee, A.H., Jr and Stern, E. (1972). Development of states in infants. In *Sleep and maturing nervous system* (ed. C.D. Clemente, D.P. Purpura, and F.E. Mayer), pp. 199–215. Academic Press, New York.

Percy, A.K., Zoghbi, H.Y., and Glaze, D.G. (1987). Rett syndrome — discrimination of typical and variant forms. *Brain and Development*, 9, 458–61.

Percy, A.K., Zoghbi, H., and Riccardi, V.M. (1985). Rett syndrome: initial experience with an emerging clinical entity. *Brain and Development*, 8, 300–4.

Perry, T.L., Dunn, H.G., Ho, H.H., and Crichton, J.U. (1988). Cerebrospinal fluid values for monoamine metabolites, gamma-aminobutyric acid, and other amino compounds in Rett syndrome. *Journal of Pediatrics*, 112, 234–8.

Rett, A. (1966). Über ein Zerebral-atrophisches Syndrom bei Hyperammon. Wien: Brüder Hollinek.

Rett, A. (1977). Cerebral atrophy associated with hyperammonämie. In *Handbook of clinical neurology*, Vol. 29 (ed. P.J. Vinken and G.W. Bruyn), pp. 305–29. North Holland Publishing Company, Amsterdam.

Riederer, P., Brucke, T., Sofic, E., Kienzl, E., Schnecker, K., and Schay, V. (1985). Neurochemical aspects of the Rett syndrome. *Brain and Development*, 7, 351–60.

Riederer, P., Weiser, M., Wichart, I., Schmidt, B., Killian, W., and Rett, A. (1986). Preliminary brain autopsy findings in progredient Rett syndrome. *American Journal of Medical Genetics* (**Suppl.** 1), 305–15.

Rosenberg, D. and Lewis, D.A. (1995). Postnatal maturation of the dopaminergic innervation of monkey prefrontal and motor cortices: a tyrosine hydroxylase immunohistochemical analysis. *Journal of Comparative Neurology*, 358, 383–400.

Sakai, K. (1984). Central mechanisms of paradoxical sleep. In *Sleep mechanisms* (ed. A. Borbély and J.L.Valatx), pp. 3–18. Springer, Berlin.

Schloon, M., O'Brien, M.J., Sholton, C.A., and Prechtl, H.F.R. (1976). Muscle activity and postural behavior in newborn infants. *Neuropediatrics*,7, 384–415.

Segawa, M. (1982). Pathogenesis of early infantile autism (in Japanese). *The Bulletin of the Japanese Association for the Scientific Study of Mental Deficiency (Tokyo)*, 4, 184–97.

Segawa, M. (1997). Pathophysiology of Rett syndrome from the standpoint of early catecholamine disturbance. *European Child and Adolescent Psychiatry*, 6, 56–60.

Segawa, M (1999). Ontogenesis of REM sleep. In *Rapid eye movement sleep* (ed. B.N. Mellick and Inoué, pp. 39–50. Narosa Publishing House, New Delhi, India.

Segawa, M. and Nomura, Y. (1990). The pathophysiology of the Rett syndrome from the standpoint of polysomnography. *Brain and Development*, 12, 55–60.

Segawa, M. and Nomura, Y. (1991). Rapid eye movements during stage REM are modulated by nigrostriatal dopamine (NS-DA) neurons? In *Basal ganglia III* (ed. G. Bermardi), pp. 663–71. Plenum Press, New York.

Segawa, M. and Nomura, Y. (1992). Polysomnography in Rett syndrome. *Brain and Development*, 14(**Suppl.**), S46–54.

Segawa, M. and Nomura, Y. (1995). Hereditary progressive dystonia with marked diurnal fluctuation and Dopa-responsive dystonia: pathognomonic clinical features. In *Age-related dopamine-dependent disorders*, Monographs in Neural Sciences (ed. M. Segawa and Y. Nomura), pp. 10–24. Karger, Basel.

Segawa, M., Nomura, Y., Hakamada, S., Nagata, E., Sakamoto, M., and Oka, N. (1986). Polysomnography-Functional topographical examination of the basal ganglia. *Brain and Development*, 8, 475–81.

Segawa, M., Nomura, Y., Hikosaka, O., Soda, M., Usui, S., and Kase, M. (1987). Roles of the basal ganglia and related structures in symptoms of dystonia. In *Basal ganglia II: structure and function* (ed. M.B. Carpenter and A. Jayaraman), pp. 489–504. Plenum Press, New York.

Swaab, D.F., Flier, E., and Partiman, T.S. (1985). Suprachiasmatic nucleus of the human brain in relation to sex, age and senile dementia. *Brain Research*, **342**, 37–44.

Takahashi, K., Shimoda, K., Yamada, N., Sasaki, Y., and Hayashi, S. (1986). Effect of dorsal midbrain lesion in infant rats on development of circadian rhythm. *Brain and Development*, **8**, 373–81.

Takeuchi, Y., Sawada, T., and Jenner, P. (1992). Early monoaminergic dysfunction. *Brain and Development*, **14**(**Suppl.** l), S131–7.

Tate, P., Skarnes, W., and Bird, A. (1996). The methyl-CpG binding protein MeCP2 is essential for embryonic development in the mouse. *Nature Genetics*, **12**, 205–8.

Uchiyama, A., Nomura, Y., and Segawa, M. (1987). Roles of cerebral basal ganglia in the modulation of body movements during sleep (in Japanese). *Clinical Electroencephalography (Osaka)*, **29**, 782–7.

Wagner, H.N., Jr (1986). Rett syndrome: positron emission tomography (PET) studies. *American Journal of Medical Genetics* (**Suppl.** 1), 211–24.

Wenk, G.L. (1995). Alterations in dopaminergic function in Rett syndrome. *Neuropediatrics*, **26**, 123–5.

Wenk, G.L. (1996). Rett syndrome: evidence for normal dopaminergic function. *Neuropediatrics*, **27**, 256–9.

Wenk, G.L. (1997). Rett syndrome: neurobiological changes underlying specific symptoms. *Progress in Neurobiology*, **51**, 383–91.

Wenk, G.L. and Hauss-Wegrzyniak, B. (1999). Altered cholinergic function in the basal forebrain of girls with Rett syndrome. *Neuropediatrics*, **30**, 125–9.

Wenk, G.L., Naidu, S., Casanova, M.F., Kitt, C.A., and Moser, H. (1991). Altered neurochemical markers in Rett's syndrome. *Neurology*, **41**, 1753–6.

Wenk, G.L., O'Leary, M., Nemeroff, C.B., Bissette, G., Moser, H., and Naidu, S. (1993). Neurochemical alterations in Rett syndrome. *Developmental Brain Research*, **74**, 67–72.

Wong, D.F., Harris, J.C., Naidu, S., Yokoi, F., Marenco, S., Dannals, R.F., *et al.* (1996). Dopamine transporters are markedly reduced in Lesch-Nyhan disease in vivo. *Proceedings of National Academy of Science USA*, **93**(11), 5539–43.

Zoghbi, H.Y., Milstien, S., Butler, I.J., Smith, E.O., Kaufman, S., Glaze, D.G., and Percy, A.K. (1989). Cerebrospinal fluid biogenic amines and biopterin in Rett syndrome. *Annals of Neurology*, **25**, 56–60.

Zoghbi, H.Y., Percy, A.K., Glaze, D.G., Butler, I.J., and Riccardi, V.M. (1985). Reduction of biogenic amine levels in the Rett syndrome. *New England Journal of Medicine*, **10**, 313, (15), 921–4.

9 The central and peripheral autonomic nervous system and possible implications in Rett syndrome patients

Annica Dahlström

Summary

The monoaminergic nervous pathways are amongst the very early systems to appear during ontogenic development. They are also the class of neurons that appear very early in phylogenesis, long before an organized nervous system can be identified. This implies that they represent systems that have been of vital importance for the ontogenic development as well as for survival of the animals during evolution. Since the monoaminergic neurons appear so early during ontogenesis, before any synaptic neurotransmission is developed, it has been proposed that the transmitters of these early systems, via release from the tips of the outgrowing axons, may have other functions than neurotransmission; thus, morphogenic or trophic effects have been proposed, both for serotonin (5-HT) and for noradrenaline (NA).

Also in the human fetus, catecholamine (CA) nerve terminals have been demonstrated in brain areas long before birth. Thus, it is possible that also in man these 'classical neurotransmitters' have non-neurotransmitter actions, and should be taken into consideration whenever defects in the development and maturation of the human brain are discussed. They may also work in consort with various neurotrophic factors, by influencing intracellular common pathways. Therefore, in this section will be described what is presently known about the 'autonomic nervous system', its ontogeny and distribution as well as physiological aspects, in order to provide a basis for further investigations and discussions concerning the basic mechanisms that may go wrong in Rett girls.

9.1 Introduction

The monoaminergic nervous systems are amongst the very early systems to appear during ontogenic development. They are also the class of neurons that appear very early in phylogenesis, long before an organized nervous system can be identified. This implies that they represent systems that have been of vital importance for the survival of animals during evolution. It is interesting to note that the cell groups of the major monoaminergic systems in mammals are located in the phylogenetically old parts of the brain, the medulla, pons and mesencephalic regions. From these locations the cells have gradually invaded the newer brain areas, including the neocortex, with axons and nerve terminals, during evolution. Since the monoaminergic neurons appear so early during ontogenesis, before any synaptic neurotransmission is developed, it has been proposed that the transmitters of these early systems, via release from the tips of the outgrowing axons, may have other functions than neurotransmission; thus, morphogenic or trophic effects have been proposed, both for serotonin (5-HT, Lauder *et al.* 1981, 1983; Lauder 1988) and for NA (Felten *et al.* 1982; Jonsson and Kasamatsu 1983; Rakic and Goldman-Rakic 1982).

Also in the human fetus, catecholamine (CA) nerve terminals have been demonstrated in several areas before birth (Olson *et al.* 1973; Choi *et al.* 1975). Thus, it is possible that also in man these 'classical neurotransmitters' have non-neurotransmitter actions, and should be taken into consideration whenever defects in the development and maturation of the human brain are discussed. They may also work in consort with various neurotrophic factors, by influencing intracellular common pathways. Therefore, in this chapter will be described what is presently known about the 'autonomic nervous system', in order to provide a basis for further investigations and discussions concerning the basic mechanisms that may go wrong in Rett girls.

The newly discovered involvement of the MECP2 gene in the Rett syndrome is very interesting, since this gene mediates transcriptional repression of other genes which may express factors that regulate trophic or modulating activities in the construction of neuronal circuits in the CNS.

9.2 The general organization of the autonomic nervous system (ANS)

The general hypothesis at the mid-century was that the ANS was organized as a syncytium, and it was not until 1946, when Nils-Åke Hillarp published his thesis (Hillarp 1946), that he could demonstrate, using a modified methylene blue staining method, that the peripheral innervation of the ANS consisted of a network of fine, varicose, nerve terminal endings. He and his collaborators (Bengt Falck in Lund and Arvid Carlsson in Göteborg) later developed the histochemical fluorescence method for demonstrating the presence and cellular localization in peripheral tissues and brain, of catecholamines (CA), including noradrenaline (NA) and dopamine (DA), as well as of serotonin (5-HT; Carlsson et al. 1962; Falck et al. 1962; Falck 1962). This method represented a true scientific revolution at the time, since, although the presence of monamines (MA) in peripheral tissues and brain was known from biochemical assays in tissue homogenates (e.g. Twarog and Page 1953; Vogt 1954; Bertler and Rosengren 1959), the exact cellular localization was only a matter of speculation. Using this histochemical fluorescence method in the early 1960s the existence of central neurons containing MA was demonstrated for the first time (Dahlström and Fuxe 1964, 1965) and the first mapping of these central neurons was carried out (e.g. Dahlström et al. 1965; Ungerstedt 1971). In the periphery the mapping of the sympathetic part of the ANS was carried out by Norberg and Hamberger (1964) and the detailed study of the pharmacology of these systems was performed (Malmfors 1965; Sachs 1970).

Hillarp demonstrated the fine nerve terminal branches of the ANS and introduced the term 'autonomic ground plexus' to describe a network type of innervation where sympathetic and parasympathetic nerve terminal branches, in an intermingled manner, surround the innervated tissue components (Hillarp 1959). Subsequently the postganglionic part of the sympathetic system, the adrenergic component, was mapped using the histofluorescence method, while the cholinergic parasympathetic part was visualized histochemically due to its content of ACh-esterase (AChE; which however, is also present in varying amounts in the adrenergic system). Later, more specific methods were used employing antisera to choline acetyltransferase (ChAT), the ACh synthesizing enzyme. The newest method to specifically study cholinergic neurons makes use of the recently developed excellent antibodies against the vesicular transporter of ACh (VAChT) as a marker (Erickson et al. 1994; Gilmore et al. 1996).

Today, the Hillarp fluorescence method is rarely used; instead immunofluorescence or immunocytochemical methods are preferred, with the use of the many specific antisera against the 'classical transmitter' 5-HT and the enzymes that control the formation of CA (tyrosine hydroxylase—TH—which converts tyrosine to DOPA; dopamine-β-hydroxylase—DBH—which converts DA to NA; and phenyl-N-methyltransferase—PNMT—that converts NA to adrenaline). Immunocytochemical methods are easier to use and give higher sensitivity, especially for 5-HT, which was difficult to study in the early days due to the rapid photodecomposition of the fluorescent product of 5-HT and formaldehyde gas.

The ANS in the periphery consists of two antagonistic systems, the parasympathetic and the sympathetic systems. In both branches of the PNS, two neurons are coupled in series. In 1948 von Euler demonstrated that NA is the sympathetic transmitter in mammals. However, there are exceptions to the 'rule' that sympathetic neurons release NA; some sympathetic neurons use ACh as mediator, and therefore the suffix -ergic was introduced, thus 'adrenergic' and 'cholinergic', respectively, for neurons releasing NA or ACh.

9.3 The peripheral ANS contains preganglionic and postganglionic neurons, two neurons coupled in series

The peripheral ANS is composed of two antagonistic divisions, each with two neurons coupled in series. The coupling from the preganglionic neuron to the postganglionic neuron takes place in a peripheral autonomic ganglion. As seen in Fig. 9.1 the preganglionic neurons of the parasympathetic division exit from the CNS from two separate levels: the brainstem (in cranial nerves III, VII, IX and X) innervating the structures of the head, the heart, and most of the GI canal, and the sacral part of the spinal cord, projecting to the urogenital tract organs and to the lowermost part of the GI canal. The sympathetic division is leaving the CNS in the thoracic and upper lumbar regions of the spinal cord. The cervical segments of the spinal cord do not harbour any ANS nerve cells (Fig. 9.1).

The classic transmitter of para- and sympathetic preganglionic neurons is ACh with coexisting peptides, for instance somatostatin (SOM), enkephalin (ENK), neurotensin or substance P (SP) (Krukoff et al. 1985). Recently it was demonstrated that about half of the sympathetic preganglionic neurons also contain nitric oxide (NO) synthase (Blottner and Baumgarten 1992), synthesizing NO, which in other parts of the CNS has been demonstrated to modulate synaptic release and also plays a role in long-term potentiation (Hope et al. 1991).

The preganglionic neurons of the parasympathetic systems, located in the brainstem nuclei, belong to the cranial nerves III, VII, IX and X. The axons of these preganglionic parasympathetic neurons are very long and the synaptic coupling to the postganglionic neuron takes place in a ganglion very close to the innervated organ, or inside it (the so-called 'intramural' autonomic ganglia). The preganglionic cell bodies of the sympathetic preganglionic neurons are located in the lateral column of the grey substance in the thoracic and upper lumbar segments of the spinal cord, and the axons leave the spinal cord together with the somatic motor axons via the ventral roots. After a short distance they leave the root, and exit via a white ramus communicans, running in a ventral direction through fine foramina in the vertebrae, to enter the paired sympathetic chain, a row of ganglia, one pair for each segment of the spinal cord. This sympathetic chain is anatomically located retroperitoneally, near the vertebral column, and these ganglia are therefore referred to as the 'paravertebral ganglia'. Some preganglionic axons synapse here on the dendrites and perikarya of the postganglionic neurons. The postganglionic axons, which are now very thin (less than 1 mm) and unmyelinated, but wrapped in Schwann cell cytoplasm, return to the spinal root via the grey ramus communicans. After this detour, the sympathetic system (now the postganglionic axons), rejoin the motor and sensory fibres in the main nerve stems and follow these distally to the innervated organs (blood vessels, sweat glands, hair follicles, endocrine organs, joints, etc.).

Some preganglionic axons do not synapse in the paravertebral ganglia, but

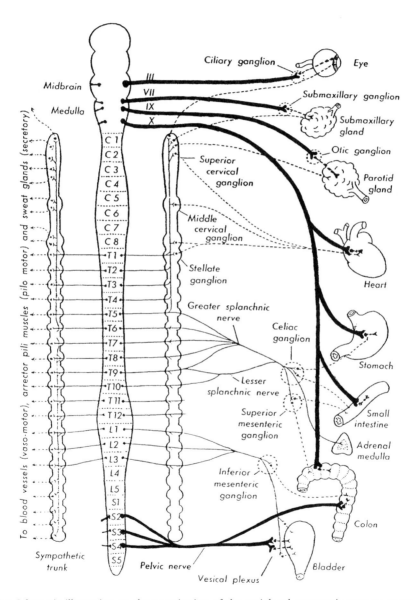

Fig. 9.1 Schematic illustration on the organization of the peripheral autonomic nervous system. The Parasympathetic system is illustrated in thick lines, the sympathetic system in thin lines. Solid lines indicate preganglionic neurons, while dashed lines represent postganglionic neurons (modified after *Bailey's textbook of histology*, 1968).

traverse the ganglia to proceed to more peripherally located ganglia, which can be found in the connective tissue anterior to the vertebral column and in front of and somewhat lateral to the main large vessels (Fig. 9.1). These ganglia are called 'prevertebral ganglia', and after coupling to the postganglionic nerve cells located here, the postganglionic axons now project to the organs to be innervated (mainly the GI tract, see Fig. 9.1). The coeliac ganglion and the superior and inferior mesenteric ganglia are prevertebral ganglia, supplying sympathetic innervation to the upper, middle and lower GI tracts. The postganglionic sympathetic fibres, as well as the preganglionic parasympathetic axons, follow the big vessels in the mesentery to the gut wall, where they branch and send nerve terminals to all layers of the gut wall (Fig. 9.2). The two systems particularly innervate the two ganglionic plexa, which form the enteric nervous system: plexus myentericus, located between the outer longitudinal and the inner circular layers of smooth muscles, and plexus submucosus located in the submucous layer close to the gut lumen. These two enteric plexa consist of groups of typically autonomic nerve cells which send axons to other groups of ganglion cells forming a true network where most neurons project in an anal direction, while some send axons in the

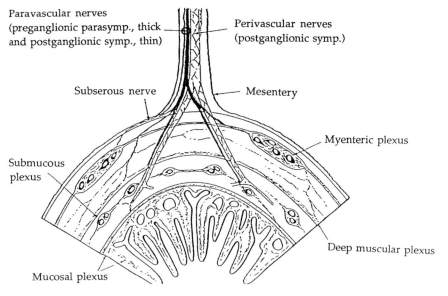

Fig. 9.2 Schematic illustration of the enteric nervous system. Incoming fibres to the gut are postganglionic sympathetic fibres with their cell bodies located in the prevertebral ganglia, and preganglionic parasympathetic fibres from the vagus nerve. These two efferent systems join the large vessels in the mesentery and enter the gut wall, where they branch and send axons to all levels of the intestinal wall. They innervate the intramural ganglia of the gut, which are located between the outer longitudinal and the inner circular layers of smooth muscles, the myenteric plexus, and in the submucous layer below the gut mucosa, the submucous plexus. The ganglionic cell bodies in these plexa send projections to other groups of cells forming a true mophologic plexus. They project mostly in an anal direction, while some neurons project orally (see Ekblad *et al.* 1987). (From Furness and Costa 1980)

oral direction. Some neurons project both anally and orally (e.g. Ekblad *et al.* 1987). These neurons, which have axons not more than 10–15 mm long, are the biological basis for the peristalsis of food.

9.4 The parasympathetic and sympathetic systems are essentially antagonistic in action

It is of course essential for the individual that the different organs can function in a balanced manner. The balanced function of the visceral organs is regulated by the para- and sympathetic systems which are essentially antagonistic to each other, but to varying extent in different tissues. In the eye, the iris is densely innervated by the two systems, and here the antagonistic actions can be nicely demonstrated physiologically and pharmacologically. Since the bulk of smooth muscles run radially to the pupilla, the pupilla widens maximally upon overactivity in the sympathetic system, at a rage or a frightening incident. This releases NA from the sympathetic nerve terminals which contracts the smooth muscles. The pupilla can also be made to widen if the parasympathetic system is blocked, for instance, by the administration of atropine to the eye, which blocks the muscarinic ACh-receptors. Normally the systems balance each other allowing the pupils to adjust in relation to the surrounding light.

In blood vessels the innervation is almost entirely sympathetic, and this division of the ANS has the main function to regulate the degree of constriction of the circular smooth muscle media of the vessels. A high sympathetic activity results in a constriction of the vessel bed, and an increase in the blood pressure. Dilation of the vessel wall seems to occur via local chemical mediators, for instance endothelin produced by the endothelium, and locally produced NO. Thus, overactivity in the sympathetic system results in constricted blood vessels, which in the lower extremities may present as reduced circulation and cold skin with a blue tinge.

The innervation to the sweat glands in the skin is mainly sympathetic. However, in the adult individual the postganglionic transmitter is not NA, but, contrary to the rule, it is ACh, with the neuropeptide VIP (which dilates blood vessels) as coexisting transmitter. The postganglionic nerve cell bodies are located in the lower sympathetic trunk ganglia, and are truly adrenergic early during development, but change transmitter (transmitter plasticity) during maturation (e.g. Landis and Keefe 1983). Overactivity in the sympathetic system will result in increased sweating, especially in the lower extremities.

In the GI canal activity in the parasympathetic system promotes efficient digestion of food, a quicker transport of the food bolus via increased peristalsis, and promotes secretion of local digestive hormones. In the normal situation the parasympathetic system dominates. In contrast, the sympathetic system is activated upon acute stress and it mainly shuts off the activity in the GI system.

The processing of food can wait while the individual takes care of the threatening situation that has caused arousal in the sympathetic system. Thus, overactivity in the sympathetic system results in slow peristalsis and even chronic constipation (although an acute emptying of the gut contents takes place in many strongly fearful situations).

9.5 The peripheral nervous system develops from the neural crest

All nerve cell bodies located outside the brain and the spinal cord are derived from the neural crest. Shortly after the closure of the middle part of the neural tube the thickened neural crest fold starts sending a train of cells peripherally to the ventral roots, to the forming sympathetic chain, the prevertebral and parasympathetic ganglia and to the gut. Many of the tissues in the head, some of the skull bones, the connective tissues and muscles develop from the cranial neural crest. Endocrine organs, like the adrenal medulla and the diffuse endocrine system (enterochromaffin cells in the GI canal, chromaffin cells in the lungs and in other places), are also of neural crest origin, as well as melanocytes in the skin. All cells (except for connective tissue cells) present in peripheral nerves and ganglia, including satellite cells and Schwann cells, originate from the neural crest (Larsen 1997, p. 86).

9.6 The preganglionic neurons are innervated by higher centres, 'the central ANS'

The central autonomic system includes, in addition to neurons using excitatory and inhibitory amino acid transmitters, the noradrenergic, adrenergic, dopaminergic and serotoninergic neurons in the brainstem and the hypothalamus. Many monoaminergic neurons send descending axons to the intermediolateral nucleus in the thoracic and lumbar parts of the spinal cord where the preganglionic neurons of the sympathetic division are located. They also innervate the nuclei of the cranial nerves, and send axons to almost all brain areas, neocortical, hippocampal and cerebellar areas included. Thus, they have a very widespread distribution and are involved in virtually all activities of the CNS.

The neuronal pathways which link central nuclei with autonomic functions with each other and with the peripheral ANS have been studied in detail during the last decade. The anatomy and chemical properties of these centres have been carefully analysed, and the afferent and efferent projections were investigated using retrograde tracing techniques in combination with immunocytochemistry. The activity of the preganglionic sympathetic and parasympathetic neurons (the vagus) that control the heart and the blood vessels is regulated by excitatory as well as inhibitory inputs originating from many areas, both spinal and supraspinal regions. The preganglionic neurons in the spinal cord are innervated by nerve terminals that are immunoreactive for a large number of different peptides as well as of coexisting monoamines. However, in a large number of investigated nerve terminals these appear to contain, in addition, an amino acid, which may act as the principal transmitter. The monoamines and peptides may in these cases serve to modulate the synapse. The origin of the afferent innervation to the preganglionic sympathetic neurons has been shown to be the rostral ventrolateral medulla, where the noradrenergic A1 cell group (Dahlström and Fuxe 1964) is located. Also the nucleus tractus solitarius and the caudal and intermedial ventrolateral medulla send axons to the spinal cord. The serotoninergic cell bodies in the caudal medulla (n. raphae obscurus and pallidus) are a major source of descending afferents to the intermediolateral nucleus in the spinal cord, synapsing with preganglionic neurons which innervate all sympathetic ganglia, as demonstrated using the transneuronal pseudorabies virus tracing technique (Strack *et al.* 1989).

Nucleus tractus solitarius is the main relay nucleus which receives afferent input from peripheral baroreceptors. It sends efferent innervation to a large number of central areas, as well as to the spinal cord, including the medullary serotoninergic raphae neurons and the noradrenergic A5 group (Dahlström and Fuxe 1964), both projecting to the preganglionic neurons in the spinal cord.

In the rostral ventral medulla a large group of nerve cells contain adrenaline (group C1) and various coexisting peptides (Hökfelt *et al.* 1984). This nucleus (corresponding to the subretrofascial nucleus) sends descending axons to the lateral grey substance innervating the sympathetic neurons. These neurons probably belong to the group of non-pacemaker sympathoexcitatory cells in the ventromedial medulla, while other, non-adrenergic, cells in the region demonstrate a pacemaker activity. In addition to projecting to the spinal cord, these adrenaline containing cells also send collaterals to supramedullary centres (Haselton and Guyenet 1989).

For an excellent review on the anatomy, transmitter content, pharmacological and neurophysiological properties of the central autonomic nuclei and their afferent and efferent projections see Dampney (1994).

The description of the central autonomic system as given above and in the review by Dampney (1994) is based on studies in rats, rabbits, and cats. Therefore, one may wonder how relevant these studies are for the human mammal. However, the monoamine containing neuronal systems have been thoroughly investigated in a number of mammalian species, including primates of the old and new world. Striking similarities in distribution and projections have been observed in all mammals studied, but also some species differences. In the primate brain, presumably very similar to the human brain, the number of both catecholamine and serotonin containing cells are greater and more widespread than in rat and cat (cf. Felten and Sladek 1983), and extend beyond the boundaries of the nuclei described for the rat (e.g. Dahlström and Fuxe 1964, 1965). This was especially the case for the serotonin cell bodies which extended far outside the identified raphae nuclei (Felten and Sladek 1983). Thus, basic information gathered from other mammals may be very relevant to the human situation with some possible variations on a common theme for the construction and function of the autonomic nervous system.

9.7 The outgrowth of nerve terminals is regulated by specific trophic factors

In 1951 Rita Levi-Montalcini reported that a substance extracted from a tumour had dramatic affects on the development of ganglionic nerve cells in culture (see Levi-Moltalcini 1987). She named this factor 'nerve growth factor' (NGF), the first in a large number of peptide factors which have now been demonstrated to be essential for the outgrowth, maintenance and survival of different types of neurons (Table 9.1). NGF belongs to the family 'neurotrophins', which is composed of NGF, brain derived nerve growth factor (BDNF), and neurotrophins 3–5 (NT 3–5). These factors appear to have specific activity on nerve cells. Also other cells in the body are dependent on similar factors, for instance members of the epidermal growth factor (EGF) family, the transforming growth factor-alpha (TGF-α), peptides in the insulin family (IGF1 and IGF II), species belonging to the fibroblast growth factor (FGF 1–9) family, the interleukins (IL 1–15) having effect on cells of the lymphoid system but also influencing nerve cells, the transforming growth factor β (TGF-β) family, with the newly discovered neuroactive member glia derived neurotrophic factor (GDNF), and the tumour necrosis factor (TNF) family. All these factors also have influence on the nervous system.

Table 9.1. Different growth factors and the types of neurons that have been shown to be responsive to the factors, either by stimulated outgrowth, survival or neuroprotection. (For a recent review of growth factors and their actions, see Neurotrophic. Factors, (eds. Loughlin and Fallon, Academic Press, San Diego)

Type of neuron	Growth factor
Sensory neurons	NGF, BDNF, NT-3, NT-4
Sympathetic neurons	NGF, bFGF, GDNF
Parasympathetic neurons	CNTF
Motoneurons	CNTF, BDNF, NT-4, IGF-I, GDNF
Basal forebrain cholinergic neurons	NGF, BDNF, bFGF
Cortical Neurons	BDNF, NT-3, NT-4
Hippocampal neurons	BDNF, NT-3, NT-4
Central noradrenergic neurons	NT-3
Dopaminergic neurons	GDNF, BDNF, NT-4, TGF a/b, aFGF, bFGF, IGF-I, activn
Striatal interneurons	BDNF, NT-3, NT-4

The neurotrophins are essential for the development, growth, and survival of neurons. Thus, NGF was early demonstrated to be vital for the development of the sympathetic adrenergic neurons, and for a subpopulation of nerve cells in sensory ganglia. A rare hereditary defect in the NGF gene leads to a special syndrome characterized by low blood pressure and lack of sensory modalities. The members of such families did not survive into old age, since one of the most important protective mechanisms, the ability to feel pain, was lacking. Other neurons are responding to other factors, and Table 9.1 gives a list of different neuron types and the growth factors they respond to.

Growth factors act on special receptors in the cell membrane. The neurotrophins bind to two classes of membrane receptors, a tyrosine kinase (Trk A, Trk B and Trk C) and a 'helper' receptor, p75NGFR. The binding to both receptors is required to obtain high-affinity binding of NGF to generate a specific physiologic response. The specific biological effects of each neurotrophin are explained by the fact that they bind to different receptors; Trk A is the functional receptor for NGF, Trk B for BDNF and NT-4, while Trk C binds NT-3. The neurotrophin receptors have one extracellular part, which defines the specificity for a specific neurotrophin, and a long intracellular part with tyrosine kinase. Upon the binding of a neurotrophin to the extracellular part of its receptor, the receptors dimerize, which causes the intracellular kinase tails to come closer, thereby activating the enzymatic activity (phosphorylating the tyrosine in the tail) and locking the enzyme in active position. The autophosphorylation of Trk then triggers a series of intracellular events, that may, for instance, signal to the nucleus to activate early (e.g. c-fos) and late genes, resulting in phenotypic effects.

Some growth factors instead activate G-protein coupled receptors, which is also the case for a large number of receptors for the classical transmitters (NA, DA, ACh), purines, and some peptides. The notion that G-coupled receptors and the G-proteins only transmit rapid effects (release of hormones, muscle contractions) is not valid; now it is known that they can mediate the same types of slow effects as classical growth factors. This may suggest that neurotransmitters may co-act with, or inter-act with, growth factors produced locally. This hypothesis may be of importance when discussing developmental aberrations in the brain, especially in view of the fact that the central monoaminergic neurons develop and release their amine very early, probably functioning as a 'morphogenesis factor' (cf. Lauder 1988) or a trophic substance before any neurotransmission is developed (see below).

All the above (and other) trophic factors must be expressed during developmental windows, in a sequenced manner, to allow a normal development of the nervous system. The genes that encode for these trophic factors and for their receptors must be expressed and repressed in a tightly regulated pattern to allow for a normal development of the nervous system. The newly discovered gene, MECP2, is considered to have an overriding influence particularly on the repression of other genes via its interaction with histone deacetylase and the corepressor SIN3A (Amir *et al.* 1999). If the repressor region in this gene is mutated, one may speculate that some specific factor(s), needed during a defined developmental window, continues to be expressed after the appropriate period, and this 'overexpression' then may result in an erroneous development of important neuronal couplings. Further investigation of the specific functions of this gene will possibly disclose one or several of the above described, or other so far unknown, growth factors, of importance for the correct development of the brain. One may hope that this will enable a treatment for girls where aberrations in the MECP2 gene have been demonstrated at a very early stage. However, here we may be faced with a factor that would need to be removed, rather than with a missing factor, that could be substituted. The development of specific antibodies, once the factor(s) of importance is (are) discovered, may, however, be a possible strategy for interference with the development of the Rett syndrome in very young girls.

9.8 Plasticity of the autonomic nervous system

Plasticity of sympathetic neurons concerns both the peripheral nerve terminal ramifications, which can be extended or retracted in relation to the need, age and status of the individual, as well as the neurotransmitter phenotype. The superior cervical ganglion (SCG), the most cranial one of the sympathetic paravertebral ganglia, has been a favourite model in the studies of neuronal functions and/or activities due to the relatively simple anatomical relationships, well-characterized target organs, large size, and accessibility. The autonomic ganglia are not basic relay stations as proposed early by Langley (1921), but are 'small brains' with the abilities of integrating exciting and inhibiting signals from the spinal cord and the targets (Elfvin 1983). In addition, many studies have shown that sympathetic neurons are not static but actively involved in adaptiveness and/or plasticities morphologically and physiologically (Purves and Njå 1978; Landis 1988).

The transmitter properties of developing and mature sympathetic neurons can be changed both *in vitro* and *in vivo* (Landis 1988). Sympathetic neurons dissociated from the rat SCG can readily be grown in cell culture. Shortly after plating, neurons attach and begin to extend processes. These neurons bear many characteristics similar to those found *in vivo* (Landis 1988). Initially these cultured neurons express typical catecholamine characteristics. However, various culture conditions can change the transmitter phenotype. The characteristics of the neurons can be regulated by hormones and growth factors. When the neurons are grown in the presence of certain types of non-neuronal cells, such as ganglionic non-neuronal cells, heart myocytes and skeletal myotubes, or in medium conditioned by non-neuronal cells, they develop cholinergic characteristics (Patterson and Chun 1977; Habecker and Landis 1994). The treatment of SCG explants with glucocorticoids prevents the development of ChAT activity in a dose-dependent fashion and increases TH activity (McLennan *et al.* 1980). The sympathetic neurons are also plastic with respect to their expression of neuropeptides. In the absence of exogenous factors, VIP and SP levels rise dramatically when either neonatal or adult ganglia are placed in explant culture (Sun *et al.* 1992). The switch from noradrenergic to cholinergic function and the increased synthesis of some neuropeptides are also observed *in vivo*. The sympathetic axons innervating rat sweat glands are initially noradrenergic, but as the sweat gland innervation matures, noradrenergic markers decrease, while cholinergic and VIP-ergic properties are acquired (Landis and Keefe 1983). An explanation is that the sweat gland releases some factor(s) that retrogradely travel to the cell body to influence the gene expression.

The neurites of ANS neurons are not immutable, even in the adult animal. Unlike the lymphatic cells, cell division has not been adopted by the nervous system as a mode to meet external challenges. Instead nerves adapt by strengthening or weakening connections. This plasticity is a major way by which the nervous system helps the animal adapt to requirements during the life of the animal. In mammals, changes in synaptic structure are ongoing throughout life (Purves *et al.* 1987; Greenough *et al.* 1986). Accumulated data suggest that selective nerve terminal expansion underlies learning and long-term memory (Greenough *et al.* 1986). The introduction of non-toxic vital fluorescent dyes has made it possible to observe the neuronal geometry and innervation of living cells *in vivo* (Purves and Voyvodic 1987; Purves *et al.* 1987). Observations of the same portion of the dendritic arbor of identified SCG cells for periods of up to three months indicate that the higher order branches of these neurons change continuously during early adult life (Purves and Voyvodic 1987). In addition, with the cell number being defined early in ontogeny, the autonomic cells seem to adjust their body size by varying the complexity of the branches of individual neurons (Purves *et al.* 1988). In the aged rat sympathetic neurons have smaller dendritic branches than at younger ages. However, infusion of NGF over the peripheral processes of the ageing neurons in SCG induces significant dendritic and cell body growth, indicating that these neurons are capable to adapt throughout life (Andrews and Cowen 1994).

Neuronal plasticity after injury has been investigated after various types of lesions. It was noticed that preganglionic denervation in newborn rats prevents the normal innervation of iris even though the ganglion itself was intact. After decentralization of the adult rat SCGs, the neuropeptides VIP, SP and galanin, that are present at low or undetectable levels, in control or normal ganglia, are increased. In contrast, NPY and TH, the rate limiting enzyme in the synthesis of NA, are decreased after decentralization (Mytilineou and Black 1976; Hyatt-Sachs *et al.* 1993; Zhang *et al.* 1996). These changes are due to removal of the preganglionic impulse flow, which normally may regulate the synthesis of the peptides (cf. Hyatt-Sachs *et al.* 1993). Consequently, TH activity was increased in SCG if the preganglionic neuron was stimulated continuously (Rittenhouse and Zigmond 1990).

In relation to neuronal plasticity we should also mention growth associated protein-43 (GAP-43), one of the best characterized growth associated proteins. GAP-43 was discovered as a growth associated protein, but it is still maintained at high level in the first few weeks of the postnatal period when most axogenesis has been completed. In addition, it is also enriched in a distinct set of neurons in the mature CNS, especially those exhibiting synaptic plasticity (Neve *et al.* 1987; Benowitz *et al.* 1988). This may suggest that the protein is also involved in synaptic plasticity or in remodelling to adapt the postnatal growth to functional modifications and for neuronal plasticity in adult animals (e.g. Gispen *et al.* 1991). GAP-43 is synthesized in the cell body and transported distally by fast axonal transport, and plays a central function in the growth cones. The protein is a substrate of protein kinase C and the phosphorylation of GAP-43 mediates several cellular functions, for instance the growth cone elongation, the dynamic regulation of cell shape, membrane adhesion and neuronal differentiation (e.g. Shea and Benowitz 1995). Thus, neurons which normally express neuronal plasticity and continuously modify their peripheral nerve terminal processes express this protein normally. The ANS neurons, as well as sensory neurons in the periphery have this capacity to modify their innervation pattern upon need, and they also normally express GAP-43. Monoamine neurons in the CNS belong to this group of normally GAP-43 expressing neurons, as well as some neurons in the hippocampus and in the neocortex of the mature CNS, especially those demonstrating synaptic plasticity (Neve *et al.* 1987; Benowitz *et al.* 1988). This suggests that the protein is also involved in synaptic plasticity and remodelling to adapt the postnatal growth to functional modifications.

Thus, the autonomic nervous system has great potential to adapt plastically also in the adult individual. Such adaptations occur as a response to extracellular factors. The regulation of extracellular factors of importance for the adaptation of the ANS in the adult individual is so far not known, but may be the target for actions of the newly discovered gene MECP2.

9.9 Monoaminergic neurons develop very early and may have trophic/morphogenetic functions in the developing individual

NA, DA and 5-HT are present very early during embryogenesis. In the chicken and mouse, 5-HT is present in the ectodermal as well as non-ectodermal tissues before neurulation, and a role for this transmitter as morphogen has been suggested (cf. Lauder 1988). In the rat, histofluorescence studies have shown that 5-HT neurons are clearly visible in the rat embryo around embryonic day (E)12,

DA neurons were detected around E13, and NA neurons could be seen around E14. When the cell bodies of the monoaminergic neurons were observed in the microscope they had already extended fibre tracts that could be traced to ascend through the met- and mesencephalon and reaching into the prosencephalon, as well as descending caudally into the myelencephalon and spinal cord. Thus, at this early stage of outgrowth of the monoamine systems they contain the complete machinery for synthesis of the transmitter, as well as metabolizing enzymes, n.b. MAO (Olson and Seiger 1972).

The birth time for these neuronal systems was investigated by Lauder and Bloom (1974). These authors studied the onset of cell differentiation in the locus coeruleus (LC), the dorsal and medial raphae nuclei and the substantia nigra (SN) using the technique of long-survival H3-thymidine autoradiography in order to date neurogenesis of these cell groups. They found that the NA cells in the LC began to differentiate around E10–13, with a peak of labelling on E12. The DA neurons in the SN showed a peak labelling on E13, while the peak of labelling in the raphae nuclei was found on E13–14. In parallel, the histofluorescence of CA and 5-HT was used to identify the labelled neuronal cells. Of special interest in this connection is that these authors also studied the date of differentiation of other neuronal groups, Purkinje cells in the cerebellum and hippocampal pyramidal and polymorph cells of areas CA3 and CA4, areas to which the NA-ergic neurons in the LC are known to project. Differentiation of these cells started at E14–15 and E13–18, respectively, with peaks of labelling of both cell types on E15, thus 3 full days after the peak of labelling of the NA neurons.

When comparing the dates for differentiation (last cell cycle) of the monoamine cell groups with the appearance of histofluorescence, indicating the presence of amines in the cells, it was observed that NA fluorescence in the cells appeared about 1 day after the peak of H3-thymidine labelling (E10–14), i.e. after the cessation of the differentiation period. In contrast, the raphae nuclei and the SN cells demonstrated histofluorescence in conjunction with, or in some cases even preceding, the onset of cell differentiation (Lauder and Bloom 1974). This is very early in brain development; the rat neuronal plate does not develop until E9, and the neural tube starts to close at E10, with closure completed by E11 (Witschi 1962; Freeman 1972). Already at E12 CA cells had extended long processes that were frequently in contact with dividing germinal cells and also with apical processes of non-dividing ventricular cells. Therefore, the temporal relation between differentiation and outgrowth of amine containing fibres from the LC and the 3 days later final differentiation event of the hippocampal neurons suggest that the LC neurons may have some significance, for instance, in the formation of synaptic contacts in these areas. Also, it has been observed that early in cortical neurogenesis CA nerve fibres are located below and above the developing cortical plate (Schlumpf et al. 1977) which is the site of genesis of cortical neurons (e.g. Shoukimas and Hinds 1978) and the first regions of cortical synaptogenesis at later stages (Lidov *et al.* 1978). It is hypothesized that monoamines may play a neurotrophic role in early ontogenesis, for instance, by providing mechanisms for specification of monoamine receptors during synaptogenesis (Olson and Seiger 1972, 1973) or supplying the motive force for morphogenic movements (Lawrence and Burden 1973).

The neocortex is profusely innervated by a network of monoamine nerve terminals in adult mammals. In the human fetus, Nobin and Björklund (1973) could detect cell bodies, fibres and nerve terminals of NA, 5-HT, and DA neurons in the 3–4 month old fetus. At this fetal stage the monoamine neurons demonstrated already an advanced development with well-characterized cell groups and principal axonal pathways. The authors compare the overall stage of development of the monoamine neurons in the 3–4 month fetus to the postnatal 1–2 weeks in the rat. The nerve terminal pattern was, however, only partially developed. The basal ganglia, the hypothalamus and the septal regions, which develop rather early, had a well-developed monoamine nerve terminal net. In contrast, the later developing areas, such as the cerebellar and cerebral cortices, which are very immature at this fetal stage, had very few nerve terminals. In an EM study Choi *et al.* (1975) could demonstrate small and large dense cored vesicles in nerve terminal endings belonging to LC neurons in 12 week old human fetuses, demonstrating that not only is NA present in the cytoplasm of the neurons, but also the storage organelles, which are presumably necessary for release of the monoamine.

Support for the hypothesis that NA and 5-HT have important functions during development of the cerebral cortex has been presented by experiments in the rat, that have been injected with neurotoxic agents. Felten *et al.* (1982) found that injection of the selective catecholamine neurotoxin 6-OH-DA to newly born rats caused an almost total disappearance of catecholamines in the rat brain (Felten *et al.* 1982). The neocortex in newborn rat pups is very immature, and the continued development of the cortex was found to be seriously disturbed in the catecholamine depleted rats, as compared to littermate controls. The pyramidal cells had a sparser dendritic arborization with fewer spines, and many apical dendrites were shorter and directed not perpendicular to the surface, but in an oblique pattern (Felten *et al.* 1982; Jonsson 1985, see Fig. 9.3). This is similar to observations of pyramidal cell abnormalities seen in the brain of Rett patients using intracellular injections of Lucifer Yellow and confocal microscopy (Belichenko *et al.* 1994, 1997). Other investigations have shown milder but still clear effects of denervation on development of the cerebral cortex of rats (Maeda *et al.* 1974; Wendlandt *et al.* 1977).

An interesting effect of neonatal 6-OH-DA lesions was that they induced an increased 5-HT innervation in most of the investigated cortical areas observed at P4 (cf. Blue *et al.* 1987). The increase was about 30% above control levels. This serotonergic hyperinnervation did not seem to be the result of a competitive ingrowth of 5-HT terminals onto sites normally occupied by NA terminals, but

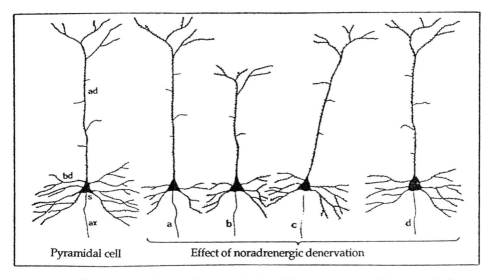

Fig. 9.3 The effect of postnatal catecholamine depletion of the development of the cortex in the rat. Denervation leads to a significant increase in pyramidal cells with abnormal appearance. (a) Reduced number of spines and reduced ramifications as well as extension of basal dendrite, (b) apical dendrite reaching the wrong level, (c) disorientation of apical dendrite, (d) rounded soma. (From Jonsson 1985).

was most notable in areas normally densely innervated by 5-HT terminals. Blue *et al.* (1987) suggest that this is due to the lack of inhibition by NA terminals on the ingrowth of 5-HT terminals. Similar 5-HT hyperinnervation has been observed in the rat striatum in animals with lesioned SN neurons (Snyder *et al.* 1986).

Thus, available experimental evidence seems to indicate that CA and 5-HT may regulate differentiation during early neurogenesis, and that NA nerve fibres, present as the earliest afferent fibres to the developing cortex, may have a distinct role in morphogenesis of e.g. the cortical pyramidal neurons, as well as a regulatory role in the subsequent 5-HT innervation of the cortex.

9.10 Gender specific development of the brain

The developing fetal brain is gender neutral during the very early period of intrauterine life. However, at a critical time, during a specific developmental window, male sexual hormones influence the continued development in gender specific patterns (Gorski *et al.* 1978). For the human child there are two developmental windows, one in the third trimester (12–22 weeks of gestation), and a second period during the first 6 weeks postnatally, when the brain is masculinized (Kelly 1991). It is not certain if there is a feminization of female brains, but behaviouristic studies in girls with Turner's syndrome (X/O, not able to produce female sex hormones) indicate that female sex hormones may play a role in feminization of the brain.

The gender specific differences in brain development are, as presently known, mainly related to a specific nucleus in the supraoptic area which is larger in males than in females, and which probably decides partner preference of the adult individual (LeVay 1994). The second difference relates to the thickness of the corpus callosum, which appears to be thicker and contains more interhemispheric connections in females than in males (Allen *et al.* 1991). This difference could be seen using MRI in the child before birth, and is thus not a result of social influence. The third difference is related to the location of speech centres in the cortex; most investigated women (studied with functional PET scanning) seem to use areas in both hemispheres for speech purposes, while most investigated men, subjected to a similar linguistic task, used only one hemisphere. Also other differences in the functional use of the brain during cognitive tasks have been described.

In female rats, the brain content of 5-HT is somewhat higher than in male rats (Hyyppä and Rinne 1971). Also the level of the serotonin metabolite 5-HIAA is higher, suggesting a higher turnover of 5-HT in females as compared with males (Simon and Vollister 1976). The levels of tryptophan, 5-HT, 5-HTP and 5-HIAA were all found to be higher in female rats. There appears, thus, to be a more developed central serotoninergic system in female as compared to male rats, but the differences show a 10–30% difference (Carlsson *et al.* 1985; Carlsson and Carlsson 1987). It is interesting to note that the CSF levels of 5-HIAA appear to vary in adult women during the menstrual cycle (Eriksson *et al.* 1994).

Thus, while the two genders have in essence similarly constructed and wired brains, there are some distinct differences, which are probably the biological basis of our different reactions and behaviours in certain situations. The fact that serotonin appears to play a more important role in female brains may be taken into consideration when Rett syndrome is discussed, especially since there are indications that 5-HT may be involved in the pathophysiology of this condition.

Also in the peripheral ANS gender differences have been observed. In many of the sympathetic ganglia testosterone influences the content of TH and of NA. Castration early after birth results in a decrease in CA content and also in cell number in most ganglia, including the SCG. At birth the number of neurons are similar, but in females a considerable number die during the first weeks after birth. They can be rescued by injections of testosterone. The functional importance is not known (Wright 1995).

9.11 Are disturbances in the ANS part of the symptomatolgy in Rett girls?

Some observations in Rett girls may indicate that the ANS system is disturbed. Thus, they often have cold and moist feet, which are smaller than for their age, and often with a blue tinge. This indicates that the blood circulation is inadequate, both for keeping skin temperature normal and for promoting normal growth. This is probably a sympathetic vasoconstriction as indicated by the observation that some girls who have undergone orthopedic surgery to correct scoliosis regain growth and normal colour and temperature of the foot on the operated side, probably due to accidental sympathectomy during operation (Hagberg, personal communication).

Rett girls very often have GI problems with chronic constipation and hard, painful feces. This may be a result of overactivity of the sympathetic system, which, as mentioned above, has an inhibitory influence on gut motility. It may also be related to a deficiency in activity of the parasympathetic system, which promotes gut motility in the normal situation.

Problems with urination may also occur; the urinary bladder, like most viscera, is supplied with both sympathetic and parasympathetic innervation. It would be of value if the clinical observation of Rett patients could regularly include special notes related to the function of the ANS. Also, a therapeutic surgical sympathectomy may be considered in view of the positive effects noted in the girls with accidental sympathectomy. It would be most valuable for the planning of efficient remedy strategies to have more information on the peripheral ANS of Rett girls in comparison with normal girls. Such information can only be obtained by investigations of tissue specimens from Rett girls investigated with immunohistochemical methods and microscopy.

Acknowledgements

The author's research is supported by the Swedish MRC (2207), The Swedish Parkinson Foundation, grants from the EC (INTAS-971–1916), and grants from the Swedish Medical Association and the Göteborg Medical Society.

References

Allen, L.S., Richley, M.F., Chai, Y.M., and Gorski, R.A. (1991). Sex differences in the corpus callosum of the living human being. *J. Neurosci.*, **11**, 933–942.

Amir, R.E., Van den Veyver, I.B., Wan, M., Tran, C.Q., Francke, U., and Zoghbi, H.Y. (1999). Rett syndrome is caused by mutations in X-linked MECP2, encoding methyl-CpG-binding protein 2. *Nature Genetics*, **23**, 185–8.

Anderson, D.J. and Axel, R. (1986). A bipotential neuroendocrine precursor whose choice of cell fate is determined by NGF and glucocorticoids. *Cell*, **47**, 1079–90.

Andrews, T.J. and Cowen, T. (1994). Nerve growth factor enhances the dendritic arborization of sympathetic ganglion cells undergoing atrophy in aged rats. *J. Neurocytol.*, **23**, 234–241.

Belichenko, P.V., Hagberg, B., and Dahlstrom, A. (1997). Morphological study of the neocortical areas in Rett syndrome. *Acta Neuropathol.*, **93**, 50–61.

Belichenko, P.V., Oldfors, A., Hagberg, B., and Dahlstrom, A. (1994). Rett syndrome: 3-D confocal microscopy of cortical pyramidal dendrites and afferents. *J. NeuroReport*, 5, 1509–13.

Benowitz, L. I., Apostolides, P., Perrone-Bizzozero, N., Finklestein, S., and Zwiers, H. (1988). Anatomical distribution of the growth associated protein Gap-43/B-50 in the adult rat brain. *J. Neurosci.*, 8, 339–352.

Bertler, Å. and Rosengren, E. (1959). Occurrence and distribution of dopamine in brain and other tissues. *Experientia (Basel)*, 15, 10.

Blottner, D. and Baumgarten, H.G. (1992). Nitric oxide synthetase (NOS)-containing sympathoadrenal cholinergic neurons of the rat IML-cell column: evidence from histochemistry, immunohistochemistry, and retrograde labeling. *J. Comp. Neurol.*, 316, 45–55.

Blue, M.E. and Molliver, M.E. (1987). 6-Hydroxydopamine induces serotoninergic axon sprouting in cerebral cortex of newborn rat. *Devel. Brain Res.*, 32, 255–69.

Bourgeois, J.P. (1997). Synaptogenesis, heterochrony and epigenesis in the mammalian cortex. *Acta Paediatr.* (**Suppl.**), 422, 27–33.

Burnstock, G. and Costa, M. (1975). *Adrenergic neurons*. John Wiley & Sons, New York.

Carlsson, A., Falck, B., and Hillarp, N.-Å. (1962). Cellular localization of brain monoamines. *Acta Physiol. Scand.* **56**(Suppl. 196), 1–27.

Carlsson, M. and Carlsson, A. (1988). A regional study of sex differences in rat brain serotonin. *Progr. Neuro-Psychopharmacol. & Biol Psychiat.*, 12, 53–61.

Carlsson, M., Svensson, K., Eriksson, E., and Carlsson, A. (1985). Rat brain serotonin: Biochemical and functionsl evidence for a sex difference. *J. Neural. Transm.*, 63, 297–313.

Choi, B.H., Antanitus, D.S., Lapham, L.W. (1975). Fluorescence histochemical and ultrastructural studies of locus coeruleus of human fetal brain. *J. Neuropathol. Exp. Neurol.*, 34, 509–16.

Dahlström, A. and Fuxe, K. (1964). Existence for the existence of monoamine containing neurons in the central nervous system. I: Demonstration of monoamines in the cell bodies of brain stem neurons. *Acta Physiol. Scand.*, **62**(Suppl. 232).

Dahlström, A. and Fuxe, K. (1965). Existence for the existence of monoamine containing neurons in the central nervous system. II: Experimentally induced changes in the intraneuronal amine levels of bulbo-spinal neuron systems. *Acta Physiol. Scand.*, **64**(Suppl. 247).

Dampney, R.A.L. (1994). Functional organization of central pathways regulating the cardiovascular system. *Physiol. Rev.*, 74, 323–64.

Edwards, R.H. (1992). The transport of neurotransmitters into synaptic vesicles. *Curr. Opin. Neurobiol.*, 2, 586–94.

Ekblad, E., Winter, C., Ekman, R., Håkansson, R., and Sundler, F. (1987). Projections of peptide containing neurons in rat small intestine. *Neuroscience*, 20, 169–88.

Elfvin Lars-Gösta (1983). *Autonomic ganglia*. John Wiley & Sons, Chichester.

Erickson, J.D., Varoqui, H., Schäfer, M.K.-H., Modi, W., Diebler, M.-F., Weihe, J.R., Eiden, L.E., Bonner, T.I., and Usdin, T.B. (1994). Functional identification of a vesicular acetycholike transporter and its expression from a "cholinergic" gene locus. *J. Biol. Chem.*, 269, 21929–21932.

Eriksson, E., Alling, C., Andersch, B., Andersson, K., and Berggren, U. (1994). Cerebrospinal fluid levels of monoamine metabolites. A preliminary study of their relation to menstrual cycle phase, sex steroids, and pituitary hormones in healthy women and in women with premenstrual syndrome. *Neuropsychopharmacology*, 11, 201–13.

Falck, B. (1962). Observations on the possibilities of the cellular localizations of monoamines by a fluorescencemethod. *Acta Physiol. Scand.*, **56**(Suppl. 197).

Falck, B., Hillarp, N.-Å., Thieme, G., and Torp, A. (1962). Fluorescence of catecholamines and related compounds condensed with formaldehyde. *J. Histochem. Cytochem.*, 10, 348–54.

Felten, D.L., Hallman, H., and Jonsson G. (1982). Evidence for a neurotropic role of noradrenaline neurons in the postnatal development of rat cerebral cortex. *J. Neurocytol.*, 11, 119–35.

Felten, D.L. and Sladek, J.R. (1983). Monoamine distribution in primate brain. V. Monoaminergic nuclei, anatomy, pathways and local organization. *Brain Res. Bull.*, **10**, 171–284.

Freeman, B.G. (1972). Surface modifications of neural epithelial cells during formation of the neural tube in the rat embryo. *J. Embryol. Exp. Morphol.*, **28**, 437-448.

Furness, J.B. and Costa, M. (1980). Types of nerves in the ebteric nervous system. *Neuroscience*, **5**, 1–20.

Gilmore, M.L., Nash, N.R., Roghani, A., Edwards, R.H., Yi, H., Hersch, S.M., and Levey, A.L. (1996). Expression of the putative vesicular acetylcholine transporter in rat brain and localization in cholinergic synaptic vesicles. *J. Neurosci.*, **16**, 2179–2190.

Gispen, W.H., Nielander H.B., De Graan, P.N.E., Oestreicher, A.B., Schrama, L.H., and Schotman, P. (1991). Role of the growth-associated protein B50/GAP-43 in neuronal plasticity. *Mol. Neurobiol.*, **5**, 61–85.

Goldstein, M., Fuxe, K. and Hökfelt, T. (1972). Characterization and tissue localization of catecholamine synthesizing enzymes. *Pharm. Rev.*, **24**, 298–309.

Gorski, R.A., Gordon, J.H., Shryne, J.E., and Southam, A.M. (1978). Evidence for a morphological sex difference within the medial preoptic area of the rat brain. *Brain Res.*, **148**, 333–346.

Greenough, W.T., McDonald, J.W., Parnisari, R.M., and Camel, J.E., (1986). Environmental conditions modulate degeneration and new dendrite growth in cerebellum of senescent rats. *Brain-Res.*, **380**, 136–43.

Habecker, B.A. and Landis, S. C. (1994). Noradrenergic regulation of cholinergic differentiation. *Science*, **264**, 1602–1604.

Hamberger, B. (1967). Reserpine-resistant uptake of catecholamines in isolated tissues of the rat. Thesis. *Acta Physiol. Scand* (**Suppl**. 295), Stockholm.

Haselton, J.R. and Guyenet, P.G. (1989). Central respiratory modulation of medullary sympathoexcitatory neurons in rat. *A. J. Physiol.*, **256**, R739–R750.

Hillarp, N.-Å. (1946). Structure and function of the synapse and the peripheral innervation apparatus of the autonomic nervous system. *Acta Anat.* (**Suppl. IV**), 1–153. Thesis, Lund's University.

Hillarp, N.-Å. (1959). Structure and function of the autonomic ground plexus. *Acta Physiol. Scand.*, **46**(**Suppl. 157**), 1–38.

Hope, B.T., Michael, G.J., Knigge, K.M., and Vincent, S.R. (1991). Neuronal NADPH diaphorase is a nitric oxide synthase. *Proc. Natl. Acad. Sci. USA*. **88**, 2811–2814.

Hökfelt, T., Everitt, B., Theodorsson-Norheim, E., and Goldstein, M. (1984). Occurrence of neurotensin-like immunereactivity in subpopulations of hypothalamic, mesencephalic and medullary catecholamine neurons. *J. Comp. Neurol.*, **222**, 543–560.

Hyatt-Sachs, H., Schreiber, R.C., Bennett, T.A., and Zigmond, R.E. (1993). Phenotypic plasticity in adult sympathetic ganglia in vivo: effects of deafferentation and axotomy on the expression of vasoactive intestinal peptide. *J. Neurosci.*, **13**, 1642–1653.

Hyyppä, M. (1972). Hypothalamic monoamines in the human fetus. *Neuroendocrinology*, **9**, 257–66.

Hyyppä, M. and Rinne, U.K. (1971). Hypothalamic monoamines after the neonatal androgenization, castration or reserpine treatment in the rat. *Acta Endocrinol.* **66**, 317–324.

Jonsson, G. (1985). Hjärnan—en dator med plastiska egenskaper. Läkartidningen 82: 3178–80.

Jonsson, G. and Kasamatsu, T. (1983). Maturation of monoamine neurotransmitters and receptors in cat occipital cortex during postnatal critical period. *Exp. Brain Res.* **50**(2-3), 449–58.

Kelley, D.D. (1991). Sexual differentiation of the nervous system. In *Principles of Neuroscience* (ed. E.R. Kandel, J.H. Schwartz, and T.M. Jessel), pp. 771-783 Appleton & Lange, Prentice-Hall Internat. Inc.

Krukoff, T.L., Ciriello, J., and Calaresu, F.R. (1985). Segmental distribution of peptide- and 5HT-like immunoreactivity in nerve terminals and fibers of the thoracolumbar sympathetic nuclei of the cat. *J. Comp. Neurol.*, **240**, 103–16.

Ladosky, W. and Gazieri, L.C.J. (1970). Brain serotonin and sexual differentiation of the nervous system. *Neuroendocrinolgy*, **6**, 168–174.

Landis, S.C. (1988). Neurotransmitter plasticity in sympathetic neurons and its regulation by environmental factors *in vitro* and *in vivo*, In *Handbook of chemical neuroanatomy*, Vol. 6: *The peripheral nervous system* (ed. A. Björklund, T. Hökfelt, and C. Owman), pp. 65–115 Elsevier Science Publishers B.V.

Landis, S.C. and Keefe, D. (1983). Evidence for neurotransmitter plasticity *in vivo*: developmental changes in the properties of cholinergic sympathetic neurons. *Dev. Biol.*, **98**, 349.

Langley, J.N., (1921). *The autonomic nervous system, Part I*. Heffer and Sons, Cambridge, England.

Larsen, W.J. (1997). *Human embryology*. Churchill Livingstone, New York.

Lauder, J.M. (1988). Neurotransmitters as morphogens. *Progr. in Brain Res.*, Ch. 2, **73**, 365–84.

Lauder, J.M. and Bloom, F.E. (1975). Ontogeny of monoamine neurons in the locus coeruleus, raphae neuclei and substantia nigra of the rat. I. Cell differentiation. *J. Comp. Neurol.*, **155**, 469–481.

Lauder, J.M., Wallace, J.A., and Krebs, H. (1981*a*). Roles for serotonin in neuroembryogenesis. *Adv. Exp. Biol. Med.*, **133**, 477–506.

Lauder, J.M., Wallace, J.A., Krebs, H., and Petrusz, P. (1981*b*). Serotonin as a timing mechanism in neuroembryogenesis. In *Progr. in Psycho-Neuro-Endocrinology* (ed. Brambilla, Racagni, and Dewied), pp. 539–56.

Lauder, J.M., Wallace, J.A., Wilkie, M.B., DiNome, A. and Krebs, H. (1983) Roles for serotonin in neurogenesis?. In *Action of neurotransmitters and hormones on the developing nervous system*, Monogr. Neurol. Sci., Vol. 9, pp. 3–10. Karger, Basel.

Lawrence, I.E. and Burden, H.W. (1973). Catecholamines and morphogenesis of the chick neuroal tube and notocord. *Am. J. Anat.*, **137**, 199–208.

Levi-Montalcini, R. (1987). The nerve growth factor 36 years later. *Science*, **237**, 1154–62.

LeVay, S. (1994). *The Sexual Brain*. Boston University Press.

Lidov, H.G.W., Molliver, M.E., and Zecevic, N.R. (1978). Characterization of monoamine innervation of immature rat neocortex. A histofluorescence analysis. *J. Comp. Neurol.*, **181**, 663–680.

Maeda, T., Tohyama, M., and Shimuzu, N. (1974). Modification of postnatal development of neocortex in rat brain with experimental deprivation of locus coeruleus. *Brain Res.*, **70**, 515–20.

Malmfors, T. (1965). Studies on adrenergic nerves. Direct observations on their distribution in an effector system, degeneration and mechanisms for uptake, storage and release of catecholamines. Thesis (Almquist & Wiksell Boktryckeri AB, Uppsala).

McAllen, R.M. (1986). Location of neurones with cardiovascular and respiratory function, at the ventral surface of the cats medulla. *Neuroscience*, **18**, 43–9.

McLennan, I.S., Hill, C.E. and Hendry, I.A. (1980). Glucocorticsteroids modulate transmitter choice in developing superior cervical ganglion. *Nature*, **283**, 206–201.

Mytilineou, C. and Black, I. B. (1976). Regeneration of sympathetic neurons: effect of decentralization. *Brain Res.*, **109**, 382–386.

Neve, R.L., Perrone-Bizzozero. N.I., Finklestein, S., Zwiers, H., Bird, E., Kurnit, D. M. and Benowitz, L. I. (1987). The neuronal growth-associated protein GAP-43 (B50, F1): use of cDNA to show the neuronal specificity, developmental regulation and regional distribution of the human and rat mRNAs. *Mol. Brain Res.*, **2**, 177–183.

Nobin, A. and Björklund, A. (1973). Topography of the monoamine neuron systems in the human brain as revealed in the fetus. *Acta Physiol. Scand.* (**Suppl.**) **388**, 1–40.

Norberg, K.-A. (1965). The sympathetic adrenergic neuron and certain adrenergic mechanisms. A histochemical study. Thesis (I. Häggströms Tryckeri AB, Stockholm).

Norberg, K.-A. and Hamberger, B. (1964). The sympathetic adrenergic neuron. *Acta Physiol. Scand.* **63** (**Suppl.** 238), 1–42.

Olson, L. (1970). Growth of sympathetic adrenergic nerves. Fluorescence histochemical studies of growing nerves in developing and adult animals with special reference to tissue transplantations. Thesis (Graficon AB, Stockholm).

Olson, L., Boréus, L., and Seiger, Å. (1973). Histochemical demonstration and mapping of 5-hydroxytryptamine and catecholamine-containing neurons in the human fetal brain. *Z. Anat. Entwicklungsgesch.*, **139**, 259–82.

Olson, L. and Seiger, Å. (1972). Early prenatal ontogeny of cantral monoaminergic neruons in the rat; fluorescence histochemical observations. *Z. Anat. Entwickl.-Gesch.*, **137**, 301–16.

Olson, L. and Seiger, Å. (1973). Late prenatal ontogeny of cantral monoaminergic neurons in the rat; fluorescence histochemical observations. *Z. Anat. Entwickl.-Gesch.*, **140**, 281–318.

Olson, L., Nyström, B., and Seiger, Å. (1973). Monoamine neuron systems in the normal and schizophrenic human brain: fluroescence histochemistry of fetal, neurosurgical and post mortem material. In *Frontiers in catecholamine research* (ed. E. Usdin and S. Snyder), pp. 1097–1100. Pergamon Press.

Patterson, P.H. and Chun, L.L.Y. (1977). Induction of acetylcholine synthesis in primary cultures of dissociated rat sympathetic neurons. I. Effects of conditioned medium. *Dev. Biol.*, **56**, 263.

Purves, D. and Njå, A. (1978). Trophic maintenance of synaptic connections in autonomic ganglia. In *Neuronal Plasticity* (ed. C.W. Cotman), pp 27–47 Raven Press, New York.

Purves, D. and Voyvodic, J.T. (1987). Imaging mammalian nerve cells and their connections over time in living animals. *TINS*, **10**, 398–404.

Purves, D., Snider, W.D. and Voyvodic, J.T. (1988). Trophic regulation of nerve cell morphology and innervation in the autonomic nervous system. *Nature*, **336**, 123–128.

Purves, D., Voyvodic, J.T., Magrassi, L., and Yawo, H. (1987). Nerve terminal remodeling visualized in living mice by repeated examination of the same neuron. *Science*, **238**, 1122–6.

Rakic, P. and Goldman-Rakic, P.S. (1982). The development and modifiability of the cerebral cortex. *Overview.Neurosci-Res-Program-Bull.*, **20**(4), 433–8.

Rittenhouse, A. R. and Zigmond, R.Z. (1990). Nerve stimulation in vivo acutely increase tyrosine hydroxylase activity in the rat superior cervical ganglion and its end organs. *Brain Res.*, **524**, 156–159.

Sachs, Ch. (1970). Noradrenaline uptake mechanisms. A biochemical and histochemical study. Thesis (Kungliga Boktryckeriet, Stockholm).

Schlumpf, M., Shoemaker, W.J., and Bloom, F.E. (1977). The development of catecholamine fibers in the prenatal cerebral cortex of the rat. *Soc. Neurosci. Abstr.*, **3**, 361.

Schoukimas, G.M. and Hinds, J.W. (1978). The development of the cerebral cortex in the embryonic mouse; An electronmicroscopic serial section analysis. *J. Comp. Neurol.*, **179**, 795–870.

Shea T. B. and Benowitz L. I. (1995). Inhibition of neurite outgrowth following intracellular delivery of anti-GAP-43 antibodies depends upon culture conditions and method of neurite induction. *J. Neurosci. Res.*, **41**, 347–354.

Simon, N. and Volicer, L. (1976). Neonatal asphyxia in the rat; greater vulnerability of males and persistent effects on brain monoamine synthesis. *J. Neurochem.*, **26**, 893–900.

Snyder, A.M., Zigmond, M.J., and Lund, R.D. (1986). Sprouting of serotininergic afferents onto striatum after dopamine-depleting lesions in infant rats; a retrograde transport and immunocytochemical study. *J. Comp. Neurol.*, **245**, 274–81.

Strack, A.M., Sawyer, W.B., Hughes, J.H., Platt, K.B., Loewy, A.D.A. (1989). General pattern of CNS innervation of the sympathetic outflow demonstrated by transneuronal pseudorabies viral infections. *Brain-Res.*, **491**(1), 156–62.

Sun, Y., Rao, M., Landis, S. and Zigmond, R. (1992). Depolarization increases vasoactive intestinal peptide- and Substance P-like immunoreactivities in cultured neonatal and adult sympathetic neurons. *J. Neurosci.*, **12**, 3717–3728.

Twarog, B.M. and Page, J.H. (1953). Serotonin content of some mammalian tissues and urine and methods for its determination. *Amer. J. Physiol.*, **175**, 157–61.

Ungerstedt, U. (1971). Stereotactic mapping of the monoamine pathways in the rat brain. Thesis. *Acta Physiol. Scand.* (**Suppl. 367**), 1–48.

Vogt, M. (1954). The concentration of sympathin in different parts of the central nervous system under normal conditions and after the administration of drugs. *J. Physiol. (London)*, **123**, 451–481.

Wendlandt, S., Crow, T.J. and Stirling, R.V. (1977). The involvement of the noradrenergic system arising from the locus coeruleus in the postnatal development of the cortex in rat brain. *Brain-Res.*, **125**, 1–9.

Willard, H.F. and Hendrich, B.D. (1999). Breaking the silence in Tett syndrome. *Nature Genetics*, **23**, 127–8.

Witschi, E. (1962) In *Growth, Biological Handbooks*, Fed. Amer. Soc. Exp. Biol., pp. 304–214.

Wright, L.L. (1995). Development and sexual differentiation of sympathetic ganglia. In *Autonomic ganglia* (ed. E.M. McLachlan), pp. 481–508. Harwood Academic Publishers.

10.1 Autonomic dysfunction and sudden death in Rett syndrome: prolonged QTc intervals and diminished heart rate variability

Daniel G. Glaze and Rebecca J. Schultz

10.1.1 Introduction

Rett syndrome girls are expected to survive into adulthood to become women with Rett syndrome. A preliminary study indicates that the survival curve for Rett syndrome (RS) follows the general female population until age 10 years. Thereafter, survival declines, most precipitously after age 20 years to 70% at age 35 years compared to 98.4% in the general US female population. However, in comparison to severely retarded individuals retaining self-feeding skills and some degree of ambulation, the survival curve for RS declines less rapidly. By age 35 years, 70% survival in RS contrasts to 27% survival for profoundly mentally retarded individuals. The majority of deaths appear to be either sudden and unexplained, or secondarily to pneumonia (DeJunco *et al.* 1992). Of the deaths reported to the International Rett Syndrome Association, 22% were sudden deaths of unknown cause without preceding acute illness (Sekul *et al.* 1994). Cardiac electrical instability is a prime suspect for causing sudden death. This paper describes electrocardiographic changes in RS and illustrates that these abnormalities occur frequently in RS. These findings provide evidence of autonomic dysfunction in RS and suggest the possibility that this may contribute to the high incidence of sudden death among RS individuals.

10.1.2 Studies designs

We evaluated corrected QT interval (QTc, Bazett's formula) and heart rate variability in RS during two studies (Sekul *et al.* 1994; Johnsrude *et al.* 1995). Study I (Sekul *et al.* 1994): 61 standard 12-lead electrocardiograms (ECGs) were obtained on 34 RS females, aged 2–22 years. Follow-up electrocardiography was performed approximately every 4–12 months, depending on patient availability and without regard to the initial ECG results. The comparison population consisted of 41 female subjects, aged 2–18 years, with no known cardiac abnormalities for whom ECG was performed for routine or preoperative screening. The ECG findings were recorded by a computer-controlled thermal digital dot array electrocardiography (Marquette Electronics, Inc., Milwaukee, Wisconsin). The QT interval, determined by the longest hand-measured QT interval in any lead, was corrected for the heart rate by the method of Bazett to yield the QTc value (Garson 1990). Study II (Johnsrude et al. 1995): QTc interval from routine ECG and heart rate variability (HRV) parameters from 24 h ambulatory monitoring were determined for 25 RS females, aged 3–27 years, and 25 age-matched female controls with no cardiac abnormalities.

10.1.3 Results

(a) *Study I*: In the earliest ECG of RS females, the QTc values were longer than in the ECG of the healthy girls (0.43±0.02 s vs 0.41±0.02 s). The QTc of RS females receiving medications (carbamazepine, phenytoin, or naltrexone) did not differ significantly from those RS females receiving no medications (0.44±0.03 s vs 0.43±0.02 s). Prolonged QTc (>0.45 s) was noted in 36% clinical stage II, 38% stage III, and 50% stage IV. The QTc intervals were significantly more prolonged across clinical stages in RS females (0.42±0.02 s RS stage II vs 0.44±0.02 s RS stage IV).

(b) *Study II*: The mean QTc interval was longer in the RS females than the control females (0.441±32 s vs 0.418±13 s). Of the RS females, significantly more had QTc > 0.450 s than control females (9 RS vs 0 controls). Diminished heart rate variability was demonstrated in RS females for: (1) mean of SD of normal RR for all 5 m segments, (2) root mean square successive differences, (3) percentage of differences between normal RR > 50 ms, and (4) high frequency power. RS females with QTc > 0.450 s and QTc < 0.450 s had similar heart rate variability parameters (see Table 10.1.1).

10.1.4 Discussion

The majority of RS individuals survive into adulthood (DelJunco et al. 1992). However, sudden, unexplained death has been noted beginning in childhood. Of the deaths reported to IRSA in individuals less than 23 years of age, 22% have been sudden, unexpected, in comparison with 2.3% in the general population up to the same age (Driscoll and Edwards 1985). Our studies were the first to

Table 10.1.1 Study II (Johnsrude et al. 1995): QTc intervals and heart rate variability in Rett syndrome patients and controls

	RS	Control	p value
Age (years)	9.1±5.8	9.1±5.7	0.490
QTc (ms)	441± 32	418±13	0.001*
Qtc > 450 ms (pts)	9	0	0.002*
Mean HR (bpm)	99±10	94±11	0.108
SDANN (ms)	74.3±28.7	102.4±38.5	0.003*
rMSSD (ms)	30.9±11.0	42.4±18.8	0.012*
pNN50 (%)	9.4±7.7	16.8±12.3	0.014*
Total power (ln ms^2)	7.54±0.54	7.59±0.74	0.768
LF power (ln ms^2)	6.66±0.60	6.57±0.76	0.628
HF power (ln ms^2)	5.33±0.82	6.11±1.00	0.005*

HR=heart rate, SDANN=mean of SD of normal RR for all 5 min segments, rMSSD=root mean square successive differences, pNN50=% of differences between normal RR>50 ms, LF=low frequency, HF=high frequency, *=$p<0.05$. RS pts with Qtc > 450 ms and Qtc < 450 ms had similar HRV parameters (p=0.203–0.950).

document that RS individuals have significantly longer QTc intervals and a higher incidence of prolonged QTc (> 0.450#s) than age-matched healthy females, and that with advancing RS clinical stage the proportion of QTc interval prolongations increases. Two subsequent studies also reported that RS females have significantly longer QTc values and an increased incidence of prolonged QTc intervals, but did not find that QTc values were prolonged across RS clinical stages (Ellaway et al. 1999; Fuster-Siebert and Castro-Gago (1995)).

Possible explanations for these findings include CNS abnormalities, a direct effect of RS on the heart, or a secondary effect of hyperventilation. Central autonomic function via neurons in the rostral ventrolateral medulla may mediate these changes (Corr et al. 1987). An imbalance in sympathetic tone is associated with QTc prolongation and an increased incidence of arrhythmias (Schwartz et al. 1992). Our study (Johnsrude et al. 1995) was the first to demonstrate diminished heart rate variability in RS individuals. A recent study also observed diminished heart rate variability and longer QTc intervals in RS females compared with an age-matched group of healthy girls (Guideri et al. 1999). These abnormalities increased with advancing RS clinical stage. There has been a growing interest in the spectral analysis of heart rate variability as a tool for noninvasive assessment of autonomic nervous system function (Task force of the European Society of Cardiology and the North American Society of Pacing and Electrophysiology 1996; Stan et al. 1994). Our RS patients showed diminished heart rate variability as indicated by lower high frequency (HF) power in comparison to age-matched controls. The HF component is believed to be medicated primarily through vagal cardiac control; the power of the HF band has been used to quantify parasympathetic activity. The ratio between low frequency and HF spectral power is generally considered to provide a good index of sympathetic modulation (Task force of the European Society of Cardiology and the North American Society of Pacing and Electrophysiology 1996). Similar findings including diminished heart rate variability, prolonged QTc interval, and decreased high frequency power have been reported in future victims of sudden infant death syndrome (Franco et al. 1999). Impairment of autonomic nervous system (ANS) control could reduce the electrical stability of the heart and precipitate sudden cardiac death. We have reported that substance P is deficient in the central nervous system of RS females (Deguichi et al. 1999). A deficiency of substance P may contribute to impairment of ANS resulting in cardiac dysautonomia. Monitoring of ECG, avoidance and/or judicious use of certain medications associated with prolongation of QT interval (e.g. cisapride, tricyclic antidepressants, among others), and use of β-blockers (e.g. propranolol) may be indicated in selected RS patients.

10.1.5 Conclusion

RS females have a high incidence of prolonged QTc and diminished heart rate variability (non-spectral parameters and high frequency power). The abnormalities likely result from disturbances of the ANS and may contribute to the high incidence of sudden death among RS females.

Rererences

Corr, P.B., Pitt, B., Natelson, B.H., et al. (1997). Sudden cardiac death: neural–chemical interactions. *Circulation*, 76, 1208–14.

Deguichi, K., Antalffy, B., Twohill, L., Chakrohorty, S., Glaze, D., and Armstrong, D. (1999). Substance P in Rett Syndrome. Relation to autonomic dysfunction. *Pediatr. Neurol.*, in press.

DelJunco, D., MacNaughton, N., Warung, S., Skencher, M., Kozinetz, C., Moore, C., Hunter, K., Percy, A., and Glaze, D. (1992). Survival in a large cohort of U.S. girls and women with Rett Syndrome. In *2nd International Workshop and Symposium on Rett Syndrome*, Orlando, Florida, 7–10 October 1992.

Driscoll, D.J., and Edwards, W.D. (1985). Sudden unexpected death in children and adolescents. *J. Am. Coll. Cardio*, 5, 118B–21B.

Ellaway, C.F., Sholler, G., Leonard, H., and Christodoulou, J. (1999). Prolonged QT interval in Rett Syndrome. *Arch. Dis. Childh.*, 80, 470–2.

Franco, P., Szliwowski, H., Dramaix, M., and Kahn, A. (1999). Decreased autonomic response to obstructive sleep events in future victims of sudden infant death syndrome. *Pediatr. Res.*, 46, 33–9.

Fuster-Siebert, M., and Castro-Gago, M. (1995). Electrocardiographic findings in Rett Syndrome. *J. Pediatr.*, 126, 506 (LTE).

Garson, A., Jr (1990). Electrocardiography. In *The science of practice of pediatric cardiology*, Vol. 2 (ed. A. Garson Jr, J.T. Bricker, and D.G. McNamara), pp. 713–67. Lea and Febiger, Philadelphia.

Guideri, F., Acampa, M., Hayek, G., Zappella, M., and Di Perri, T. (1999). Reduced heart rate variability in patients affected with Rett Syndrome. A possible explanation for sudden death. *Neuropediatrics*, 30, 146–8.

Johnsrude, C., Glaze, D.G., Schultz, R.J., and Friedman, R. (1995). Prolonged QT intervals and diminished heart rate variability in patients with Rett Syndrome (abstract). *PACE: Pacing and Electrophysiology*, **18**, 889.

Schwartz, P.J., Bonazzi, O., Locati, E., *et al.* (1992). Pathogenesis and therapy of the idiopathic long QT syndrome. *Ann. NY Acad. Sci.*, **644**, 112–41.

Sekul, E.A., Moak, J.P., Schultz, R.J., Glaze, D.G., Dunn, J.K., and Percy, A.K. (1994). Electrocardiographic findings in Rett Syndrome: an explanation for sudden death. *J. Pediatr.*, **125**, 80–2.

Stan, P.K., Bosner, M.S., Klerger, R.E., and Conger, B.M. (1994). Heart rate variability: a measure of cardiac autonomic tone. *Am. Heart J.*, **127**, 1376–81.

Task force of the European Society of Cardiology and the North American Society of Pacing and Electrophysiology. (1996). Heart rate variability: standards of measurement, physiological interpretation and clinic use. *Circulation*, **93**, 1043–65.

10.2 Feeding in Rett syndrome

Richard Morton

Oral motor abilities closely parallel general neurological changes in Rett syndrome (Mortan et al. 1997a). Normal infants begin to make lateral movements of the tongue for chewing at around 8 months, but this is delayed in Rett syndrome. Regression in feeding occurs around 14 months with generalized regression; only half are able to chew before this occurs and some lose the ability at this time. Most individuals with Rett are therefore left with an immature suckle feeding pattern and can only manage mashed solids. If chewing is maintained, it is always poor and suckling remains dominant. This is characterized by poor bolus formation with solids and instead of a discrete oral swallow, there are repetitive undulations of the mid and posterior tongue which are ineffective in pushing the food bolus into the pharynx. There is also a poor seal between the posterior tongue and soft palate, so liquids escape uncontrolled into the pharynx where food collects until sufficient to provoke a pharyngeal swallow. This type of immature swallowing is present whenever development is sufficiently delayed, but in Rett there are other characteristic abnormalities which appear to increase with age, irrespective of neurological status. Movements of the mid and posterior tongue become excessively slow and even when the pharynx is full, a delay occurs before swallowing. As individuals become older therefore, the time taken to swallow a mouthful of food increases. Some acquire the novel technique of 'back flip', in which the anterior tongue folds back on itself to push the food bolus past the static posterior segment and into the pharynx.

While the majority of feeding problems occur in the oral phase of the swallow, those with severe neurological impairment and poor mobility also have pharyngeal problems. These consist mainly of poor pharyngeal motility, resulting in food residue remaining after the swallow, which can be aspirated. Similar oral and pharyngeal problems are present in quadriplegic cerebral palsy.

Adaptation in breathing is needed to cope with the long delays before a swallow, during which food collects in the pharynx (Morton et al. 1997b). Apnoea usually occurs until the swallow, and sometimes afterwards, even in individuals who do not apnoea at other times. When the time to swallow is very prolonged, usually in older individuals, breathing can take place meanwhile. Those who have reasonable tone and mobility manage to breathe gently without aspirating. However, this cannot be achieved in those severely affected, who usually apnoea until the swallow for protection. If they do try and breathe, it is sharp and uncontrolled, and often results in aspiration before the swallow. Such severely affected individuals can therefore aspirate both before and after a swallow; they often have chest infections and may need gastrostomy feeds. In some milder cases, even without aspiration, feeding is so slow that gastrostomy feeding may be needed.

References

Morton, R.E., Bonas, R., Minford, J., Kerr, A., and Ellis, R.E. (1997*a*). Feeding ability in Rett Syndrome. *Developmental Medicine and Child Neurology*, **39**, 331–5.

Morton, R.E., Bonas, R., Minford, J., Tarrant, S.C., and Ellis, R.E. (1997*b*). Respiration patterns during feeding in Rett Syndrome. *Developmental Medicine and Child Neurology*, **39**, 607–13.

10.3 Oropharyngeal dysfunction and upper gastrointestinal dysmotility, a reflection of disturbances in the autonomic nervous system in Rett syndrome

Kathleen J. Motil, Rebecca J. Schultz, Daniel G. Glaze, and Dawna Armstrong

10.3.1 Introduction

Feeding impairment frequently complicates the clinical course of females with Rett syndrome (RS) (Budden 1986, 1995; Morton *et al.* 1997; Rice and Haas 1998; Thommessen *et al.* 1991, 1992). The neurophysiologic mechanisms that account for this abnormality have not been elucidated fully (Motil *et al.* 1999). This paper describes the functional characteristics of the oropharynx and upper gastrointestinal (UGI) tract in RS females and illustrates the pervasive nature of swallowing dysfunction and UGI dysmotility in this disorder. These findings raise the possibility that disturbances in the autonomic nervous system (ANS) may be causally related to the abnormalities of the UGI tract and, hence, the feeding impairment of RS females.

10.3.2 Study design

Thirty-four RS females, aged 2.3–40.1 years, who were classified as stage III (50%), IV (41%), or atypical (9%) in the progression of their disorder (The Rett Syndrome Diagnostic Working Group 1988; Hagberg and Witt Engerström 1986), were evaluated because they had a history of eating difficulty, emesis, eructation, or irritability, with or without feeding (Table 10.3.1). Oropharyngeal and UGI function was assessed fluoroscopically by a swallowing function study ($n=20$) using barium-laced liquid and solid meals of various consistencies (Logemann 1986; Mirrett *et al.* 1994) and a UGI series ($n=31$), respectively (see Table 10.3.2) (Dodds 1993).

Table 10.3.1 Characteristics of subjects with Rett syndrome

Number	34
Age (years)	13.1±8.9
Rett stage (III:IV:atypical)	17:14:3
Height (cm)	120.9±20.2
(Z-score)[a]	-2.35±1.81
Weight (kg)	27.2±11.7
(Z-score)[a]	-1.29±1.84
Body mass index (kg/m^2)	17.6±4.0
(%ile)[b]	38±34
Muscle tone (hypotonic:normal:hypertonic)	9:11:14

[a]Hamill *et al.* (1976). [b]Hammer *et al.* (1991).

Table 10.3.2. Feeding abnormalities of RS subjects determined by videofluoroscopic swallowing function study

Feeding Abnormality	Food Consistency			
	Liquid		Solid	
	Thin (n=20) (%)	Thick (n=16)[a] (%)	Pudding (n=19)[a] (%)	Cookie (n=17)[a] (%)
Oral preparatory phase				
Poor bolus formation	85	81	84	59
Oral transit phase				
Stasis on tongue surface	75	69	74	35
Reduced posterior oral containment	80	69	78	41
Weak base of tongue retraction	37	37	28	12
Pharyngeal transit phase				
Diffuse falling over base of tongue	80	76	84	69
Pooling in valleculae	57	75	74	35
Pooling in pyriform sinuses	50	44	26	24
Laryngeal penetration/aspiration during swallow	60	37	11	0
Residue in valleculae	76	87	79	59
Residue in pyriform sinuses	30	56	47	29

[a] Thick liquid not offered to four subjects; pudding not offered to one subject; solid food offered to two subjects, but no attempts to chew or swallow were made, solids not offered to one subject.

10.3.3 Results

Ninety-five per cent of all RS females had abnormalities throughout the oral preparatory, oral transit, and pharyngeal transit phases of swallowing function. At least 80% displayed poor bolus formation, stasis on the tongue surface, and reduced posterior oral containment because of reduced posterior tongue and soft palate apposition, and 37% displayed weak base of tongue retraction when consuming thin liquids. Eighty per cent demonstrated diffuse falling of thin liquid over the base of the tongue before swallowing. At least 50% displayed pooling of thin liquid in the vallecular and pyriform sinuses because of a delay in swallowing. Sixty per cent demonstrated laryngeal penetration of thin liquid during swallowing. All of these abnormalities persisted when the females consumed a thick liquid or pudding, but were less frequent when a cookie was consumed. Liquid and solid food residues of all consistencies persisted in the vallecular and pyriform sinuses after swallowing in at least 50% and 25% of the females, respectively.

Twenty-one (68%) females displayed abnormal UGI function. Esophageal dysmotility, characterized by the absence of primary or secondary waves, delayed emptying, atony, the presence of tertiary waves, or spasm was found in 11 (39%) females. Gastroesophageal reflux (GER) was present in 11 (35%) females and one individual had nasopharyngeal reflux. Gastric dysmotility, characterized as decreased peristasis or atony, was present in six (20%) females and duodenal dysmotility was present in one individual.

10.3.4 Discussion

Feeding impairment, characterized as chewing or swallowing difficulties, choking, and nasal regurgitation, has been described in RS females (Budden 1986; Budden 1995; Morton *et al.* 1997; Rice and Haas 1998; Thommessen *et al.* 1991, 1992). Our report, however, is the first to document not only the magnitude of oromotor dysfunction, but also the extensive involvement of the UGI tract in RS females. Oropharyngeal dysfunction was found in 95% of the RS females evaluated, while UGI dysmotility was present in 68%. The most common abnormalities included poor tongue mobility, reduced oropharyngeal clearance before and after swallowing, laryngeal penetration during swallowing, esophageal dysmotility, and GER. These findings underscore the possibility of a causal relationship between abnormalities in oropharyngeal and UGI function and feeding impairment.

Oropharyngeal and UGI function is controlled, in part, by the enteric nervous system (ENS) (Goyal and Hirano 1996). The excitatory motor neurons of the ENS project to the circulatory muscle of the UGI tract where the release of neurotransmitters such as acetylcholine and substance P results in peristaltic activity of the muscle (Goyal and Hirano 1996). Although the ENS can function independently, the CNS coordinates the function of the ENS through the parasympathetic and sympathetic pathways of the ANS (Gelshon *et al.* 1994). Of interest to us is the finding that substance P is deficient in the CNS of RS females (Deguchi *et al.* 1999; Matsuishi *et al.* 1997). We speculate that substance P may also be deficient in the

ENS, resulting in the functional disturbances of the oropharynx and UGI tract in RS females.

10.3.5 Conclusion

Oropharyngeal dysfunction and UGI dysmotility are pervasive findings in RS and may reflect disturbances of the ANS in this disorder.

Acknowledgements

This work is a publication of the USDA/ARS Children's Nutrition Research Center, Department of Pediatrics, Baylor College of Medicine, and Texas Children's Hospital, Houston, TX, and has been funded in part with federal funds from the US Department of Agriculture Agricultural Research Service, under Cooperative Agreement Number 58-6250-6-001, the National Institutes of Health Program Project Grant Number P01 HD 24234, and the National Institutes of Health, Clinical Research Centers Branch, Grant Number MO1 RR-00188. The content of this publication does not necessarily reflect the views or policies of the US Department of Agriculture, nor does mention of trade names, commercial products, or organizations imply endorsement by the US government.

References

Budden, S.S. (1986). Rett syndrome: studies of 13 affected girls. *American Journal of Medical Genetics*, 24, 99–109.
Budden, S.S. (1995). Management of Rett syndrome: a 10 year experience. *Neuropediatrics*, 26, 75–7.
Deguchi, K., Antalffy, B., Twohill, L.J., Chakroborty, S., Glaze, D., and Armstrong D. (2000). Decreased substance P immunoreactivity in Rett syndrome. (2000). *Pediatric Neurology*, 22, 259–66.
Dodds, W.J. (1993). Esophagus and esophagogastric region including diaphragm. In *Practical Alimentary Tract Radiology* (ed. A.R. Margulis and H.J. Burhenne), pp. 78–91. Mosby Year Book, St Louis, Missouri.
Gelshon, M.D., Kirchgessner, A.L., and Wade, P.R. (1994). Functional anatomy of the enteral nervous system. In *Physiology of the gastrointestinal tract*, (3rd edn). (ed. L.R. Johnson), pp. 381–422. Raven Press, New York.
Goyal, R.K. and Hirano, I. (1996). The enteric nervous system. *New England Journal of Medicine*, 334, 1106–15.
Hagberg, B., Witt Engerström, I. (1986). Rett syndrome: a suggested staging system for describing impairment profile with increasing age towards adolescence. *American Journal of Medical Genetics*, 24(Suppl. 1), 47–59.
Hamill, P.V.V., Drizd, T.A., Johnson, C.L., Reed, R.B., and Roche, A.S. (1976). *NCHS growth charts*. Monthly Statistics Report. (HRA) 76-1120. Vol. 25(3): Supp. United States Department of Agriculture/Public Health Service/Health Resources Administration, Rockville, Maryland.

Hammer, L.D., Kraemer, H.C., Wilson, D.M., Ritter, P.L., and Dombusch, S.M. (1991). Standardized percentile curves of body-mass index for children and adolescents. *American Journal of Diseases of Children*, **145**, 259–63.

Logemann, J.A. (1986). *Manual for the videofluorographic study of swallowing*, College Hill Press, San Diego, California.

Matsuishi, T., Nagamitsu, S., Yamashita, Y., Murakami, Y., Kimura, A., Sakai, T., *et al.* (1997). Decreased cerebrospinal fluid levels of substance P in patients with Rett syndrome. *Annals of Neurology*, **42**, 978–81.

Mirrett, P.L., Riski, J.E., Glascott, J., and Johnson, V. (1994). Videofluoroscopic assessment of dysphagia in children with severe spastic cerebral palsy. *Dysphagia*, **9**,174–9.

Morton, R.E., Bonas, R., Minford, J., Kerr, A., and Ellis, R.E. (1997). Feeding ability in Rett syndrome. *Developmental Medicine and Child Neurology*, **39**, 331–5.

Motil, K.J., Schultz, R.J., Browning, K., Trautwein, L., and Glaze, D.G. (1999). Oropharyngeal dysfunction and gastroesophageal dysmotility are present in girls and women with Rett syndrome. *Journal of Pediatric Gastroenterology and Nutrition*, **29**, 31–7.

Rice, M.A., Haas, R.H. (1988). The nutritional aspects of Rett syndrome. *Journal of Child Neurology*, **3(Suppl.)**, S35–42. for Rett syndrome. *Annals of Neurology*, **23**, 425–8.

The Rett Syndrome Diagnostic Criteria Work Group. (1988). Diagnostic criteria for Rett Syndrome. *Annals of Neurology*, **23**, 425–8.

Thommessen, M., Heiberg, A., Kase, B.F., Larsen, S., and Riis, G. (1991). Feeding problems, height and weight in different groups of disabled children. *Acta Paediatrica Scandinavia*, **80**, 527–33.

Thommessen, M., Kase, B.F., and Heiberg, A. (1992). Growth and nutrition in 10 girls with Rett syndrome. *Acta Paediatrica*, **81**, 686–90.

10.4 Possible link between skeletal and electrocardiographic abnormalities and autonomic dysfunction in Rett syndrome

Helen Leonard, Susan Fyfe, and Carolyn Ellaway

Population-based radiological studies of the hands and feet have identified features possibly relevant to the underlying mechanism of this disorder. Abnormalities present included a short fourth metatarsal (previously found clinically by Kerr *et al.* 1993, 1995) and negative ulnar variance (Glasson *et al.* 1998). At least one of these was present in over half of girls five years and older with Rett syndrome. Compared with controls bone age was more advanced but tended to normalize with age (Leonard *et al.* 1999). Using available population standards, Z-scores for bone lengths of the metacarpal and phalangeal hand bones were also derived and compared with controls. Overall bones were longer in Rett syndrome in girls under five years. However, the reverse occurred at other ages, and, in girls aged over 11 years, bone lengths were nearly two standard deviations below the norm. Neurobiological research on NMDA receptors has suggested that excitatory neurotransmission is enhanced early in the disease and that age related changes occur (Blue *et al.* 1999). Could the age related changes in hand growth also reflect these effects?

Julu *et al.* (1997) conclude that vagal tone in Rett syndrome is at an immature level and that sympathetic activity is unrestrained. Both prolonged rate corrected QT intervals (QTc) (Ellaway *et al.* 1999) and reduced heart rate variability (Guideri *et al.* 1999) have been found in Rett syndrome compared with healthy controls of similar age. Of interest therefore is the recognized association between imbalance in sympathetic tone and QTc prolongation and increased incidence of arrhythmias (Schwartz *et al.* 1992). The possibility of developmental arrest of the cardiac conduction system in Rett syndrome has also been mooted (Kearney *et al.* 1997). Alternatively central autonomic function via neurons in the rostral ventro-lateral medulla may mediate the changes.

Although not as a radiological investigation, Schultz *et al.* (1998) have also examined hand and foot growth. They calculated Z-scores for hand and foot length and found evidence to suggest deceleration of both foot and hand growth with the former present even after adjusting for height-age. They hypothesized that this effect might be mediated through excessive sympathetic vasomotor tone. In support of this theory was the finding that blood supply and growth in the affected limb improved after an accidental unilateral sympathectomy ('Dahlstrom 1998' in Witt Engerström and Kerr 1998). The osteopenia, which we found by measuring the cortical thickness of the second metacarpal (Leonard *et al.* 1999), might be occurring partly as a result of a similar mechanism.

In addition to the effect on blood supply there may be a direct effect of sympathetic innervation on bone growth and density. Both noradrenergic neurons (Bjurholm *et al.* 1988) and vasoactive intestinal peptide (VIP)-immunoreactive sympathetic postganglionic neurons have been found in both periosteum and bone (Hohmann *et al.* 1986). VIP is a strong inducer of bone resorption (Sisask *et al.* 1996). Hohmann *et al.* (1986) found that sympathetic chain ganglionectomy caused loss of VIP-immunoreactive neurons in rib periosteum. These findings may help to explain the excessive sympathetic influence on bone growth and demineralization in Rett syndrome. Mutations in the MECP2 gene, which has an important role in gene silencing, have been found in a proportion of cases of Rett syndrome (Amir *et al.* 1999). The relationship between the downstream effects of this gene and the disturbance of sympathetic activity remains to be elucidated.

References

Amir, R. E., Van den Veyver I.B., Wan M., Tran C.Q., Francke, U., and Zoghbi, H.Y. (1999). Rett syndrome is caused by mutations in X-linked MECP2, encoding methyl-CpG-binding protein 2. *Nature Genetics*, **23**, 185–188.

Bjurholm, A., Kreicbergs, A., Terenius, L., Goldstein, M., and Schultzberg, M. (1988). Neuropeptide Y-, tyrosine hydroxylase- and vasoactive intestinal polypeptide-immunoreactive nerves in bone and surrounding tissues. *Journal of the Autonomic Nervous System*, **25**(2–3), 119–25.

Blue, M.E., Naidu, S., and Johnston, M.V. (1999). Altered development of glutamate and GABA receptors in the basal ganglia of girls with Rett syndrome. *Experimental Neurology*, **156**(2), 345–52.

Ellaway, C.J., Sholler, G., Leonard, H., and Christodoulou, J. (1999). Prolonged QT interval in Rett syndrome. *Archives of Diseases in Children*, **80**, 470–2.

Glasson, E. J., Bower, C., Thomson, M.R., Fyfe, S., Leonard, S., Rousham, E., *et al.* (1998). Diagnosis of Rett syndrome: can a radiograph help?. *Developmental Medicine and Child Neurology*, **40**, 737–42.

Guideri, F., Acampa, M., Hayek, C., Zappella, N., and Di Perri, T. (1999). Reduced heart rate variability in patients affected with Rett syndrome. A possible explanation for sudden death. *Neuropediatrics*, **30**, 146–8.

Hohmann, E.L., Elde, R.P., Rysavy, J. A., Einzig, S., and Gebhard, R.L. (1986). Innervation of periosteum and bone by sympathetic vasoactive intestinal peptide-containing nerve fibers. *Science*, **232**(4752), 868–71.

Julu, P. O.O., Kerr, A.M., Hansen, S., Apartopoulos, F., and Jamal, G.A. (1997). Functional evidence of brain stem immaturity in Rett syndrome. *European Child and Adolescent Psychiatry*, 6(**Suppl. 1**), 47–54.

Kearney, D., Armstrong, D.L., and Glaze, D.G. (1997). The conduction system in Rett syndrome. *European Child and Adolescent Psychiatry*, 6(**Suppl. 1**), 78–9.

Kerr, A., Robertson, P., and Mitchell, J. (1993). Rett Syndrome and the fourth metatarsal. *Archives of Diseases in Children*, 8, 433.

Kerr, A., Mitchell, J.M., and Robertson, P.E. (1995). Short fourth toes in Rett Syndrome: a biological indicator. *Neuropediatrics*, 26, 72–4.

Leonard, H., Thomson, M.R., Glasson, E.J., Fyfe, S., Leonard, S., Bower, C., *et al.* (1999). A population based approach to the investigation of osteopenia in Rett syndrome. *Developmental Medicine and Child Neurology*, 41, 323–8.

Leonard, H., Thomson, M., Glasson, E., Fyfe, S., Leonard, S., Ellaway, C., *et al.* (1999). Metacarpophalangeal pattern profile and bone age in Rett syndrome: further radiological clues to the diagnosis. *American Journal of Medical Genetics*, 83, 88–95.

Schultz, R., Glaze, D., Motil, K., Herbert, D. and Percy, A. (1998). Hand and foot growth failure in Rett syndrome. *Journal of Child Neurology*, 13(2): 71–4.

Schwartz, P. J., Bonazzi, O., Locati, E., Napolitano, C., and Sala, S. (1992). Pathogenesis and therapy of the idiopathic long QT syndrome. *Annals of the New York Academy of Sciences*, 644, 112–41.

Sisask, G., Bjurholm, A., Ahmed, M., and Kreicbergs, A. (1996). The development of autonomic innervation in bone and joints of the rat. *Journal of the Autonomic Nervous System*, 59(1–2), 27–33.

Witt Engerström, I. and Kerr, A. (1998). Workshop on Autonomic Function in Rett Syndrome. Swedish Rett Centre, Froson, Sweden. *Brain and Development*, 20, 325–6.

10.5 The electroencephalogram in Rett syndrome

R.A. Cooper

The electroencephalogram (EEG) has been extensively studied in Rett syndrome (RS) and many abnormalities have been described (Hagberg et al. 1983; Verma et al. 1986; Niedermeyer et al. 1986; Glaze et al. 1987; Ishizaki 1989; Robb et al. 1989; Cooper et al. 1998). None of these show an EEG pattern which is diagnostic of Rett disorder and the term 'typical' is misleading. The EEG can, however, be of considerable help in the differential diagnosis of RS taken together with clinical evidence.

Few EEGs are taken in the pre-regression stage (Hagberg stage I; see Chapter 1) but there is a suggestion of some immaturity and lack of reactivity. More work needs to be done in this area. During pre-regression, and apart from infantile autism, the EEG is much more likely to be normal than in developmental defects, prenatal infections, metabolic disorders such as gangliosidoses, and lipofuchsinoses as well as in Angelman's syndrome. Careful correlation of the clinical picture with EEG patterns and additional Evoked Potential studies are likely to provide an answer (Harden and Pampiglione 1982; Pampiglione and Harden 1984; Cooper et al. 1998). During regression (Hagberg stage II) there is clear evidence of evolving abnormality. In early regression (within six months of onset) the EEG may be within normal limits or show some immaturity and slight slowing. In a recent study (Cooper et al. 1998) only 6 of 18 records were abnormal. All of these showed epileptogenic activity. In the same study, in late regression and early post-regression (six months from onset of regression until age six) the EEG became grossly abnormal in the majority: 92% of 72 EEGs. Abnormalities included absence of an age dependent dominant post-central rhythm, excess θ or δ slowing, which may be random, generalized and/or paroxysmal, and various forms of epileptogenic activity. At this time, EEG changes will be less marked than those seen in two conditions which may cause confusion clinically, namely acute encephalitis and lead poisoning. On the other hand, the EEG in RS and

Angelman's syndrome may be similar except for the characteristic changes on eye closure in the latter (Williams and Frias 1982; Pampiglione and Martinez 1983; Boyd *et al.* 1988) (see Table 10.5.1).

In later post-regression (after six years; Hagberg stages III and IV) occasional normal records are described. In recent studies of this stage 49 records of 72 patients were abnormal. They often showed persistent, mainly unreactive 'monorhythmic' θ (Ishizaki 1992). During this stage there is no notable EEG pattern distinguishing RS from other similar disorders. Epileptogenic activity is common and of varied form, but none is that of true primary generalized epilepsy. Nor, in a recent survey (Cooper *et al.*) of 150 records of classic RS, was there evidence of hypsarrhythmia, although this pattern has been recorded (Glaze *et al.* 1987). There are occasionally repetitive spike discharges similar to those seen in spongiform encephalopathy (Hagne *et al.* 1989; Cooper *et al.* 1998). In 59 of 78 RS patients, 46 showed epileptogenic activity. In 6 of the 59 patients epileptogenic activity, seen on the EEG, preceded the onset of seizures. Of the 78 patients 18 reported no seizures but had epileptogenic activity on their EEG.

Andreas Rett (Rett 1966, 1977) reported periods of reduced awareness, which Kerr (1992) named 'vacant spells'. These are brief recurrent events, stereotyped in any one patient, occurring inappropriately and raising the question of a minor seizure (Cooper *et al.* 1998). The EEG is of considerable value in these patients since none of the girls in whom vacant spells occurred during prolonged EEG recording showed any evidence of seizure activity during the vacant spell suggesting that anticonvulsant medication for vacant spells alone is not indicated (Kerr *et al.* 1990).

Continuous EEG recording with video, respiratory movements and blood gas monitoring over prolonged periods provides evidence of a fluctuating level of clinical and EEG (neurophysiological) arousal/non-arousal (Cooper *et al.* 1998). Periods of hyperventilation, increased movement, anxiety and sometimes agitation are associated with decreased abnormality (Kerr *et al.* 1990). The absence of normal often paroxysmal slowing with hyperventilation, notable in normal childhood, is particularly striking. Periods of clinical quiet, often withdrawal, and sleep are associated with increased abnormality particularly in overnight sleep when abnormality may be so marked as to make staging impossible (Aldrich *et al.* 1990; Segawa and Nomura 1992*a, b;* Cooper *et al.* 1998). This oscillation of both behavioural and EEG arousal/non-arousal suggests a fluctuating disturbance of neurochemical substances especially the monoamines (Pelligra *et al.* 1992; Percy 1992; Takeuchi *et al.* 1992).

These clinical and EEG findings suggest both cortical pathology and midbrain/brainstem impairment. Both are supported by the work of Armstrong (1995), Armstrong *et al.* (1995), Bauman *et al.* (1995) and Julu *et al.* (1998). EEG investigation in RS provides help in diagnosis and management and also in many other aspects of RS enquiry: genetic, autonomic, neuropathological and

Table 10.5.1 Number of patients, number reporting seizures and EEG characteristics in different phases (*note*: several patients were recorded in more than one group).

Phase	Cases	Patients reporting past seizures No. (%)	No. of records	EEGs					
				Abnormal records			Sleep records		
				Total No. (%)	With epileptogenic activity No. (%)		Total No. (%)	Abnormal increase in sleep No. (%)	
Pre-regression	1	1	1[a]	1	1		1	1	
Early regression	18	2	18	6	6		4	1	
Late regression/early post-regression	37	24(65)	59	44(75)	37(84)		20(34)	16(80)	
Late post-regression	49	38(76)	72	66(92)	47(71)		30(42)	22(73)	

[a]febrile convulsion
Reproduced with permission of the European Journal of Paediatric Neurology © European Paediatric Neurology Soc. 1998

neurochemical. The recent genetic breakthrough is a dramatic step forward but it is most likely that full a understanding of the phenotype of Rett disorder will arise from the combined work of many specialties.

Acknowledgements

I would like to acknowledge the help received from families and girls with Rett syndrome, from the many physicians who have willingly contributed information, from Jean Hyslop and the Department of Medical Illustration at the Royal Hospital for Sick Children, Glasgow. I am also very grateful to the National, the UK and the International Rett Syndrome Associations, the Quarriers's Homes and the green Trust through Mr and Mrs Nicholas Moore, all of whom helped to fund the various projects.

References

Aldrich, M.S., Garofalo, E.A., and Drury, I. (1990). Epileptiform abnormalities during sleep in Rett syndrome. *Electroencephalography and Clinical Neurophysiology.*, 75, 365–70.

Armstrong, D.D. (1995). The Neuropathology of the Rett syndrome — overview. *Neuropediatrics*, 26, 100–4.

Armstrong, D, Dunn, J.K., Antalffy, B., and Trevedy, R. (1995). Selective dendritic alterations in the cortex of

Rett syndrome. *Neuropathology and Experimental Pathology*, 54, 195–201.

Baumann, M.I., Kemper, T.L., and Arin, D.M. (1995). Microscopic observations of the brain in Rett syndrome. *Neuropediatrics*, 26, 105–8.

Boyd, S.G., Harden, A. and Patton, M.A. (1988). The EEG in early diagnosis of Angelman (Happy Puppet syndrome) *Neuropaediatrics*, 147, 508–13.

Cooper, R.A., Kerr, A.M., and Amos, P. (1998). Rett syndrome: critical examination of clinical features, serial EEG and video-monitoring in understanding and management. *European Journal of Paediatric Neurology*, 2, 127–35.

Glaze, D., Frost, J., Renner, H.Y. and Percy, A.K. (1987). Rett syndrome: correlation between electroencephalographic characteristics with clinical staging. *Arch. Neurol.* 44, 1053–56.

Hagberg, B., Aicardi, J., Dias, K., and Ramos, O. (1983). A progressive syndrome of autism, dementia, ataxia and loss of purposeful hand use in girls with Rett syndrome: report of thirty-five cases. *Annals of Neurology*, 14, 471–9.

Hagne, I., Witt Engerström, I., and Hagberg, B. (1989). EEG development in Rett syndrome: study of thirty cases. *Electroencephalography and Clinical Neurophysiology.*, 72, 1–6.

Harden, A. and Pampiglione, G. (1982). Neurophysiological studies (EEG/ERG/VEP/SEP) in children in so-called neuronal ceroid lipofuscinosis (Batten's disease) In *Ceroid lipofuscinosis* (ed. D. Armstrong, N. Coppang, and J.A. Rider). Elsevier, Amsterdam.

Ishizaki, A., Inoue, I., Sadaki, H. and Fukuyama, Y. (1989). Longitudinal observation of electroencephalograms in the Rett syndrome. *Brain Development and Child Neurology*, 11, 407–12.

Ishizaki, A. (1992). Electroencephalographic study of the Rett syndrome with special reference to the monorhythmic theta activities in adult patients. *Brain Development and Child Neurology*, 14(s) 31–6.

Julu, P.O.O., Kerr, A.M., Hansen, S., et al. (1998). Functional evidence of brainstem immaturity, in press.

Kerr, A.M., Southall, D.F,. Amos, P., et al. (1990). Correlation of electroencephalogram, respiration and movements in the Rett syndrome. *Brain Development and Child Neurology*, 12, 61–8.

Kerr, A.M. (1992). A Review of the respiratory disorder in the Rett Syndrome. *Brain and Development.* 14(5), 43–45.

Niedermeyer, E., Rett, A., Renner, H. et al. (1986). Rett syndrome and the electroencephalogram. *Am. J. Genet*, 24, 195–99.

Niedermeyer, E. and Naidu, S. (1990). Further EEG observations in children with the Rett syndrome. *Brain Development and Child Neurology*, 12, 533–54.

Pampiglione, G. and Harden, A. (1984). Neurophysiological investigations in GMI and GM2 gangliosidosis. *Pediactrics*, 16S, 74–84.

Pampiglione, G. and Martinez, A. (1983). Evolution of Angelman syndrome. Follow-up of three new cases. *Electroencephalography and Clinical Neurophysiology*, X, 72.

Pelligra, R., Norton, R.D., Wilkinson, R., et al. (1992). Rett syndrome: stimulation of endogenous biogenic amines. *Neuroppediatrics*, 23, 131–7.

Percy, A.K. (1992). Neurochemistry of the Rett syndrome. *Brain Development and Child Neurology*, 145 57–62.

Rett, A. (1966). Uber ein eigernartiger hirnatropisches Syndrome bei Hyperammonamie im Kindersalter. *Weiner Medischiner Wochenschrift*, 115, 713–76.

Rett, A. (1977). Cerebral atrophy associated with hyperammonaemia In *Handbook of clinical neurology* (ed. P.J. Winken and G.W. Bruyn). North Holland, Amsterdam.

Robb, S.A., Harden, A., and Boyd, S.G. (1989). Rett syndrome: an EEG study in fifty-two girls. *Neuropaediatrics*, 20, 192–5.

Santavuori, P. (1998). Neuronal ceroid-lipofuscinosis. *Brain Development and Child Neurology (Tokyo)*, 10, 80–3.

Segawa, M. and Nomura, Y. (1992a). Pathophysiology of the Rett syndrome from the standpoint of polysomnography. *Brain Development and Child Neurology*, 12, 55–60.

Segawa, M. and Nomura, Y. (1992b). Polysomnography in the Rett syndrome. *Brain Development and Child Neurology*, 145, 45–54.

Takeuchi, Y., Sawada, T., and Jenner, P. (1992). *Brain Development and Child Neurology*, 14SS, 131–7.

Verma, M.P., Chedda, R.L., Nigro, M.A., and Har, Z.H. (1986). Encapalographic findings in Rett syndrome. *Electroencephalography and Clinical Neurophysiology*, 64, 394–401.

Williams, C.A. and Frias, J.L. (1982). Angelman ('Happy Puppet') syndrome. *American Journal of Genetics*, 11, 453–60.

10.6 Electromagnetic stimulation of motor neurons

U.M. Fietzek, F. Heinen, U. Ziemann, H. Petersen, K. Hühn, J. Schulte-Mönting, H.-J. Christen, R. Korinthenberg, and F. Hanefeld

Transcranial magnetic stimulation (TMS) provides information on the excitation of motor neurons and the propagation within the fast corticospinal efferents. Besides the conduction time along the corticospinal axon, the central motor conduction time (CMCT) measured by TMS includes transmission times at the spinal and cortical level. In addition, there is substantial evidence that the transcranial magnetic pulse of a round magnetic coil reaches the cortical Betz' cells by a trans-synaptic pathway. This interneuronal pathway might be altered in specific pathological states, such as the Rett syndrome (RS). Previously, the central motor conduction times were described to be abnormally short in RS, but only small groups or older patients were investigated (Eyre *et al.* 1990; Heinen and Korinthenberg 1996; Guerrini *et al.* 1998; Nezu *et al.* 1998). This study included 29 patients (2–38 years) diagnosed with classic RS. The results were compared to the data of 75 normal, healthy subjects (4 weeks – 29 years).

We used the MagStim 200® stimulator and the round coil for transcranial cortical as well as for cervical spinal root stimulation. Motor evoked potentials (MEP) were detected on the first dorsal interosseus muscle. Signals were amplified and recorded using a Nicolet Compass® myograph (high-pass filter 10 Hz, low-pass filter 2.5 kHz). TMS registration was performed with the subjects in a sitting position. Patients were to perform a traction manoeuvre or asked to squeeze the fingers of one of the investigators, thus ensuring that measurements were done under the facilitated preinnervation condition. The shortest reproducible latency of four MEP was considered to be the global conduction time. The peripheral conduction time was measured as the longest reproducible latency of four MEP. The CMCT was the difference of both latencies.

The CMCT in the younger patients with RS was measured with distinctly shorter latencies in comparison to normal control persons. The maturation profile demonstrated an increasing rather than a declining CMCT, as was seen for normal subjects. The difference in CMCT seen between the investigated groups was particularly evident for the time period between two and five years.

A shortened CMCT may theoretically be explained through mechanisms at the spinal segment or at the motor cortex. With respect to the first possibility, it could be argued that since similar facilitated preinnervation conditions were used for all subjects, there were always some spinal motor neurons at the firing threshold. Therefore, the CMCT measured during the muscle contraction eliminates such group differences in the summation time at the spinal motor neuron.

The other possibility considers abnormal motor cortical excitability as being responsible for the short CMCT in RS. This is supported by the following circumstantial evidence: (i) Giant somato-sensory potentials have been assessed only in patients younger than 8 years(Yoshikawa *et al.* 1991). (ii) Over-expression of the NMDA receptor has been demonstrated for young patients with RS (Blue et al. 1999). (iii) Rarefication of the dendrite trees in layer V was described and could be related to an altered transsynaptic route of the magnetic pulse. Therefore, TMS could activate the corticospinal neurons in RS more directly than in age matched controls, either through direct excitation of the corticospinal neurons or through a reduced number of interneurons.

References

Blue, M.E., Naidu, S., and Johnston, M.V. (1999). Development of amino acid receptors in frontal cortex from girls with Rett syndrome. *Annals of Neurology*, 45, 541–5.

Eyre, J.A., Kerr, A.M., Miller, S., O'Sullivan, M.C., and Ramesh, V. (1990). Neurophysiological observations on corticospinal projections to the upper limb in subjects with Rett syndrome. *Journal of Neurology, Neurosurgery, and Psychiatry*, 53, 874–9.

Guerrini, R., Bonanni, P., Parmeggiani, L., Santucci, M., Parmeggiani, A., and Sartucci, F. (1998). Cortical reflex myoclonus in Rett syndrome. *Annals of Neurology*, 43, 472–9.

Heinen, F., and Korinthenberg, R. (1996). Does transcranial magnetic stimulation allow early diagnosis of Rett Syndrome? *Neuropediatrics*, 27, 223–4.

Nezu, A., Kimura, S., Takeshita, S., and Tanaka, M. (1998). Characteristic response to transcranial magnetic stimulation in Rett syndrome. *Electroencephalography and Clinical Neurophysiology*, 109, 100–3.

Yoshikawa, H., Kaga, M., Suzuki, H., Sakuragawa, N., and Arima, M. (1991). Giant somatosensory evoked potentials in the Rett syndrome. *Brain and Development*, 13, 36–9.

11 The morphological substrate for communication

Pavel V. Belichenko

11.1 Brief review of language representation in the neocortex

11.1.1 Language representation in human neocortex

It is a consistent finding in the study of human language brain areas that 90–95% of right-handed people have a left dominant language hemisphere while the majority of left-handed people do not have a right dominant hemisphere (Milner 1974; Hecaen et al. 1981; Beaton 1997; Moffat et al. 1998; Tzourio et al. 1998).

The neocortical areas, Broca's motor speech areas 44, 45 and Wernicke's sensory speech area 22 are known to play an important role in human language processing (for review see Mesulam 1990). There are a few major and several minor factors which influence speech dominance. Chief factors bearing on interhemispheric asymmetry include handedness, sex, age, use of language and cultural background (Galaburda and Sanides 1980; Bogolepova 1994, 1996; Glezer et al. 1994; Witelson et al. 1995; Moffat et al. 1998).

Asymmetry of the planum temporale (the superior surface of the temporal lobe) has been studied in relation to handedness and gender (Beaton 1997; Moffat et al. 1998). Magnetic resonance imaging (MRI) demonstrates a strong left dominance of the planum temporale in subjects with left hemisphere speech representation regardless of handedness; however there was no consistent planum temporale asymmetry among subjects with right hemisphere speech dominance (Moffat et al. 1998). These results suggest that reversed speech lateralization is not necessarily accompanied by reversal of planum temporale asymmetry (Moffat et al. 1998). According to Beaton (1997) the frequency of right asymmetry was higher than expected judging from the proportion of right hemisphere speech representation in the general population whereas the frequency of leftward asymmetry was less than expected from the proportion of the population with left hemisphere speech. Beaton (1997) suggests that morphological asymmetry may relate more to handedness than to language lateralization.

There are indications that certain human talents such as outstanding musical or literature abilities are associated with increased asymmetry of the neocortex (Bogolepova 1994; Schlaug et al. 1995a, b). People with exceptional literary talents have been shown to have peculiarities of neuronal orientation including an increase in the pyramidal cell/glial cell index and neuronal regrouping in cortical layers III and IV of areas 44 and 45 (Bogolepova 1994). Other human talents such as musical ability have also been associated with left-right differences in brain structure and function (Schlaug et al. 1995a). *In vivo* MRI morphometry of the brain in musicians showed stronger left asymmetry of the planum temporale than was found in non-musicians or musicians without perfect pitch (Schlaug et al. 1995a).

11.1.2 Functional imaging of speech processing

Great progress has been made during the last decade in the study of language representation in the human neocortex using functional positron emission tomography (fPET), functional magnetic resonance imaging (fMRI) and transcranial magnetic stimulation (TMS) (Petersen et al. 1988; Zatorre 1992; Klein 1995; Fiez et al. 1996; Price et al. 1996; Kim et al. 1997). This data supports previous clinical observations and has shown significant involvement of areas 44 and 45 in speech production, and involvement of areas 22 and 40 in speech recognition (Creutzfeldt et al. 1989; Fiez et al. 1996; Price et al. 1996).

PET studies by Buckner et al. (1995) were designed to determine whether there are hemispheric differences in prefrontal cortex activation during two different motor speech tasks and sex differences in the same tasks. Activation was mainly found in the left inferior prefrontal cortex (near Brodmann's areas 44 or 45) in both tasks and for both gender groups; activation in the right prefrontal cortex was slight or absent (Buckner et al. 1995). Activation in the left anterior prefrontal cortex (near Brodmann's areas 10 or 46) was only observed during verb generation, pointing to functional differences between the left inferior prefrontal cortex and the more anterior prefrontal cortex (Buckner et al. 1995). The left inferior prefrontal areas were activated by tasks that require high-level word retrieval and production processes (Buckner et al. 1995). These areas were distinct from the more anterior areas, which were not always activated by such tasks. No differences in activation of different neocortical areas were detected between gender groups; however intensity of activation in male subjects was greater than in female subjects during verb generation (Buckner et al. 1995). At the present time this subdivision of prefrontal areas is important because previous descriptions of human functional anatomy have often been based on activation within over-large regions of the neocortex.

Tzourio *et al.* (1998) analysed the patterns of activation and deactivation during speech processing and silent rest from PET studies of healthy controls selected on the basis of their handedness. The results showed temporal activation mainly in the left hemisphere in right handers and also activation in Broca's area and the medial frontal area. Right lateralized deactivation was also observed in the parietal and inferior temporal gyrus. In left handers, temporal activation was more symmetrical than parietal and inferior frontal deactivation and activation was seen additionally in Broca's area and the medial frontal gyrus (Tzourio *et al.* 1998). Comparing activation of the neocortex in right- and left-handed people, larger activations were found in right handers in the left planum temporale and the temporal pole, while left handers activated an additional right middle temporal region. In left-handed people, high individual variability of functional dominance was demonstrated, with two people left dominant, two symmetrical and one showing a right lateralization of temporal activation. From this study Tzourio *et al.* (1998) concluded that there was no relationship between functional dominance and handedness score and suggested greater participation of the right hemisphere in language processing in left-handed people.

PET studies of Murphy *et al.* (1997) demonstrated areas associated with articulation and breathing, without language processing. They found bilateral activation in the sensorimotor and motor cortex, together with activation in the thalamus, cerebellum, and supplementary motor area. In these conditions there was no activation in Broca's area, so the specificity of Broca's area for speech processing was supported by this modern method.

The resolution of the modern fMRI makes it possible to distinguish activation in two cortical areas approximately 1.1 mm apart (Kim *et al.* 1997). Using fMRI to study the motor speech area (area 44) in late bilingual people (those who learned a second language after their native tongue), Kim *et al.* (1997) found that the morphological representation in the neocortex was different for the new language as compared to the native language during internal speech tasks. However in early bilingual people there was no morphological separation in representation of languages in the motor speech areas. In both early and late bilingual people the sensory speech area (area 22) showed little or no separation of activity during an internal speech task (Kim *et al.* 1997). On the other hand Klein (1995) showed no differences in activation of separate speech areas in the inferior frontal gyrus during multi-language tasks.

11.1.3 Morphological studies of the speech areas

Cytoarchitecture: In spite of the progress in functional imaging which has demonstrated lateralization of motor and sensory speech functions to the left hemisphere in right handers, relatively little is known about the morphological basis of that specialization.

Hayes and Lewis (1993, 1995) reported that in Nissl-stained sections from control human brains, the mean cross-sectional area of the largest layer III pyramidal neurons in area 45 was significantly greater in the left hemisphere than in the right. In contrast to area 45, there was no interhemispheric difference in the mean cross-sectional area of the largest layer III pyramids in primary motor cortex (Hayes and Lewis 1995). In addition, in area 46, a region of prefrontal association cortex not known to be functionally lateralized, the mean soma size of the largest layer III pyramidal neurons was significantly smaller in the left hemisphere than in the right (Hayes and Lewis 1995). These findings demonstrate that layer III of Broca's area contains a distinctive subpopulation of neurons which may play an important role in the specific functional architecture of this region (Hayes and Lewis 1995).

Gender differences in the morphology of speech areas should be noted. For example, women have a greater density of neurons in layers II and IV of the auditory association cortex as compared to men; however no differences were found between the sexes in the morphology of layers III, V, VI (Witelson *et al.* 1995).

I have found no morphological data about asymmetry in sensory areas 22 and 40.

Dendritic architecture: In the dominant hemisphere, neurons had a longer total dendritic length and more complicated dendritic branches than neurons in corresponding areas of the contralateral hemisphere (Seldon 1981a, b, 1982; Scheibel *et al.* 1985; Jacobs and Scheibel 1993; Hayes and Lewis 1996). A larger proportion of the length on the left (dominant) side was made up of higher order dendritic branches whereas lower order segments predominated on the right. The pattern was partially reversed in non-right-handed subjects (Scheibel *et al.* 1985). Hayes and Lewis (1996) could not find any interhemispheric differences in quantitative parameters of the geometry of dendrites of the giant pyramidal neurons in the left and right hemispheres.

According to Jacobs *et al.* (1993) the classical Wernicke's and Broca's speech areas were characterized by different dendritic patterns as compared to primary motor cortex. It has been suggested that distal (fourth order and above) basal dendritic branches matured ontogenetically later than proximal (first, second, and third order) dendrites (Jacobs *et al.* 1993). In primary motor cortex, proximal dendritic segments were longer than distal segments, and this relationship was reversed in association cortical areas (Jacobs *et al.* 1993). Fourth order segments had significantly more dendritic spines than third order segments in all areas (Jacobs *et al.* 1993).

Postnatal development of the motor speech area shows an increase in number and length of the developing distal order segments of dendrites in layer V pyramidal neurons and possibly shortening of the proximal segments of these dendrites (Simonds and Scheibel 1989). Initially after birth, dendrites on the right side have significantly longer total segment length and individual segment length. By the first year of life, the total length of dendrites and distal segment length in the left hemisphere are significantly larger than in the right one, and this relationship is true for more mature (42–72 months) brain (Simonds and Scheibel 1989).

Neurochemistry: Little is known about neurochemical asymmetry in speech related neocortical areas. In superior temporal gyri higher levels of choline acetyltransferase were shown in the left (dominant) hemisphere (Amaducci *et al.* 1981). The pattern of acetylcholinesterase staining in both hemispheres of the posterior temporal areas (areas 22, 40) was the same (Hutsler and Gazzaniga 1996). However large acetylcholinesterase-rich pyramidal neurons in layer III were bigger on the left (dominant) hemisphere compared to the right, within different neocortical areas. This was not limited only to speech areas (Hutsler and Gazzaniga 1996). Non-phosphorylated neurofilament protein was found in the large layer III pyramids in area 45 in both hemispheres but the mean cell body area of the largest labelled neurons was significantly greater in the left (dominant) hemisphere than in the right (Hayes and Lewis 1995). Calcium binding proteins (parvalbumin, calretinin, and calbindin) were studied in relation to functional lateralization (Glezer *et al.* 1994). The degree of immunoreactivity was associated with handedness, especially for the parvalbumin positive cells (Glezer *et al.* 1994).

Configuration of corpus callosum: The corpus callosum (CC) is important to this chapter, as it is the largest connection between the functionally asymmetric cerebral hemispheres. It is composed of several functionally and morphologically distinct parts, genu, body and splenum, which are involved in handedness, age, sex, and the acquisition of knowledge (for review see Koshi *et al.* 1997).

The relationships between morphology of the CC and age, gender, handedness, education, and cranial size have been studied with MRI (Hopper *et al.* 1994; Parashos *et al.* 1995; Ferrario *et al.* 1996; for review see Beaton 1997). It should be appreciated that there is great individual variability. The variability coefficient was 20% in total callosal area and from 19% to 40% in the CC subareas (Parashos *et al.* 1995). Increasing age and smaller cranial area were both associated with smaller total and subareas of the CC but there was no association with sex or education (Parashos *et al.* 1995). The relative effects of age and cranial size varied across regions and were most prominent for the anterior region (Parashos *et al.* 1995). However age and cranial size together explained less than half the variance in regional callosal size (Parashos *et al.* 1995).

In the adult brain there is conflicting evidence relating to handedness and gender differences in CC structure (Hopper *et al.* 1994; Ferrario *et al.* 1996; for review see Beaton 1997). There is inconclusive data that asymmetry is reduced in females as compared to males (for review see Beaton 1997).

The morphometric data supporting a sex difference in CC organization is conflicting. Some studies showed sexual dimorphism in interhemispheric relations in humans (Zaidel *et al.* 1995). Examination of CC midsagittal morphology in left-handed and right-handed males, using MRI, showed that left-handed subjects with left hemisphere speech functions had a larger CC than either left-handed subjects with right hemisphere speech functions or right-handed subjects (Moffat et al. 1998). Morphologically, the posterior region of the female CC was larger than its corresponding region in the males in an elderly group, indicating sex-related differences in the callosal shape and size (Davatzikos et al. 1996). Contrary to previous data, left handers did not show larger CC measurements compared to right handers (Jancke et al. 1997). Increased interhemispheric communication may be required when the neural systems underlying speech and handedness are represented in opposite hemispheres (Moffat et al. 1998).

Using high-resolution *in vivo* MRI morphometry in a large number of healthy young adults, Steinmetz et al. (1992, 1995) showed that the size of the CC was larger in women than in men, with no correlation with handedness. In another study, no sex difference was found in the human CC and its seven subareas on midsaggital MRI morphometry (Constant and Ruther 1996; Ferrario et al. 1996). No significant correlation was found between CC area and either cerebral hemispheric area or cranial capacity (Constant and Ruther 1996). The only apparent influence of sex was on the CC ratios, which were larger in women (Jancke et al. 1997). However, smaller brains had larger CC ratios, mainly independent of sex (Jancke et al. 1997). Jancke et al. (1997) suggest that the previously described sex differences in CC anatomy may be better explained by an underlying effect of brain size, with larger brains having relatively smaller CC. This lends empirical support to the hypothesis that brain size may be an important factor influencing interhemispheric connectivity and lateralization (Jancke et al. 1997).

A significant effect of age has been demonstrated in adults (Hopper et al. 1994; Ferrario et al. 1996; Jeeves and Moes 1996). However, the shape of the CC within age and sex groups in childhood was more homogeneous than in adulthood (Ferrario et al. 1996). Hopper et al. (1994) found the body of the CC to decrease in size with age and to be larger in right-handed persons. The cross-sectional areas of the genu, splenium, and CC, overall, do not vary significantly with respect to age, gender, or handedness (Hopper et al. 1994). Jeeves and Moes (1996) found the size of the CC to decrease consistently with age, particularly in the anterior region.

Many papers are concerned with heterogeneity of development of the CC (de Azevedo et al. 1997; Koshi et al. 1997; for review see Gelot et al. 1998). In normal brain CC development includes three steps (Gelot et al. 1998). The first step is callosal neuron differentiation with growth of the future callosal axon and this occurs during neuronal migration to the cortical plate. The second step is callosal axon guidance towards its specific target which includes crossing the midline, target recognition and synapse formation. Within the second step, during 12–22 post-ovulation weeks there is progressive invasion of axons by callosal growth cones from the dorsal part of lamina reuniens and the three parts of CC (truncus, rostrum and splenum) appear (Gelot et al. 1998). The third step is synapse remodelling by synaptic activity, giving rise to axonal elimination, morphologically presented as a transitory thinning of CC (Gelot *et al.* 1998). Maturation of CC is completed after the age of 5 years and corresponds to axonal elimination and myelination of the remaining axons (Gelot *et al.* 1998; Heinen *et al.* 1998).

The anatomy of the human fetal CC was studied in midsagittal sections of formalin fixed brains by Koshi *et al.* (1997). The length of CC and width of its genu, body, and splenum showed no significant sex difference. There was a significant absolute increase in callosal length and genu width with gestational age but the body and splenum widths remained the same (Koshi *et al.* 1997).

Language processing in asymmetrically organized cortical areas (area 44 and area 22) inhibits the reciprocal transcallosal exchange of information in favour of the lateralized processing (Karbe *et al.* 1998). The important role of collateral inhibition for transcallosal information exchange was shown by Karbe *et al.* (1998). Using MRI and PET in a study of functional activity of CC during speech processing they found a significant negative correlation between task-induced metabolic changes in the callosal midbody and isthmus and in areas of language processing in the left area 44 and in the right area 22.

There is some evidence from the literature to indicate an effect of experience on the size of the CC. The midsagittal area of the CC was studied by MRI morphometry in professional musicians and in age-, sex- and handedness-matched controls (Schlaug *et al.* 1995b). The anterior half of the CC was significantly larger in musicians who had begun musical training before 7 years old (Schlaug *et al.* 1995b).

There is some neurophysiological evidence to show variations related to age, gender and sex differences in the CC (Corsi-Cabrera *et al.* 1989; Jeeves and Moes 1996; Polich *et al.* 1998). Elderly subjects showed a significant difference in simple reaction times to unstructured stimuli compared to younger subjects, with elderly females contributing the greatest increase (Jeeves and Moes 1996). No significant sex differences were found for younger subjects (Jeeves and Moes 1996). The relationship of EEG activity to sex showed that interhemispheric correlation in the α band was significantly higher in women than in men at central, parietal and occipital derivations (Corsi-Cabrera *et al.* 1989). Significant correlations were found between verbal, spatial and abstract scores and interhemispheric correlation, positive for women with abstract and spatial aptitudes in the central cortex, and negative for men with spatial, abstract and verbal scores in most areas recorded (Corsi-Cabrera *et al.* 1989). This male-female difference suggests different cerebral functional organization, women showing less hemispheric differentiation than men (Corsi-Cabrera *et al.* 1989). The amplitude of the P300 event-related potential was greater in left-handed than in right-handed people at anterior and central electrode sites during auditory and visual tasks (Polich *et al.* 1998). The P300 latency was shorter across all task conditions for left- than for right-handers (Polich *et al.* 1998). Task difficulty did not affect P300 handedness, although smaller P300 components were obtained for males than for females (Polich *et al.* 1998).

11.1.4 Stagnation of hemispheric differentiation occurs

There is little data on the earliest appearance of interhemispheric asymmetry but by the end of the eighth month most children show handedness (Stroganova *et al.* 1998). Physiological data from 11 months old infants showed that right hand preference strongly predicted asymmetry in motor function (Stroganova *et al.* 1998).

The data about lateralization of the function are incomplete and conflicting; however, lateralization of some of the common functions can be found in Table 11.1.

Table 11.1 Interhemispheric lateralisation of main functions

Function	Left hemisphere	Right hemisphere
Vision	Letters, words	Complicated geometrical patterns
		Face recognition
Hearing	Sounds, related to language	Non-language sound. Music
Somatosensory system	?	Tactile recognition of complicated pattern
		Alphabet of Braille
Motor system	Complicated free movement	?
Memory	Verbal memory	Visual memory
Language	Speech. Reading. Writing. Arithmetic	
Space ability		Geometry. Mentally movement of object

11.2 Rett syndrome and speech processing: morphological aspects and hypothesis

Lack of communication is a major social problem for people with RS. Major disturbances in motor behaviour have been described (Budden *et al.* 1990; see also Chapter 1). The early clinical features of RS have been analysed in an attempt to identify the anatomic-functional systems involved in the pathological process. The initial phase is characterized by impaired motor function and stereotyped orofacial and hand movements which may result from impaired complex motor processing due to dysfunction of the basal ganglia system (Leontovich *et al.* 1999). In the next phase decreased speech processing and self-initiated action may result from dysfunction of the neocortical motor areas.

My working hypothesis concerning speech communication in people with Rett syndrome is that the profound motor disturbances interfere with speech processing and that this disturbance chiefly affects motor speech production and to a lesser extent sensory speech recognition.

My arguments are based on anatomical, functional and neurophysiological data.

From the anatomical point of view, the motor speech areas 44 and 45 are situated very close to the area of hand representation in the area 6 of motor cortex (see map in Penfield and Rasmussen, 1950 and Fig. 11.1) so that disruption of the motor cortex might be expected to have both direct and indirect effects on the motor speech areas. On the basis of dendritic morphology, Jacobs et al. (1993) suggested ontogenetically later development of the classical Broca's and Wernicke's speech areas than of the primary motor cortex, so that primary abnormal development of the motor cortex might be expected to disturb the normal morphological relationships between the speech areas.

Hypoperfusion was found in the frontal lobes and parts of the midbrain in RS at of 3–4 years of age (Bjure et al. 1997). Armstrong et al. (1998; Chapter 3) showed that the neocortical distribution of the dendritic alterations in the RS is specifically frontal, motor and limbic cortices.

From the functional point of view, there is data to support a reciprocal relationship between the speech-related neocortical areas and motor neocortical areas. Motor speech areas (Broca's areas) are not only activated during speech processing. A recent PET study showed that these areas become active also during hand or arm movements (Schlaug et al. 1994) and during the task of imagining of

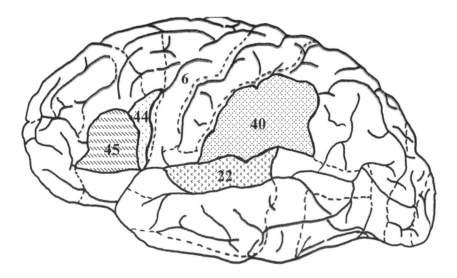

Fig. 11.1 Localization of speech-related cortical areas in the left hemisphere of the human brain. Note motor speech areas 44 and 45, sensory speech areas 22 and 40 and hand area 6.

hand movement and hand rotation (Bonda et al. 1996). Schlaug et al. (1994) studied brain areas activated during right-hand finger movements. Using PET techniques in humans they found consistent task-specific activation in the contralateral sensorimotor cortex and additional specific activation at sites in the medial and lateral premotor areas (44, 45), the parietal, and cingulate areas and the subcortical structures including the basal ganglia of both cerebral hemispheres. The observed patterns of activity were related to movement rate and accuracy in individual subjects (Schlaug et al. 1994). Bonda et al. (1996) studied the brain areas activated during hand-space mental representation tasks using PET in humans. In their experiments, subjects had to decide whether it was the left or the right hand which was presented. To do this task subjects had to think about moving position of an arm to adopt the position of the experimenter's arm. Increased activity was seen in the caudal superior parietal cortex, including the intraparietal sulcus and the adjacent medial parietal cortex (Bonda et al. 1996). Using a different approach, Topper et al. (1998) aimed to see if activation of the motor systems for arm movements (which are phylogenetically older) can facilitate language processes. In right-handed subjects, focal transcranial magnetic stimulation (TMS) was applied to the left motor cortical area for proximal arm muscles and the effect was compared with TMS of Wernicke's area. In this study TMS of the motor cortex and the non-dominant temporal lobe had no effects, TMS of Wernicke's area decreased picture naming latencies significantly (Topper et al. 1998).

It has been demonstrated that speech affects the excitability of the neocortical motor arm areas (Tokimura et al. 1996; Wildgruber et al. 1996; Topper et al. 1998). In a study by Tokimura et al. (1996) single TMS stimuli were delivered randomly over the hand area of the left or right motor cortex in normal subjects. Electromyographic responses were recorded in the relaxed first dorsal interosseous muscle while the subjects read aloud a piece of text, read silently, spoke spontaneously or made sounds without speaking. In all subjects it was only during reading aloud that a significant increase was recorded in the size of responses evoked in the dominant hand with a smaller effect registered in the non-dominant hand (Tokimura et al. 1996). Wildgruber et al. (1996) used fMRI during a speech task to evaluate lateralization of speech production at the level of the Rolandic cortex. During automatic speech strong functional activation was found in the left lower primary motor cortex. Non-speech tongue movements produced symmetrical activation within the same area. In contrast singing produced a predominant right-sided activation of the Rolandic region. Based on this study they suggested that functional lateralization of speech production therefore seems to include the precentral gyrus as well as Broca's area (Wildgruber et al. 1996).

Recently, Rizzolatti and Arbib (1998) suggested an elegant hypothesis, explaining an important relationship between primary motor cortex and motor speech areas. They studied the 'mirror neurons' system (neurons which discharge both when an animal manipulates things and also when it watches the experimenter executing similar actions). They proposed that 'such an observation/execution matching system provides a necessary bridge from 'doing' to 'communicating', as the link between actor and observer becomes a link between the sender and the receiver of each message'. TMS and PET experiments support their hypothesis and suggest that a mirror system for gesture recognition is also present in humans and includes motor speech areas (for review see Rizzolatti and Arbib 1998).

The physiological argument draws on data from Niedermeyer and Naidu (1998) who explain the clinical phenomena of RS on the basis of hyperexcitability of the motor cortex. Using TMS in cases with RS such cortical hyperexcitability was also found already during the early stages of RS (Eyre *et al.* 1990; Heinen *et al.* 1997; Chapter 10.6). Such motor cortex dyscontrol may result from dysfunction of the frontal area which in RS was also smaller in size than other cerebral regions (Niedermeyer and Naidu 1998). Niedermeyer and Naidu (1998) explained the motor disturbance in RS as the expression of disorganized prefrontal/premotor function.

11.3 Communication in RS: review and comments

Several papers have been devoted to the study of communication and behavioural skills in females with RS (Budden *et al.* 1990; Woodyatt and Ozanne 1992, 1997; Zappella 1992, 1997; Tams-Little and Holdgrafer 1996; von Tetzchner *et al.* 1996; von Tetzchner 1997; Gillberg 1997; Burford and Trevarthen 1997; Chapters 1 and 12). Loss of communication is a sign of the onset of regression (stage II) and is followed by alteration in oral-motor function and respiration correlated with the evolution of the disorder (Budden *et al.* 1990; Chapter 1). Zappella (1992) found that only 3% of classic RS girls had the ability to speak in fully formed phrases.

Tams-Little and Holdgrafer (1996) retrospectively studied pre-linguistic and linguistic communication development from birth to 24 months in people with RS and found limited use of communicative gestures. No child exceeded single word use and most had begun to regress. Pre-regression delay was obvious along with poor intentional gestural communication as precursor to single word use (Tams-Little and Holdgrafer 1996). The majority of females with RS displayed no behaviours which could be interpreted as showing an intention to communicate (von Tetzchner *et al.* 1996; von Tetzchner 1997). Girls with RS were a comparatively homogeneous group demonstrating similar cognitive patterns and fewer communicative behaviours, communicative functions, and total numbers of inferred communicative acts than a non-RS group (Woodyatt and Ozanne 1997). Fewer girls with RS were intentionally communicating to communicative partners (Woodyatt and Ozanne 1997). The RS girls retained the preverbal communication seen in normal infants (Burford and Trevarthen 1997). Such communication had characteristic rhythmic patterns and phrases, mutual imitation, reciprocal emotional phases and rudimentary oral, vocal and gestural expressions (Burford and Trevarthen 1997; Chapter 12). After passing the critical stage of RS, they retained positive orientation to human faces and eyes with smiling (Burford and Trevarthen 1997). Detailed analyses showed that the girls can employ rhythms and phrases of conversation, sometimes showing a sense of humour and sensitivity to playful teasing (Burford and Trevarthen 1997). They respond to repeated patterns of expression in rhythmic/prosodic play and to certain forms in music (Burford and Trevarthen 1997).

Since in normal subjects there is a relationship between handedness and speech dominance (Milner 1974; Hecaen *et al.* 1981; Beaton 1997; Moffat *et al.* 1998), it is interesting to consider some facts, relating to the RS.

Firstly, almost all RS girls under 7 years who grasp objects are left-handed (Nomura *et al.* 1984; Olsson and Rett 1986). Such left-handedness in RS up to age 7 comes from a functional lateralization of the neocortex similar to normal infants up to age 1. However on examination of children over 7 Olsson and Rett (1986) reported that almost all of those patients who grasped objects preferred the right hand. They proposed that due to the severe developmental arrest in RS the right shift in handedness is delayed and suggested that the central nervous system regression was more pronounced in the right than in the left hemisphere, (but see also Chapter 1).

A change in hand dominance may have an important influence on speech, since morphologically there are no speech dominant areas in the right hemisphere and this leads to suspicion that the mechanism for determination of the dominant hemisphere is not functioning normally in the RS.

Karbe *et al.* (1998) suggested two strategies which the brain adopts to recover from post-stroke aphasia: the structural repair of primarily speech-relevant regions and the activation of compensatory areas. They studied cortical metabolic recovery in aphasic stroke patients using PET at rest and during word repetition. The left supplementary motor area showed the most prominent compensatory activation in the subacute state of stroke. The brain also recruited right-hemispheric regions for speech processing when the left speech areas were permanently impaired (Karbe *et al.* 1998). It is interesting to understand the compensatory events in RS cases.

Secondly, it is interesting to note that in almost half of the girls with RS, the hand stereotypy is asymmetrical and not midline (Elian and Rudolf 1996). These authors reported that in girls with strong handedness the hand most affected by stereotypy was also used for purposeful tasks. Emotional and mental states as well as the respiratory pattern significantly influenced the hand movements (Elian and Rudolf 1996; Chapter 1).

Thirdly, since the same anatomical structures (mouth, tongue, etc.) are used for speech processing and for other physiological acts it is relevant that feeding abilities are affected in RS, where there are reduced movements of the mid and posterior tongue with premature spill-over of food and liquid from the mouth into the pharynx (Morton *et al.* 1997). These authors also showed delayed pharyngeal swallow (Morton *et al.* 1997; Chapters 1 and 10.2, 3).

Additional factors which might influence speech in RS are masseteric hypertrophy, bruxism, and severe wasting (Peak *et al.* 1992). Also many PET studies indicate activation of the putamen in speech processing (Klein *et al.* 1994). Klein *et al.* (1994) suggested that this region plays a specific role in articulation of a second language. A role for the putamen in articulation is also supported by 'foreign accent syndrome', which can occur after damage to the left putamen (Klein *et al.* 1994). Recently Leontovich *et al.* (1999) showed morphological alterations in different subcortical areas, including the putamen, in RS girls.

Some evidence gives hope that there is potential for communication in girls with RS, since no abnormality has been shown in the peripheral sensory system. Females with RS have good function of the afferent visual pathways (Saunders *et al.* 1995 and Chapter 14.2). Hearing sensitivity and the functional integrity of the eighth nerve and auditory brainstem pathways were not affected (Stach *et al.* 1994). However abnormality of some components of auditory evoked potentials suggests the presence of alteration in central auditory areas (Stach *et al.* 1994). Some publications have shown communication with girls through the visual system as in the eye-pointing method of Jensen and Skogstrom (1997) and by means of music (Wesecky 1986; Wigram 1997; Chapter 13). Even severely disabled people with RS do respond to music and they showed a good understanding of rhythm and melodies (Wesecky 1986).

11.4 Presentation of a morphological study

11.4.1 Aim of the study

The aim of the study was to find possible morphological substrates for the well-known functional asymmetry between the hemispheres in control human neocortical areas associated with language functions and to use this data for comparison with RS cases. Careful analysis of previous *in vivo* fPET imaging data and EEG data, identifying speech specific activated areas, gave us the idea to concentrate our attention on studying motor speech areas 44 and 45, and sensory speech areas 22 and 40 (Creutzfeldt *et al.* 1989; Fiez *et al.* 1996; Price *et al.* 1996 and see Fig. 11.1). We were interested in (a) cytoarchitectonic variation, and (b) morphology and distribution of synapses in these areas, using interhemispheric asymmetry in speech neocortical areas as a measure of speech development in RS. If the same pattern of interhemispheric asymmetry is present in RS as in controls we will have an indirect understanding of how the speech centres are developed in RS.

11.4.2 Patient data and tissue fixation

Fourteen RS cases, aged 4–30 years (mean 13,3 +/–1,8), mainly stage III-IV and 11 control cases, aged 4–59 years (mean 33,2 +/–6,3), without a previous history of neurological disease were included in this study. This study protocol was approved by the ethical committee in the Brain Research Institute (Moscow, Russia). Handedness information was not available in some control cases; however the hemispheric differences in size of the planum temporale showed the typical pattern for left dominant language hemisphere. Autopsy material was obtained from the left and/or right neocortical areas and fixed in 4% paraformaldehyde in 0.1 M phosphate buffer (PB).

11.4.3 Methods

Cytoarchitecture of the cortex: Serial sections from each cortical area and each case were stained with Nissl method and analysis of the cytoarchitecture was performed. Additionally, on Nissl-stained sections, the cell bodies of the largest pyramidal neurons ($n=30$) in deep layer III were drawn using the camera Lucida on an 'Ortholux' microscope (Leitz, Germany) at 400x magnification. The area of cell bodies was calculated from the drawings using the 'A.S.M.' system (Leitz, Germany).

Indirect immunofluorescence: Two or three sections from each cortical area and each case were incubated for indirect immunofluorescence using rabbit anti-synaptophysin (p38) (donated by G. Wilkin, UK), dilution 1:3000 as previously described (Belichenko *et al.* 1996a). After preincubation in 5% non-fat milk in PB saline (PBS), the primary incubation was carried out overnight (4ºC) in a free floating condition. The sections were then rinsed in PBS (20 min, three changes) and incubated for 3 hr at room temperature with biotinylated goat anti-rabbit IgG (1:200; Vector Labs, Burlingame, CA) and rinsed again with PBS (20 min, three changes). After further incubation with FITC-conjugated streptavidin (1:200; Amersham, Buckinghamshire, UK) for 1 hr at room temperature and rinsing, the sections were mounted on a microscope glass slide and coverslipped with glycerol in PB. As a control for specificity of the primary antibody, sections were incubated with normal rabbit serum instead of specific antiserum during the first incubation. In such control sections immunofluorescence was negative, but lipofuscin autofluorescence was strongly present.

Confocal microscopy imaging: Immunofluorescence-stained sections were scanned in a BioRad MRC-600 or MRC-1024 confocal microscope, employing an argon/krypton mixed gas laser as previously described (Belichenko *et al.* 1996a). The superimposition of immunofluorescence and lipofuscin fluorescence on the screen was made by merging the two images from the same focal level. In some sections, 3-D reconstructions and rotations were computed using a Silicon

Graphics IRIS work station with VoxelView/GT program (Vital Images, Fairfield, Inc., UK).

Quantitative analysis of p38: The quantitative analysis of p38-immunoreactivity (IR) and lipofuscin was carried out on single confocal images using 'Pixel Anatomy' software, as described previously (Belichenko *et al.* 1996a). Briefly, three steps were carried out for every confocal image. As a first step, background fluorescence was estimated by analysing the distribution of the pixel intensities in the image areas that did not contain any immunolabelled objects (the background threshold). This background was subtracted by setting the baseline of pixel intensities to the background value. In the second step, every image scanned for lipofuscin was subtracted in the pixel-by-pixel manner from the paired image of the same area scanned for p38-IR and lipofuscin. In the third step, an arbitrarily outlined polygon was chosen for quantification of p38-IR and lipofuscin, in an image area without artefacts. In the polygon area chosen for analysis the relative area (%) of immunolabelled pixels with an intensity value above background was calculated. The data was statistically processed with StatView software. Non-parametric two-way analysis of variance (ANOVA) was used, and $p<0.05$ was considered significant.

11.4.4 Results

Cytoarchitecture of the brain neocortical areas, related to speech processing: Quantitative analysis of distribution of the cells according to their neuronal radius in four control cases showed greater soma size in deeper sublayer III^3 in area 44, and in sublayers III^1 and III^2 in area 45 (Fig. 11.2). This closely matches previously published data on the cytoarchitectonic analysis (Hayes and Lewis 1993, 1995). These interhemispheric differences in soma size were a good morphological measure of remaining speech processing in RS girls.

In sensory speech areas 22 and 40 smaller soma size in sublayer III^1 in area 22 and in all sublayers III in area 40 should be noted (Fig. 11.2).

The area of cell bodies of the largest neurons was calculated for deeper sublayers III. The relationship in three control cases (not used in Fig. 11.2) showed an interhemispheric difference in motor speech areas 44 (Fig. 11.3(a)). In all three RS cases the area of cell bodies of largest neurons was significantly reduced (15–30% less) compared to control cases (Fig. 11.3(a)). However interhemispheric differences in both motor speech areas 44 and 45 could be seen in all RS (Fig. 11.3(b)). There were great individual variations among the RS cases (Fig. 11.3(b)). In RS case 2 the largest layer III^3 neurons in the left area 45 were smaller than those in the right hemisphere, and in RS case 3 the reverse situation was found (Fig. 11.3(b)). It is interesting to note that the RS case 2 had left hand dominance

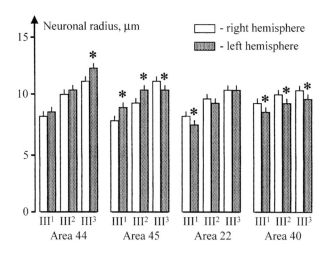

Fig. 11.2 Quantitative analysis of the neuronal radius distribution in layer III in the left and right human neocortical areas related to the speech processing in control cases. The radius of neurons was counted separately in different sublayers of layer III in right (empty bars) and left hemisphere (shadowed) in four control cases. Results are presented as the mean of neuronal radius (y-axis) +/− S.E.M. * = $p<0.05$, significantly different from the right hemisphere. Note the increased neuronal radius in motor speech areas 44 and 45 in the left hemisphere. (small figures 1, 2, 3 indicate subdivisions of layer III)

whereas RS case 3 had right hand dominance. Unfortunately handedness in RS case 1 was not known.

Synaptic architecture of the brain: Synaptic architecture was studied in control and RS cases using synaptophysin immunoreactivity (p38-IR) as a marker for synaptic vesicle proteins. There was high individual variability in interhemispheric distribution of p38-IR in control speech areas (Fig. 11.4). In some control cases the density of p38-IR structures (boutons) was higher in the left than in the right hemisphere (Fig. 11.4, case no. 1). In the other control cases this relationship was reversed (Fig. 11.4, case no. 2). The average distribution of p38-IR in all control cases was shown in Fig. 11.5. Only in area 45 there was a significant interhemispheric difference in p38-IR distribution. In the RS cases p38-IR was low in all the investigated speech areas as compared to control cases (Fig. 11.5); however some interhemispheric differences in p38-IR could be seen in RS cases (Fig. 11.5). In a further study I intend to use factor analysis of p38-IR among individual control and RS cases in order to further examine the relationships between the morphological and clinical data.

11.4.5 Discussion of morphological results

In deep layer III of area 44 and area 45 neuronal size was greater in the left than in the right hemisphere in some control cases. Previous studies of area 45 also

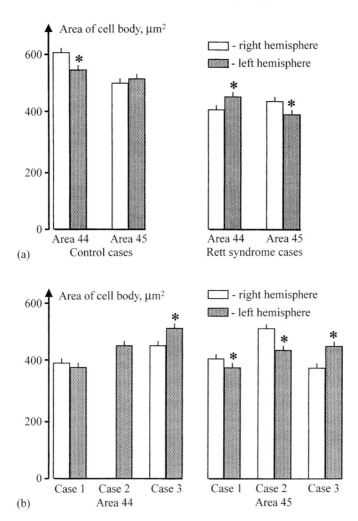

Fig. 11.3 Quantitative analysis of the cell body area distribution in the deeper layer III in the left and right human neocortical areas related to speech processing. (a) Interhemispheric differences of the area of cell body in three control and 3 RS cases. (b) Individual variability of area of cell body within interhemispheric differences in three RS cases. The area of cell body of biggest neurons in deeper layer III (90 cells in each case) was counted separately in right (empty bars) and left (shadowed) hemisphere. Results are presented as the mean of cell body area (y-axis) +/− S.E.M. * = $p<0.05$, significantly different from the right hemisphere. Note the interhemispheric differences in area of cell body of biggest layer III[3] pyramidal neurons in motor speech areas in control and RS cases.

indicate that pyramidal cells have larger cell bodies in the left hemisphere (Hayes and Lewis 1993, 1995; Scheibel *et al.* 1985; Bogolepova 1996). I do emphasize that there is very high individual variability in the speech centres. In four of our control cases the radius of the cell bodies in layer III of areas 44 and 45 was greater in the left hemisphere than in the right (see Fig. 11.2), and in three other control cases the area of cell bodies was greater in the right than in the left area 44 but the same

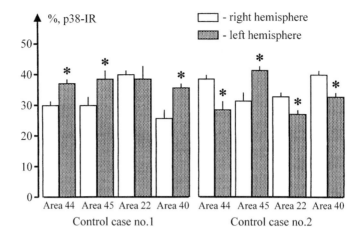

Fig. 11.4 Quantitative analysis of the synaptophysin immunoreactivity (p38-IR), from confocal images, in layers II-III in the right (empty bars) and left (shadowed) human neocortical areas related to the speech processing in two control cases. The p38 antigen was visualized by confocal microscope imaging after immunofluorescence incubation with p38 antibody. The relative areas (%, y-axis) of pixels with intensity value above a background threshold were calculated. Results are presented as the mean of p38-IR per case in $n=9$ optical fields (y-axis) +/− S.E.M. * = $p<0.05$, significantly different from the right hemisphere. Note the variability of p38-IR distribution in these two cases.

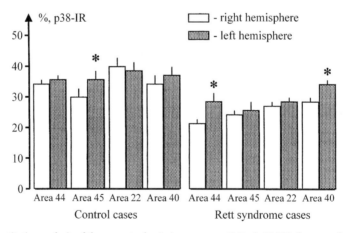

Fig. 11.5 Quantitative analysis of the synaptophysin immunoreactivity (p38-IR), from confocal images, in layers II-III in the right (empty bars) and left (shadowed) neocortical areas related to the speech processing in control and RS cases. The p38 antigen was visualized by confocal microscope imaging after immunofluorescence incubation with p38 antibody. The relative areas (%, y-axis) of pixels with intensity value above a background threshold were calculated. Results are presented as the mean of p38-IR per case in $n=18$ optical fields (y-axis) +/− S.E.M. * = $p<0.05$, significantly different from the right hemisphere. Note the general decrease of p38-IR in RS compared to control cases and existence of interhemispheric variability within RS cases.

in area 45 (see Fig. 11.3(a)). Hayes and Lewis (1993) also found greater areas of cell bodies in the left area 45 in five control cases but no differences in two control cases. I also found great individual variability in hemispheric differences of cell body areas in speech centres among RS cases (see Fig. 11.3(b)). Since in the left-handed RS case 2 the size of biggest layer III[3] neurons was in right area 45 and in right-handed RS case 3 the reverse was found (see Fig. 11.3(b)), it is possible that the asymmetry of motor speech areas relates to handedness but this requires further study.

In this study the pattern of p38-IR within the investigated areas varied among the individual controls. However, fPET study of activation in the parietal lobes during word processing has also shown individual variability (Price *et al.* 1996).

In RS cases p38-IR was low in all the speech areas as compared to control cases. This accords with our previously published data in which we found low p38-IR in frontal, motor and visual cortices in RS (Belichenko *et al.* 1996*b*). However the reductions in the number of dendrites and in the number of spines were the main features in the neocortex of RS cases (Armstrong 1992; Armstrong *et al.* 1995, 1998; Belichenko *et al.* 1994; Belichenko and Dahlstrom 1995). This indicates the importance of changes in both the pre-synaptic and the post-synaptic structures in the RS cases.

Although in the RS cases the neuronal size is less than in controls in all the investigated speech areas (see Fig. 11.3(a)) it is fascinating to note that inter-hemispheric differences were indeed present (see Fig. 11.3(b)). There are three interpretations that can be applied to these findings in RS. Firstly, the reduced cell size in RS may reflect the lack of normal speech in RS patients. Secondly, the cell size differences in RS may relate to the microcircuitry of intracortical and cortico-cortical connections which depend upon existing speech and hand dominance. Thirdly, the asymmetry in synaptic distribution (p38-IR in this study) may relate to the actual number of contacts betweens neurons, without alteration in the number of neurons available for contact.

As was shown by Price *et al.* (1996) in their fPET study, while language areas in the left hemisphere are activated, corresponding areas in the right hemisphere are normally inhibited by word stimuli (Price *et al.* 1996). Such a reciprocal relationship between the two hemispheres requires an anatomical pathway to correlate neuronal activities.

Two important statements can be made from the morphological study comparing speech areas in RS and controls. From the RS/control differences I have shown in cell body areas and the distribution of synapses, it is clear that hemispheric differences are indeed present in the RS, both at neuronal and at synaptic level. This leads to the conclusion that the morphological basis for speech processing is present in this disorder. This should encourage the development of strategies to improve speech in RS. Since there is wide individual variability of higher functions, including language ability, factor analysis of our data would help us further to correlate the morphological and clinical findings. Recent data suggests the existence of a critical period during which primary language proficiency must be attained if normal lateralization of language function is to occur (Simonds and Scheibel 1989). It is probable that the main motor disturbance in RS takes place in such a critical period. It will be valuable if early diagnosis of RS becomes possible from the study of speech and communication from home videos.

11.5 Conclusions

A strong reciprocal motor-speech relationship in normal subjects has been demonstrated morphologically and physiologically (Schlaug *et al.* 1994; Bonda *et al.* 1996; Tokimura *et al.* 1996; Wildgruber *et al.* 1996; Topper *et al.* 1998). In RS dysfunction of the motor cortex is found at the clinical and neurophysiological levels (Niedermeyer and Naidu 1998). Niedermeyer (1998) suggests that in RS the motor cortical dyscontrol is mainly due to primary frontal lobe dysfunction. I suggest that the neurological profile concerning speech processing in RS may result from progressive alteration of the motor system. Present morphological data supports the existence of interhemispheric differences in RS and the possibility for the use of this phenomenon in improving communication in girls with the RS.

11.6 Future perspectives

A morphological study of speech processing in RS girls is now in progress in our laboratory. We plan to study in more detail the interhemispheric differences in cytoarchitecture of speech areas in RS and to correlate with clinical data. I hope to find support for our hypothesis that the RS girls have better understanding of speech than the capacity for producing it. Some important questions relating to the processing of speech remain to be answered:

(1) Is there a characteristic asymmetry of motor and sensory speech areas in RS?
(2) Are there similar morphological alterations in other disorders involving speech, such as infantile autism?
(3) How may the existing morphological capacities of the speech areas in RS be used to improve communication?

A possibility for improvement of communication in RS is suggested by the study of Epstein (1998) who demonstrated that TMS may result both the inhibition and facilitation of speech and may influence speech areas directly or indirectly through intracortical networks. Recent results showed that TMS of

Wernicke's area facilitated speech processing due to a general preactivation of language-related neuronal networks (Topper *et al.* 1998); however TMS over the left inferior frontal region blocked speech output in normal subjects (Epstein 1998). On the other hand speech output also facilitated motor responses to TMS in the dominant hemisphere (Epstein 1998). Such new techniques may provide important insights into the organization of remaining speech processing and improving communication in RS.

Acknowledgements

This work was done in collaboration with Dr Andrey I. Khrenov (Brain Research Institute, Moscow, Russia), Prof. Dawna Armstrong (Department of Pathology, Baylor College of Medicine, Houston, Texas, USA), Dr Alison Kerr (Department of Psychological Medicine, Glasgow University, Glasgow, Scotland), Prof. Marco R. Celio (Institute of Histology and General Embryology, Fribourg University, Fribourg, Swiss), and Prof. Annica Dahlstrom (Department of Anatomy and Cell Biology, Goteborg University, Goteborg, Sweden). The author wishes to thank Prof. Benght Hagberg and Ms Kathy Hunter for assistance in collecting the clinical data. This work was partly supported by the Russian Fund for Fundamental Investigation (RFFI 98–04–49550), INTAS grant no. 1916–97, IRSA grant.

References[1]

Selected References Related to the study of speech processing

[1] The list provides selected references related to the study of speech processing.

Amaducci, L., Sorbi, S., Albanese, A., and Gainotti, G. (1981). Choline acetyltransferase (ChAT) activity differs in the right and left human temporal lobes. *Neurology*, **31**, 799–805.

Armstrong, D.D. (1992). The neuropathology of the Rett syndrome. *Brain Dev.*, **14**, S89–98.

Armstrong, D.D., Dunn, K., Antalffy, B., and Trivedi, R. (1995). Selective dendritic alterations in the cortex of Rett syndrome. *J. Neuropathol. Exp. Neurol.*, **54**, 195–201.

Armstrong, D.D., Dunn, K., and Antalffy, B. (1998). Decreased dendritic branching in frontal, motor and limbic cortex in Rett syndrome compared with trisomy 21. *J. Neuropathol. Exp. Neurol.*, **57**(11), 1013–7.

Beaton, A.A. (1997). The relation of planum temporale asymmetry and morphology of the corpus callosum to handedness, gender, and dyslexia: a review of the evidence. *Brain Lang.*, **60**(2), 255–322.

Belichenko, P.V., Oldfors, A., Hagberg, B., and Dahlstrom, A. (1994). Rett syndrome: 3-D confocal microscopy of cortical pyramidal dendrites and afferents. *NeuroReport*, **5**, 1509–13.

Belichenko, P.V. and Dahlstrom, A. (1995). Studies on the 3-dimensional architecture of dendritic spines and varicosities in human cortex by confocal laser scanning microscopy and Lucifer Yellow microinjections. *J. Neurosci. Meth.*, **57**(1), 55–61.

Belichenko, P.V., Fedorov, A.A., and Dahlstrom, A. (1996a). Quantitative analysis of immunofluorescence and lipofuscin distribution in human cortical areas by dual-channel confocal laser scanning microscopy. *J. Neurosci. Meth.*, **69**, 155–61.

Belichenko, P.V., Hagberg, B., and Dahlstrom, A. (1996b). Morphological study of the neocortical areas in Rett syndrome. *Acta Neuropathol.*, **93**, 50–61.

Bjure, J., Uvebrant, P., Vestergren, E., and Hagberg, B. (1997). Regional cerebral blood flow abnormalities in Rett syndrome. *Eur. Child Adolesc. Psychiatry*, **6**(**Suppl. 1**), 64–6.

Bogolepova, I.N. (1994). The cytoarchitectonic characteristics of the speech center of the brain in gifted people in the plan to study individual variability of human brain structure. *Morfologiia*, **106**(4–6), 31–8.

Bogolepova, I.N. (1996). Features of the architectonics of motor speech fields of the brain of gifted people in relation to the study of the individual variability of the structure of the human brain. *Neurosci. Behav. Physiol.*, **26**(2), 189–93.

Bonda, E., Frey, S., and Petrides, M. (1996). Evidence for a dorso-medial parietal system involved in mental transformations of the body. *J. Neurophysiol.*, **76**(3), 2042–8.

Buckner, R.L., Raichle, M.E., and Petersen, S.E. (1995). Dissociation of human prefrontal cortical areas across different speech production tasks and gender groups. *J. Neurophysiol.*, **74**(5), 2163–73.

Budden, S., Meek, M., and Henighan, C. (1990). Communication and oral-motor function in Rett syndrome. *Dev. Med. Child Neurol.*, **32**(1), 51–5.

Burford, B. and Trevarthen, C. (1997). Evoking communication in Rett syndrome: comparisons with conversations and games in mother-infant interaction. *Eur. Child Adolesc. Psychiatry*, **6**(**Suppl. 1**), 26–30.

Constant, D. and Ruther, H. (1996). Sexual dimorphism in the human corpus callosum? A comparison of methodologies. *Brain Res.*, **727**(1–2), 99–106.

Corsi-Cabrera, M., Herrera, P., and Malvido, M. (1989). Correlation between EEG and cognitive abilities: sex differences. *Int. J. Neurosci.*, **45**(1–2), 133–41.

Creutzfeldt, O., Ojemann, G., and Lettich, E. (1989). Neuronal activity in the human lateral temporal lobe. I. Responses to speech. *Exp. Brain Res.*, **77**(3), 451–75.

Davatzikos, C., Vaillant, M., Resnick, S.M., Prince, J.L., Letovsky, S., and Bryan, R.N. (1996). A computerized approach for morphological analysis of the corpus callosum. *J. Comput. Assist. Tomogr.*, **20**(1), 88–97.

deAzevedo, L.C., Hedin-Pereira, C., and Lent, R. (1997). Callosal neurons in the cingulate cortical plate and subplate of human fetuses. *J. Comp. Neurol.*, **386**(1), 60–70.

Elian, M. and de M. Rudolf, N. (1996). Observations on hand movements in Rett syndrome: a pilot study. *Acta Neurol. Scand.*, **94**(3), 212–4.

Epstein, C.M. (1998). Transcranial magnetic stimulation: language function. *J. Clin. Neurophysiol.*, **15**(4), 325–32.

Eyre, J.A., Kerr, A.M., Miller, S., O'Sullivan, M.C., and Ramesh, V. (1990). Neurophysiological observations on corticospinal projections to the upper limb in subjects with Rett Syndrome. *J. Neurol. Neurosurg. Psychiatry*, **53**, 874–9.

Ferrario, V.F., Sforza, C., Serrao, G., Frattini, T., and Del Favero, C. (1996). Shape of the human corpus callosum in childhood. Elliptic Fourier analysis on midsagittal magnetic resonance scans. *Invest. Radiol.*, **31**(1), 1–5.

Fiez, J.A., Raichle, M.E., Balota, D.A., Tallal, P., and Petersen, S.E. (1996). PET activation of posterior temporal regions during auditory word presentation and verb generation. *Cereb. Cortex*, **6**, 1–10.

Galaburda, A.M. and Sanides, F. (1980). Cytoarchitectonic organization of the human auditory cortex. *J. Comp. Neurol.*, **190**, 597–610.

Gelot, A., Esperandieu, O., and Pompidou, A. (1998). Histogenese du corps calleux. *Neurochirurgie*, **44**(**Suppl. 1**), 61–73.

Gillberg, C. (1997). Communication in Rett syndrome complex. *Eur. Child Adolesc. Psychiatry*, **6**(**Suppl. 1**), 21–2.

Glezer, I.I., Witelson, S.F., and Kigar, D.L. (1994). Immunocytochemistry of calcium-binding proteins reveals functional lateralization in human brain. *Abstr. Soc. Neurosci.*, pp. 1425.

Hayes, T.L. and Lewis, D.A. (1993). Hemispheric differences in layer III pyramidal neurons of the anterior language area. *Arch. Neurol.*, **50**, 501–5.

Hayes, T.L. and Lewis, D.A. (1995). Anatomical specialisation of the anterior motor speech area: hemispheric differences in magnopyramidal neurons. *Brain Lang.*, **49**, 289–308.

Hayes, T.L. and Lewis, D.A. (1996). Magnopyramidal neurons in the anterior motor speech region. Dendritic features and interhemispheric comparisons. *Arch Neurol.*, **53**(12), 1277–83.

Hecaen, H., De Agostini, M., and Monzon-Montes, A. (1981). Cerebral organization in left-handers. *Brain Lang.*, **12**, 261–84.

Heinen, F., Glocker, F.X., Fietzek, U., Meyer, B.U., Lucking C.H., and Korinthenberg, R. (1998). Absence of transcallosal inhibition following focal magnetic stimulation in preschool children. *Ann. Neurol.*, **43**(5), 608–12.

Heinen, F., Petersen, H., Fietzek, U., Mall, V., Schulte-Monting, J., and Korinthenberg, R. (1997). Transcranial magnetic stimulation in patients with Rett syndrome: preliminary results. *Eur. Child Adolesc. Psychiatry*, **6**(**Suppl.1**), 61–3.

Hopper, K.D., Patel, S., Cann, T.S., Wilcox, T., and Schaeffer, J.M. (1994). The relationship of age, gender, handedness, and sidedness to the size of the corpus callosum. *Acad Radiol.*, **1**(3), 243–5.

Hutsler, J.J. and Gazzaniga, M.S. (1996). Acetylcholinesterase staining in human auditory and language cortices: regional variation of structural features. *Cereb. Cortex*, **6**, 260–70.

Jacobs, B., Schall, M., and Scheibel, A.B. (1993). A quantitative dendritic analysis of Wernicke's area in humans. II. Gender, hemispheric, and environmental factors. *J. Comp. Neurol.*, **327**, 97–111.

Jacobs, B. and Scheibel, A.B. (1993). A quantitative dendritic analysis of Wernicke's area in humans. I. Lifespan changes. *J. Comp. Neurol.*, **327**, 83–96.

Jancke, L., Staiger, J.F., Schlaug, G., Huang, Y., and Steinmetz, H. (1997). The relationship between corpus callosum size and forebrain volume. *Cereb. Cortex*, **7**(1), 48–56.

Jeeves, M.A. and Moes, P. (1996). Interhemispheric transfer time differences related to aging and gender. *Neuropsychologia*, **34**(7), 627–36.

Jensen, M. and Skogstrom, K. (1997). Rett syndrome: a useful and simple visual communication aid for daily use. *Eur. Child Adolesc. Psychiatry*, **6**(**Suppl. 1**), 38.

Karbe, H., Thiel, A., Weber-Luxenburger, G., Herholz, K., Kessler, J., and Heiss, W.D. (1998). Brain plasticity in poststroke aphasia: what is the contribution of the right hemisphere?. *Brain Lang.*, **64**(2), 215–30.

Kim, K.H.S., Relkin, N.R., Lee, K-M., and Hirsch, J. (1997). Distinct cortical areas associated with native and second languages. *Nature*, **388**, 171–4.

Klein, D. (1995). The neural substrates underlying word generation: A bilingual functional-imaging study. *Proc. Natl. Acad Sci. USA*, **92**, 2899–2903.

Klein, D., Zatorre, R.J., Milner, B., Meyer, E., and Evans, A.C. (1994). Left putaminal activation when speaking a second language: evidence from PET. *NeuroReport*, **5**(17), 2295–7.

Koshi, R., Koshi, T., Jeyaseelan, L., and Vettivel, S. (1997). Morphology of the corpus callosum in human fetuses. *Clin. Anat.*, **10**(1), 22–6.

Leontovich, T.A., Mukhina, J.K., Fedorov, A.A., and Belichenko, P.V. (1999). Morphological study of the entorhinal cortex, hippocampal formation, and basal ganglia in Rett syndrome patients. *Neurobiol. Dis.*, **6**, 77–91.

Mesulam, M.M. (1990). Large scale neurocognitive networks and distributed processing for attention, language and memory. *Ann. Neurol.*, **28**, 597–613.

Milner, B. (1974). Hemisphere specialization: scope and limits. In *The neurosciences: third study program*, (ed. F.O. Schmitt and F.G. Worden), pp. 75–89. MIT Press, Cambridge, MA.

Moffat, S.D., Hampson, E., and Lee, D.H. (1998). Morphology of the planum temporale and corpus callosum in left handers with evidence of left and right hemisphere speech representation. *Brain*, **121 (Pt. 12)**, 2369–79.

Morton, R.E., Bonas, R., Minford, J., Kerr, A., and Ellis, R.E. (1997). Feeding ability in Rett syndrome. *Dev. Med. Child Neurol.*, **39**(5), 331–5.

Murphy, K., Corfield, D.R., Guz, A., Fink, G.R., Wise, R.J., Harrison, J., and Adams, L. (1997). Cerebral areas associated with motor control of speech in humans. *J. Appl. Physiol.*, **83**(5), 1438–47.

Niedermeyer, E. (1998). Frontal lobe functions and dysfunctions. *Clin. Electroencephalogr.*, **29**(2), 79–90.

Niedermeyer, E. and Naidu, S.B. (1998). Rett syndrome, EEG and the motor cortex as a model for better understanding of attention deficit hyperactivity disorder (ADHD). *Eur. Child Adolesc. Psychiatry*, **7**(2), 69–72.

Nomura, Y., Segawa, M., and Hasegawa, M. (1984). Rett syndrome — clinical studies and pathophysiological consideration. *Brain Dev. (Tokyo)*, **6**, 475–86.

Olsson, B. and Rett, A. (1986). Shift to righthandedness in Rett syndrome around age 7. *Am. J. Med. Genet.* (**Suppl. 1**), 133–41.

Parashos, I.A., Wilkinson, W.E., and Coffey, C.E. (1995). Magnetic resonance imaging of the corpus callosum: predictors of size in normal adults. *J. Neuropsychiatry Clin. Neurosci.*, **7**(1), 35–41.

Peak, J., Eveson, J.W., and Scully, C. (1992). Oral manifestation of Rett's syndrome. *Br. Dent. J.*, **172**(6), 248–9.

Penfield, W. and Rasmussen, T. (1950). *The cerebral cortex of man.* Macmillan Publishing Company.

Petersen, S.E., Fox, P.T., Posner, M.I., and Raichle, M.E. (1988). Positron emission tomographic studies of the cortical anatomy of single world processing. *Nature*, **331**, 585–9.

Polich, J. and Hoffman, L.D. (1998). P300 and handedness: on the possible contribution of corpus callosal size to ERPs. *Psychophysiology*, **35**(5), 497–507.

Price, C.J., Wise, R.J.S., and Frackowiak, R. (1996). Demonstrating the implicit processing of visually presented words and pseudowords. *Cereb. Cortex*, **6**, 62–70.

Rizzolatti, G. and Arbib, M.A. (1998). Language within our grasp. *Trends Neurosci.*, **21**(5), 188–94.

Saunders, K.J., McCulloch, D.L., and Kerr, A.M. (1995). Visual function in Rett syndrome. *Dev. Med. Child Neurol.*, **37**(6), 496–504.

Scheibel, A.B., Paul, L.A., Fried, I., Forsythe, A.B., Tomiyasu, U., Wechsler, A., Kao, A., and Slotnick, J. (1985). Dendritic organization of the anterior speech area. *Exp. Neurol.*, **87**(1), 109–17.

Schlaug, G., Knorr, U., and Seitz, R. (1994). Inter-subject variability of cerebral activations in acquiring a motor skill: a study with positron emission tomography. *Exp. Brain Res.*, **98**(3), 523–34.

Schlaug, G., Jancke, L., Huang, Y., and Steinmetz, H. (1995*a*). In vivo evidence of structural brain asymmetry in musicians. *Science*, **267**(5198), 699–701.

Schlaug, G., Jancke, L., Huang, Y., Staiger, J.F., and Steinmetz, H. (1995*b*). Increased corpus callosum size in musicians. *Neuropsychologia*, **33**(8), 1047–55.

Seldon, H.L. (1981*a*). Structure of human auditory cortex. I. Cytoarchitectonics and dendritic distribution. *Brain Res.*, **229**, 277–94.

Seldon, H.L. (1981*b*). Structure of human auditory cortex. II. Axon distribution and morphological correlates of speech perception. *Brain Res.*, **229**, 295–310.

Seldon, H.L. (1982). Structure of human auditory cortex. III. Statistical analysis of dendritic trees. *Brain Res.*, **249**, 211–21.

Simonds, R.J. and Scheibel, A.B. (1989). The postnatal development of the motor speech area: a preliminary study. *Brain Lang.*, **37**(1), 42–58.

Stach, B.A., Stoner, W.R., Smith, S.L., and Jerger, J.F. (1994). Auditory evoked potentials in Rett syndrome. *J. Am. Acad. Audiol.*, **5**(3), 226–30.

Steinmetz, H., Jancke, L., Kleinschmidt, A., Schlaug, G., Volkmann, J., and Huang, Y. (1992). Sex but no hand difference in the isthmus of the corpus callosum. *Neurology*, **42**(4), 749–52.

Steinmetz, H., Staiger, J.F., Schlaug, G., Huang, Y., and Jancke, L. (1995). Corpus callosum and brain volume in women and men. *Neuroreport*, **6**(7), 1002–4.

Stroganova, T.A., Orekhova, E.V., and Posikera, I.N. (1998). The emergence of hand preference as a sign of asymmetry in motor control in 11-months-old infants. Abstr. In *XVth Biennial ISSBD Meetings*, Berne, Switzerland, 1–4 July 1998, p. 128.

Tams-Little, S. and Holdgrafer, G. (1996). Early communication development in children with Rett syndrome. *Brain Dev.*, **18**(5), 376–8.

Tokimura, H., Tokimura, Y., Oliviero, A., Asakura, T., and Rothwell, J.C. (1996). Speech-induced changes in corticospinal excitability. *Ann. Neurol.*, **40**(4), 628–34.

Topper, R., Mottaghy, F.M., Brugmann, M., Noth, J., and Huber, W. (1998). Facilitation of picture naming by focal transcranial magnetic stimulation of Wernicke's area. *Exp. Brain Res.*, **121**(4), 371–8.

Tzourio, N., Crivello, F., Mellet, E., Nkanga-Ngila, B., and Mazoyer, B. (1998). Functional anatomy of dominance for speech comprehension in left handers vs right handers. *Neuroimage*, **8**(1), 1–16.

von Tetzchner, S., Jacobsen, K.H., Smith, L., Skjeldal, O.H., Heiberg, A., and Fagan, J.F. (1996). Vision, cognition and developmental characteristics of girls and women with Rett syndrome. *Dev. Med. Child Neurol.*, **38**(3), 212–25.

von Tetzchner, S. (1997). Communication skills among females with Rett syndrome. *Eur. Child Adolesc. Psychiatry*, **6**(**Suppl. 1**), 33–7.

Wesecky, A. (1986). Music therapy for children with Rett syndrome. *Am. J. Med. Genet.* (**Suppl. 1**), 253–7.

Wigram, T. (1997). Meaning in music: non-verbal communication in music therapy for girls with Rett syndrome. *Eur. Child Adolesc. Psychiatry*, **6**(**Suppl. 1**), 61–3.

Wildgruber, D., Ackermann, H., Klose, U., Kardatzki, B., and Grodd W. (1996). Functional lateralization of speech production at primary motor cortex: a fMRI study. *Neuroreport*, **7**(15–17), 2791–5.

Witelson, S.F., Glezer, I.I., and Kigar, D.L. (1995). Women have greater density of neurons in posterior temporal cortex. *J. Neurosci.*, **5**(**Pt. 1**), 3418–28.

Woodyatt, G.C. and Ozanne, A.E. (1992). Communication abilities in a case of Rett syndrome. *J. Intellect Disabil. Res.*, **36**(**Pt. 1**), 83–92.

Woodyatt, G. and Ozanne, A. (1997). Rett syndrome (RS) and profound intellectual disability: cognitive and communicative similarities and differences. *Eur. Child Adolesc. Psychiatry*, **6**(**Suppl. 1**), 31–2.

Zaidel, E., Aboitiz, F., and Clarke, J. (1995). Sexual dimorphism in interhemispheric relations: anatomical-behavioral convergence. *Biol. Res.*, **28**(1), 27–43.

Zappella, M. (1992). The Rett girls with preserved speech. *Brain Dev.*, **14**(2), 98–101.

Zappella, M. (1997). The preserved speech variant of the Rett complex: a report of 8 cases. *Eur. Child Adolesc. Psychiatry*, **6**(**Suppl. 1**), 23–5.

Zatorre, R.J. (1992). Lateralization of phonetic and pitch discrimination in speech processing. *Science*, **256**, 846–9.

12 Early infant intelligence and Rett syndrome

Colwyn Trevarthen and Bronwen Burford

Abstract

The developmental psychobiology of Rett syndrome may explain how a young child who is severely reduced in voluntary activity, intelligent response to experience and learning, and who lacks speech, can have appeared normal in early infancy, when many psychological capacities are already functional, before the development of language. A defect in the regulatory mechanisms of the brainstem that begins in the embryo appears to be responsible for dysregulation of neocortical mechanisms at a critical stage in late infancy. Examination of home movies of 12 infants aged 7–12 months shows that there are subtle signs before regression.

12.1 Introduction: how does the developmental process go off track in Rett Syndrome?

Newborn infants have clear manifestations of purposeful intelligence (Trevarthen *et al.* 1981). Their motives direct their attentions to particular objects. They show clear preferences for human stimuli, in touch, hearing, olfaction, taste and sight. They can mirror intimate communications of caregivers. Coordinated timing of body movements and emotional expressions in rhythmic patterns, alertness to expressions of the human voice, eyes, face and hands, and the production of complementary or imitative expressions in precise intercoordination with those of a partner, testify to complex adaptive functions of the core emotional processes in the infant brain. Sympathetic emotions appear to be adapted to guide cognitive growth, and the learning of cultural skills (Aitken and Trevarthen, 1997; Papousek and Bornstein 1992; Papousek and Papousek 1987; Reddy *et al.* 1997; Schore 1994;

Stern 1985; Trevarthen 1979, 1993*b*, 1998). These are a foundation on which more complex understanding and skill in acting are developed through both differentiation and learning.

The developmental anatomy of the human embryo brain (O'Rahilly and Müller 1994) indicates that formation of the neocortex, which is believed to be where all higher levels of intelligent function are built up in postnatal life, is dependent on neurochemical factors transmitted from subcortical neurons (Trevarthen 1997; Trevarthen and Aitken 1994). A reticular intrinsic motive formation (IMF) in the brainstem core, laid down in the first trimester of gestation, regulates neocortical morphogenesis in the foetus, and continues to direct neocortical development, cognition and learning through postnatal brain maturation (Trevarthen and Aitken, loc. cit.). Gene-regulated body-mapping of motive systems in the brain and of rhythmic time-patterns imposed on neuronal group activity would appear to be a principal guide for the primary organization of action, thought and intersubjective communication through infancy and early childhood. This intrinsic regulation generates and constrains all plastic responses of the brain to experience of the environment. It is also capable of triggering neurodevelopmental disorders that can seriously compromise psychological growth.

Developments in Rett syndrome confirm the idea that causes of behavioural regression, which is coincident with arrest of cortical growth in late infancy, involve the subcortex. The brain may function near normally in earliest months, as in other conditions, including autism, giving the impression that the infant's sociability, playfulness and alertness are as they should be. Gradually, however, signs appear that the organization of posture, investigative curiosity and coordination of voluntary, visually guided motor activity is failing.

By the end of the first year of infancy a girl developing Rett disorder is clearly falling behind. This comes at a crucial time when an infant is normally making strides to more systematic combinatory operations of manipulation, with sequential focus of attention on goals selected from memory, and to cooperative awareness with attention to the interests and actions of other persons. At 1 year, joint attention and gestures and vocalizations of 'protolanguage' (Halliday 1975) guide the child to language and other meaningful behaviours (Bruner 1983; Locke 1995), beginning the first active period of cultural learning by mimesis (Donald 1991). In the second year the devastating effects of Rett syndrome on voluntary action, learning of skills and arbitrary conventions and creative communication by gesture and speech are clear. The girl who has Rett syndrome appears to lose all but automatic 'mirror' reactions to the present behaviours of other persons and aimless or self-directed gestures, as her cerebral cortex ceases to differentiate. Nevertheless, evidence that some voluntary expressions, desires and preferences can be elicited by carefully paced interrogation, and that the rhythms and prosody of speech, song or music can excite facial and vocal expression of emotions and sympathetic rhythmic movements of the body and limbs, would indicate that a sensitivity to the foundational motives of communication remains intact from infancy, beneath the vacant gaze, 'empty' smile and confusing involuntary stereotypies of movement.

Gene regulation and epigenetic constraints of motive systems, and changes in their adaptation to environmental affordances, have a definite intrinsic timetable in childhood. Pathology can affect different cerebral mechanisms in the embryo, foetus and infant, setting up catastrophic states at different ages in the future, precipitating different developmental disorders of communication, voluntary action and reasoning about experience (Tager-Flusberg 1999). The unique intersubjective impulses in human development entail new vulnerability for brain disorders affecting communication and cognition, and these higher order psychological effects are associated with varying degrees of failure in sensory, motor and autonomic function, the causes of which must also be sought subcortically.

Effective facilitation of communication and motivation in Rett syndrome engages and supports the residual impulses for action and intersubjective response that were present and functioning when the affected child was an infant (Burford and Trevarthen 1997). Such support requires that a partner sensitively adjusts his/her movements and expressions to the girl's limited capacities for mirroring and adjusting purposes, complementing the fragile 'zone of proximal development' of the child (Vygotsky 1962). In particular, methods that employ rhythmic movement and/or music can give substantial aid with problems of attentional inflexibility, motor discoordination and emotional confusion. Such methods of interpersonal guidance or therapy have the power to give organization to motive processes and autonomic self-regulations that have become weakened and disordered as a result of insufficient or unbalanced maturation of key monoamine systems of the reticular core of the brain (Wigram and De Backer 1999).

In normal infant development, sympathetic communication has, of course, key importance. In newborns, rhythmic coordination of body parts, imitations, and expressions of emotion precisely intercoordinated with a partner testify to motive integrations of subcortical origin, and maternal responses have powerful effects on the autonomic regulations of the infant. They certainly can affect the development of the infant's brain (Schore 1994). The brainstem core, organized in the embryo and regulating foetal neurogenesis, becomes an IMF regulating postnatal brain maturation with caregivers' aid (Trevarthen and Aitken 1994). Physiological controllers in the hindbrain and cerebellum are integrated with expressive and receptive mechanisms of the midbrain, diencephalon, basal ganglia and limbic system. All these structures play a part in activating and modulating the functions of the growing neocortex, as they regulate the anatomical elaboration of cell migrations and interconnections forming neocortical tissues in the embryo.

The neurobiology of Rett syndrome indicates that failure of cognitive and linguistic developments is a consequence of dysfunction of brainstem monoaminergic regulators (Chapter 7). Near normal behavioural development in the earliest months indicates that core functions of motivation and socio-emotional response may be more intact than normally appears, and that more organized behaviour may be evoked by contingent and appropriately supportive stimulation. Persons with Rett syndrome respond by orienting and expressing pleasure to 'emotional narratives' of nursery rhymes, musical games and songs. Therapies that incorporate rhythms of body movement, speech prosody and music, seek to support retained motives for purposeful action and communication. They may help counteract dysregulations of autonomic state, attention, motor coordination and emotion.

12.1.1 Infant motives and the developing brain

The development of an infant shows periods of rapid change in psychological interests and abilities that allow one to chart a sequence of developmental stages. Changes in perceptual orienting and attending, in the coordination of intentional movements and in emotional changes give evidence of intrinsic regulatory processes that undergo periodic, discontinuous transformations. These developmental steps can presumably be identified with changes in activity of interacting cells in neurochemical systems of the brainstem and their effects at target sites among cortical cells. Both these brain regions change in structure and activity under the influence of genes which are expressed at particular ages. An examination of the relationship between 'periods of rapid developmental change' and so-called 'difficult periods', when the infant is more demanding of maternal attention, suggests that there are cycles alternating between more adventurous experience-seeking *ergotropic* phases, when new skills and knowledge are being gained, and more 'nurturant' or self-regulating *trophotropic* episodes that monitor and balance internal physiological states (Trevarthen, 2001; Trevarthen and Aitken, 2000).

At present, efforts to correlate a flood of new findings on change in cells and tissues of the brain, neurochemistry of transmitters and their receptors, and metabolic activity of neural tissue recorded by functional brain scanning are hampered by inadequate descriptions of age-related psychological changes, and by conceptions of cortical network development that direct attention away from the likely morphogenetic control processes originating in the brainstem.

A survey of evidence on the time of emergence of intrinsic regulatory systems in the brainstem of the human embryo, and comparison with the anatomy and physiological role of the sub-cortical Emotional Motor System (Holstege *et al.* 1997), which affects both autonomic and motivational control and reinforcement of learning and the acquisition of motor skills through postnatal life, leads to the hypothesis that monoamine neurons mediate in transactions between brain activity, the body and the external environment (Trevarthen, 2001). This, one may presume, will also be the system that determines the equilibrium and periodic transformations of balance between ergotropic and trophotropic functions in motivation for behaviour through the life cycle. Comparison with abnormal developmental trajectories should help confirm or infirm this model of the process regulating the changes and the role of different neuron populations.

Developing brain systems of an infant generate selective interneuronal connections first by an intrinsic process, then, at a precise stage of their maturation in relation to other systems of the intensely interconnected CNS, they become ready to receive support from specific forms of environmental input, especially in the form of both physiological and psychological (emotional) support from parental caregiving. Growth of the brain of a human infant and development of self-regulation of brain activity states are sensitive to contingent responses of a caregiver to the infant's expressions of emotional state or need (Aitken and Trevarthen, 1997; Trevarthen, 2001). From birth the more immediate input from the mother, through body contact, movement, and breast milk, a complex of stimulation and nourishment which sedates or activates the infant and assists development of regular motive state transitions, is facilitated or guided by psychological responses to the mother's vocalisations and eye contact with her (Schore 1994; Zeifman *et al.* 1996). Both physiological and psychological regulation depend on maternal sensitivity and measured responsiveness to the infant's signals in a mutual 'co-regulating' system. The effects of 'kangarooing' in intensive care, a procedure whereby premature infants are given body contact, warmth and vibratory and acoustic stimulation from the parent's voice by being placed against the chest beneath the clothes, prove the benefit of intimate and affectionately responsive mothering with all these features, even for neonates born up to 3 months before term (van Rees and de Leeuw 1993).

Desire for human contact achieved through mutual looking with the eyes, vocalizing and listening with the ears, or touching with the hands and soft parts of the body is thus an innate regulator of an infant's development, not a learned ability or need.

A large part of an infant's brain, in subcortical and limbic regions, is adapted to regulation from the stimuli of mothering. Maternal care is essential to autonomic as well as psychological (motoric and cognitive) growth in infancy (Panksepp *et al.* 1997). Evolution of a special visceral efferent mechanism coordinates the infant's looking, listening, respiration, heart activity and other visceral activities (Porges 1997) with effects on voluntary motor coordination and consciousness (Panksepp 1998). Development of comprehension of meaning in the human community by integration of personal investigative curiosity with self-other interaction extends the integration of motives and physiological state-regulation with emotional expression and the construction of conscious and purposeful behaviours. This development is postnatal and involves maturation of prefrontal and temporal neocortex in an intimate two-way relation with the earlier maturing brainstem and limbic systems (Dawson and Fisher 1994; Trevarthen and Aitken 1994).

12.2 The path to meaning in human society: motives for learning by communicating

The story of psychological development through the two years of infancy is made more comprehensible by these psychobiological considerations. A totally naive but purposefully active subject, who is adapted to elicit and respond to parental care and the rudiments of companionship, develops into a toddler with intelligent grasp of many human needs and interests. In year 1, the infant shows motives adapted to generate, on the one hand, autonomous investigative learning and, on the other hand, intersubjective communication with the motives and interests of familiar persons (Trevarthen, 1998). Such persons, for their part, are attracted to the infant and motivated to provide both nurture of the infant's state regulations, ensuring the infant has necessary protection, nourishment, comfort and rest, and partnership in joint activities and attention to shared goals. Parenting responds to highly specific and clearly manifested needs of the infant, and it changes when these needs change. In other words, the parent adapts to internally generated changes in the infant's motives and self-regulatory states.

In the past three decades psychological research has accumulated a rich array of facts concerning the needs of infants and the preferences and aversions that guide infant experience (Trevarthen *et al.,* 1981; Trevarthen and Aitken, 2000). With the demise of the behaviourist model of the infant as a learning machine, the cognitive approach concentrates on evidence of perceptual discrimination of objects, selective orienting to perceptual information and the development of coherent representations of reality that are competent to direct emerging motor skills. While enriching our concepts of the primary mental functions that assimilate information and generate concepts, this cognitive model tends to leave the nature of the infant's intrinsic motives for different kinds of experience relatively obscure. Nevertheless, it is now clearly established that a fundamental guiding principle in infant cognitive growth is provided by motives that immediately recognize and seek to interact with the psychological activities of another person's mind (Stern 1985; Papousek and Papousek, 1987; Trevarthen 1998, 1999*a*; Aitken and Trevarthen, 1997). These intersubjective motives change, as do those that govern the infant's engagements with physical objects and events that offer no psychologically active response.

Motives for praxic investigation and manipulative mastery of objects and those adapted to intersubjective communication with persons both depend on anticipatory 'motor images' that *cause* perceiving as much as sensory information does (Jeannerod 1994). Major developmental changes are characterized by shifts in the balance of these two kinds of experience-seeking motive—'object-directed' and 'person-directed'. By the end of infancy a coordinated 'secondary intersubjectivity' enables fluent 'person-person-object' coordination in cooperative awareness with 'joint attention' (Trevarthen and Hubley 1978). For example, a normally developing 1-year-old makes rapid shifts between focusing awareness on objects of visual or auditory exploration, or on the things taken in hand for tactile exploration and manipulative operations, and such intersubjective acts as making eye-to-eye contact, smiling, pointing, vocalizing and gesturing in a 'protolinguistic' way, 'showing off' and laughing at jokes, to all of which family members are likely to respond immediately, with intermodal 'affect attunement' (Stern *et al.* 1985). A number of re-orientations of interest can be made without the infant losing track of the overall purpose of his/her activity. Emotions of curiosity, surprise and self-gratification or impatience and irritation with things are integrated with those of affectionate joy and pride, suspicious shame, fear or anger, and playful humour, which regulate communication and relationships with persons (Stern 1993, 1999). This integration of purposes allows the consolidation of companionship in which the child begins to learn arbitrary customs and meanings, opening the way to the learning of language and other elaborated cultural forms of shared knowledge and skill.

Infants are very alert socially before 9 months, and can be proficient in many games learned in play with familiar persons. At 6 months they are beginning to have effective control of bimanual manipulative intentions, as well as quick recognition of many categories of auditory and visual experience, especially as these may contribute to consciousness of other persons and what they are doing. The baby's social awareness is characterized by new imitativeness, interest in other infants and in mirror images of the self, and 'showing off' behaviour that are highly responsive to other persons' attentions (see Fig. 12.1). But an infant younger than about 36 weeks after a full-term birth, is not willing and able to accept another's initiatives in expressed purposes as a request or instruction for a particular act. Cooperation in a task comes rather suddenly around 9 months. By what steps is this crucial stage in human psychological growth achieved?

12.2.1 Summarizing what normally develops in Year 1 and when it appears

The most important changes in an infant's psychological abilities and reactions to other persons over the first year can be summarized as follows (Trevarthen *et al.* 1981; Trevarthen 1998; Trevarthen and Aitken, 2000).

(1) Vision develops quickly after birth. Newborns show awareness of a person by orienting to look towards sounds of the voice, and can fixate on the region of the eyes. They can imitate seen facial expressions, head movements and gestures of the hands. In the first few weeks, improvement in visual accommodation, orienting and fixation, with expansion of the ability to coordinate successive foci of visual attending in an intelligent 'scan' of an object or situation, to grasp its 'affordances' for purposeful action, transforms the way the infant reacts to, and experiences, persons and things. After 12 weeks, there

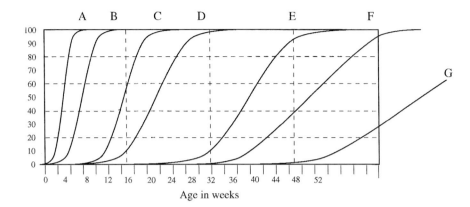

A Regulation of sleep, feeding and breathing. Innate 'pre-preaching'. Imitation of expressions.

B Fixates eyes with smiling. Protoconversations. Mouth and tongue imitations give way to vocal and gestural imitations. Distressed by 'still face' test.

C 'Person–person' games, mirror recognition. Smooth visual tracking, strong head support, reaching and catching.

D Accurate reach and grasp. Binocular stereopsis. Manipulative play with objects. Interest in surroundings increases. Imitation of clapping and pointing. Development of 'person–person–object' games.

E Playful, self-aware imitating. Showing off. Stranger fear. Strong focus on manipulation. Babbling and rhythmic banging objects. Crawling and sitting, pulling up to stand.

F Cooperation in tasks; follows instructions and pointing. Makes declarations with 'joint attention'. Protolanguage. Clowning. Combining objects and 'executive thinking'. Begins to categorize experiences.

G Self-feeding with hand. Beginning if mimesis of purposeful actions, and cultural learning.

Fig. 12.1 Important transitions in the first year.

begins a transformation in the depth and range of an infant's curiosity for things in the space outside the body, and this seems to be driven largely by internally generated developments in visuo-motor systems, including the rather sudden maturation of the cortical circuits of binocular stereoptic depth detection at around 20 weeks. This development is, of course, dependent upon concurrent maturation of motor mechanisms that aim the two eyes conjugately, and that synchronize accommodation of their lenses to focus on stimuli at different distances.

(2) Hearing begins weeks before birth. Foetuses can learn to recognize their mother's voice. Newborns imitate simple vocal sounds, and they make 'pleasure' vocalizations adapted to speech vowels, and rudimentary articulation movements of 'pre-speech'. At about 4–6 weeks there is a conspicuous advance in visually elicited smiling, though even premature infants show well-developed smiles to a voice or vibratory or tactile contact with a person. After 6 weeks, encounters with a sympathetic other develop into intimate 'protoconversations', coordinating voice, facial expression and gesture in

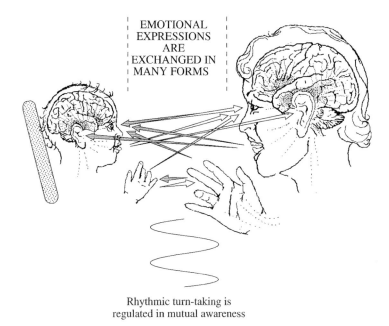

Fig. 12.2 2 month-old and mother in protoconversation.

reciprocal and mutually compatible interactions with Coordinated Interpersonal Timing (CIT) (Beebe *et al.* 1985; Jaffe *et al.* 1999) (Fig. 12.2). Infants participate in these exchanges with the finely regulated rhythms and melodies of the adult's affectionate baby talk or 'motherese'.

(3) Efficient antigravity support of the head, arms, trunk, hips and finally legs matures by a succession of stages: holding the head up to look about; reaching and grasping, tracking and catching; sitting and leaning; rolling over; crawling; standing and walking. The physical 'dynamic system' comprising the growing skeleto-muscular system, its receptors, which are sensitive to mechanical forces in the body and limbs, in interaction with activity produced in the motor centres of the CNS, generates a sequence of revolutions or 'catastrophes' in motor competence.

(4) Aiming the hands to a distant object seen (or imagined) can be observed in the form of 'pre-reaching' in the neonate stage. This develops into accurate reaching and grasping, and effective manipulation, exploring and transforming of objects in the hand, after the emergence of strong antigravity support at 16–20 weeks. Fine controlled manipulation develops after this, through the last half of the first year. Similarly hand-to-mouth coordination can be observed in foetuses many weeks before birth, but is not efficient until after 4 months. Visual guidance of hand use undergoes major development around the middle of the first year.

(5) After 3 months there is marked development in the range of an infant's vocal expressions that convey transient emotions and readiness for communication. Lively 'games' develop with familiar partners around the middle of the first year, becoming rhythmic narratives with features of 'communicative musicality' that are practised and learned as habitual routines in family friendships. Infants at this stage respond strongly to a mother's singing, joining in with the timing and prosodic expressions (Malloch 1999; Trevarthen 1999*b*). They are especially responsive to vowels at the termination of phrases of an utterance or melody, and often imitate these sounds. The baby has fluent transitions in interest and an ability to assume control of the contact; for example, taking a proactive role in teasing games. The routines of 'person-person games', in which the infant's voice, face, body and hands are reacted to or manipulated by the mother, become increasingly combined with object play as the baby withdraws attention from the mother to attempt to look at, listen to or grasp and manipulate objects (Trevarthen and Hubley, 1978). A 6-month-old is very quick to manage these changes, and parents respond by developing more lively and sustained interactive 'person-person-object games'.

(6) The preference for a mother's voice which a newborn can show begins a process of recognition that reinforces an affectionate bond. Attachment relationships of trust in which pride in playfully acquired skills and expressions is defended against the fear and shame occasioned by the incomprehension of strangers, become very strong after 6 months, when infants are said to manifest clear 'self-awareness' for the first time (Schore 1994; Stern 1985).

(7) Comprehending shared attentions and intentions in joint exploration and cooperative task performance shows a conspicuous emergence at 9 months, the change identified as Secondary Intersubjectivity, which motivates efficient person-person-object awareness (Trevarthen and Hubley 1978). This is the time when infants begin to point and vocalize 'declarative' pronouncements with expressive modulation in 'protolanguage' (Halliday 1975; Locke 1995). By 1 year an infant confides expression of purposes and ideas to others by coordinating signals of emotion and volition (smiles, frets, pointing, reaching for, etc.) with attentions to their interest, and responses to the sympathetic quality of their interest and emotions.

What is constructed and what grows?
Newborn infants, as we have pointed out, show the outlines of many psychological purposes, although they lack the discrimination and motor power to execute them effectively. A neonate can mark intersubjective contacts by smiling, eye-seeking, touching with the hands and vocalizing; imitating vocalizations, face expressions, gestures of hands and fingers; coordinating interactive sequences with turn-taking on a beat and phrasing; scanning surroundings by rhythmic conjugate steps of the

eyes coupled to head rotations; making purposeful movements of mouthing and sucking; reaching to grasp (pre-reaching); stepping alternately or kicking (Trevarthen 1997).

Motor coordination expressing primary motives directed to the outside world, for reaching and for communication, seems to be a key intrinsic or biological factor in determining the important transitions in the first year that are summarized in Fig. 12.1. A second factor is the dynamic balance between the environment-directed assertive and investigative *ergotropic* activities, on the one hand, and self-regulating nurturance-seeking *trophotropic* behaviours, on the other, the latter integrated with autonomic state-control (Hess 1954). When young infants are perturbed by unresponsive or non-contingent and emotionally inappropriate mothering, they demonstrate disordered movements and may make automatic repetitive self-touching, hand-to-hand clasping, forced hand-regard, etc., as well as well-coordinated expressions of avoidance and distress (Murray and Trevarthen 1985; Trevarthen 1993*a*). These automatisms may have important relation to ritualistic motor patterns in both Rett syndrome and autism.

At this point, it is important to clarify in what ways Rett syndrome differs from autism (Trevarthen *et al.* 1998). Both conditions appear in late infancy after an early period of apparent normality. Both show subtle signs of disintegration of purposeful action and selective awareness around the end of the first year. In the initial phase of Rett syndrome the signs of emotional irritability and distress, and social avoidance resemble autism, but thereafter the characteristic unwillingness to identify with the interests and expressions of another person that define autism are missing from the girl with Rett syndrome. Indeed, while her intelligence and capacity for voluntary use of her hands decline, and she loses what progress she made towards speech, she keeps a positive orientation to the face, eyes and voice of a person who seeks to make contact. Her distinctive hand movements do not resemble the flapping and fiddling which occupy some autistic children when they are most withdrawn.

Until such time as a reliable genetic or phenotypic marker is found that will enable detection of a predisposition to the condition in foetal or newborn stages, it will be important to relate the findings from chance documents, such as home movies, recording the earliest signs of abnormal development in Rett syndrome to the transitions and 'difficult periods' of normal infancy. These periodic phases of instability and developmental change give us evidence of significant shifts in the ergotropic/trophotropic equilibrium which occur with advances in perceptual, motor and cognitive processes. However, 'regression periods' reported for normal development (van de Rijt-Plooij and Plooij 1992) are quite different from the period of regression in Rett syndrome which traumatically descends on Rett infants and their families. Are there clues before the onset of this catastrophic change that the infant is experiencing developmental problems?

We report the results of a preliminary study undertaken by Bronwen Burford in collaboration with Alison Kerr. Videos taken by parents in the UK are being subjected to microanalysis by methods that have proved immensely fruitful in recent decades in charting developments in infancy and the environmental factors that are important to its normal flourishing.

12.3 Early communication and the Rett disorder: clues to disruption

Subtle signs of disruption in development have been detected in retrospective analysis of home videos taken during early infancy, providing evidence of the much earlier onset of the disorder than has been accepted (Kerr and Stephenson 1986; Kerr et al. 1987). These studies noted that the girls showed excessive patting and arm waving, jerky coordination and poor hand skills in the pre-regression period. It is striking that the early signs seen on the videos were rarely recognized by families at the time. However, parents who subsequently watched pre-regression videos of their own or other children were able to recognize such features. They reported that they had in fact registered them, but their child's bright appearance and desire for human contact had quelled their doubts.

It is not surprising that parents usually report the pre-regression period as having been 'trouble-free' in contrast to the regression phase, though in retrospect some parents do report on concerns about their child's development before the onset of regression. Leonard and Bower (1998) found that of the 127 parents in Australia they questioned about early development, 59 had harboured concerns about their daughter during the first six months of life. The fact that the children do make some progress during the pre-regression phase gives assurance to parents that 'all is well'. As indicated Kerr's video studies, home videos taken before the child's problems were recognized, are valuable sources of information about the aspects of development that do make some progress and those which indicate that there is a problem.

What should we expect to see on video recordings of young infants at play and in social exchanges? As explained above, we should see lively and robust social interactions that are frequently initiated and actively driven by the infant and also great curiosity and exploration of new objects and surroundings. We should also see an increasingly mobile infant who exploits new motor skills to explore her environment at ever increasing distances and with greater independence.

12.3.1 Infant videos: searching for clues

A recent detailed survey by Burford of 12 randomly selected home videos[1] of infants (aged 7–12 months) suggests that problems are subtly indicated at 7

---

[1] All video records are from Dr A.M. Kerr's collection of infant home videos of girls with a subsequent diagnosis of Rett syndrome.

months, detectable by the time the infant reaches 9–10 months and more clearly evident by the first birthday. The videos were all taken in the family home and showed the infants in situations where they had opportunities for play and social exchanges during everyday family events and gatherings. All the video material available for each infant within this age range was examined and on most videos there was a minimum of 10 minutes of material suitable for analysis. Observations were collected using the Video Logger, a computerized system of video analysis developed by Macleod and Burford (see Macleod *et al.* 1993 for details of this system).

At this stage the observations from the survey must remain speculative and descriptive until systematic, detailed analyses have been conducted on a larger sample, including younger infants, and the tapes have been subjected to the scrutiny of independent raters.[2] A second note of caution must be sounded in declaring behaviours to be 'absent' simply on the basis of their non-appearance during video recording. Nevertheless, in the 12 videos included in this initial survey some striking absences and limitations, which appear genuine, were repeatedly noted in crucial developmental behaviours:

- no active exploration of toys and objects
- no shared attention between objects and adult
- little evidence of hand-eye coordination
- few attempts to explore surroundings
- inappropriate repetition of social responses
- lack of animation and expressive body movement
- easily distracted by voices and movements of others
- minimal leg movement

In addition, there was evidence of hand movements with qualities typical of the characteristic Rett hand movements in four of the girls and of the striking opening and closing of the hand to grasp objects noted by (Kerr *et al.* 1987; Kerr 1995). Other observations include a distinctive staring into space and periods of almost statue-like stillness, glimpses of which can be seen in the sequences between 7 and 10 months, becoming more marked at 12 months. More extensive analysis is required before the potential significance of these observations can be properly assessed.

How then can parents fail to notice such deficiencies? In fact, it is unsurprising that few parents express misgivings about their child's development during the

---

[2] An ESRC-funded research project to study pre-regression infant videos, to be conducted by Burford, Kerr and Macleod, will begin in late 1999.

first year. On first observing the videos the infants do appear to meet normal expectations. They can appear alert and engaged: smiling, laughing, squealing with delight, flapping their arms in excitement, vocalizing, watching the events around them, holding and playing with toys, and responding with pleasure to social overtures from family members and friends. Some can be seen crawling, pulling up to standing, walking with support and walking independently within the normal timescale of development. On closer inspection, however, clues that 'all is not well' can be detected. A typical example of a 7-month-old baby (E) who seems busy and engaged with toys and people offers an illustration. E nearly always has a toy in her hand and appears to handle and manipulate the toys. However, her activity lacks variety and purpose. Observations over a 1 hour period are characterized by constant but unvaried hand activity over and around the toys but no purposeful exploration or examination:

E is sitting on the floor surrounded by toys and objects, all within reach. She is constantly 'busy', batting/patting toys with one hand, picking up toys, and occasionally mouthing them. She rarely looks at the toys. She holds the same toy in her other hand for over 15 min but pays no attention to it. She is immediately responsive whenever her mother calls to her from behind the camera. She looks down at the pile of toys around her, always at the same spot, but rarely looks at the toy she is holding or handling. Occasionally she becomes animated and waves her arms up and down, but there is little leg movement. She looks around and watches what is going on around her and shows interest in another child nearby, watching what he is doing.

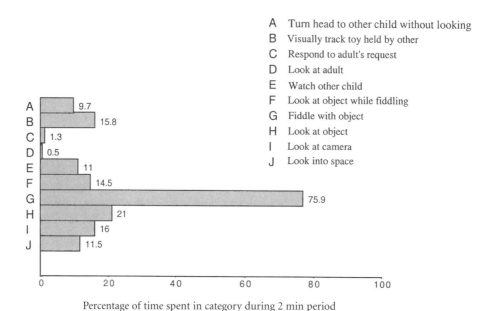

Fig. 12.3 Child E, 7 months: distribution of activities.

Figure 12.3 shows a 2 min extract from the same section of video in greater detail which is illustrative of the 1 h period. Her non-exploratory handling is labelled 'fiddle with object'.

E's activities give an illusory appearance of purpose; she is always 'doing something', looking around, looking at others, and gives a ready response to her mother. However, she did not seek to explore the toys or her surroundings although she appeared to have some interest in them. She did not look at the toy in her hand, explore its surfaces, or test its possibilities, but her hands were constantly passing over toys and it is easy to see how this gives an appearance of purpose to adults.

Examples of a further two infants give a similar picture—S aged 7 months and Y aged 10 months (shown in Fig. 12.4 and 12.5 respectively). Each short time period is typical of the pattern of behaviours observed overall for each infant. Although the categories of activities and behaviours are different for each of the infants, a greater proportion of time is allocated to non-investigative activities in all three examples. A disproportionate amount of passive, reactive activity and behaviour is typical of the picture gained from all 12 infants. However, it cannot be said that the infants lack interest in objects, their surroundings or people, but they demonstrate this more often by passive watching than actively participating.

Child S (shown in Fig. 12.4) also demonstrated an unvarying fixed smile. In Fig. 12.4 she smiles throughout the sequence, as indeed she does in much of her home video material from the age of 2 months onwards. When her smiling is tracked using a potentiometer little variation is seen in its intensity; it remained at the same intensity for 17 s, then changed to a slightly higher intensity for the remainder of the sequence. Seventeen seconds is an unduly long period to show no fluctuation in the intensity of an expressive behaviour. In infants with Rett syndrome the readiness to smile and its unvaried nature raises suspicions; it seems stereotypical and does not appear finely tuned to what is happening.

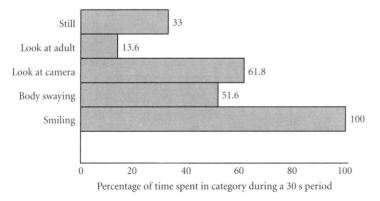

Fig. 12.4 Child S, 7 months: distribution of activities.

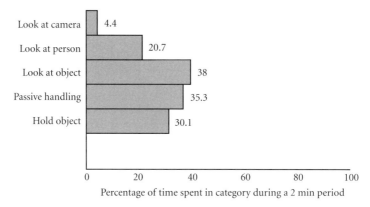

Fig 12.5 Child Y, 10 months: distribution of activities.

Many infants appeared too easily distracted. In one scene a child can be seen constantly turning her head from one person to another immediately they begin to speak or make a move, even when not directed at her, and her attention is easily taken away from the toys beside her. Turning to the voices and activity of those around them seemed too immediate, which raises questions about the extent to which the infants were absorbed in a task or engaged with a person.

The Rett infants' behaviours seem to offer a sufficient smokescreen which covers developmental limitations effectively, but closer examination may give a different picture. Passive holding or patting and passing hands over toys and objects without clear purpose can easily be mistaken for purposeful play when viewed within the context of everyday family life. In similar vein, infants who can pull to standing, crawl and walk with support do not use these new motor skills to explore more widely. Anomalies may make appearances (e.g. the child sitting with control and balance suddenly and without reason topples over, making no attempt to right herself), but are not sufficiently frequent or striking to draw attention.

As might be expected, the extent to which possible warning signs are evident varies between infants, with some infants giving only subtle indications (e.g. occasional trouble grasping objects but usually managing to accomplish the task) while others exhibit more obvious signs (e.g. constant repetitive finger movements). Two children in the sample raised instant concerns. One child, aged 7 months, had a blank face, stared, did not show interest in the other children and adults present, and had repetitive finger movements. Another, aged 9 months, held a constant unvarying smile, a wide-eyed look, had a poor hand grasp, and displayed a hand clasping motion and frequent bouts of rocking. There was no footage of the second child between 7 and 9 months, though recordings at an earlier age also raise doubts about her development even as early as 2 months.

In the videos some infants showed marked changes between 11 months and 12 months. At 11 months one infant can be seen sitting in a swing, holding on with both hands, smiling and vocalizing to the camera. Also at 11 months she can be seen clapping hands in imitation. Yet one month later the picture is beginning to change, showing evidence of disengagement from other people and lack of interest in surroundings. She shows a poor grasp, lacks animation, stares into the distance, her eyes 'looking through' those around her. Another infant who was very active at 11 months laughing, crawling, pulling herself up to standing, peering into the camera appears quiet and disengaged during her first birthday party. She has a distant look, a blank face and is less steady on her feet. She does not respond to social overtures from others. It is possible that the infants were simply in a quieter mood or affected by noise and excitement. The second infant though did show a similar pattern a few days later in a quieter situation. Although she is physically active and babbling in the later scene she still does not show the engagement typical of her recordings at a younger age.

However, most infants still give the appearance of being engaged with the social world. The 12-month episodes mostly focused on the first birthday. The immediate impression one gains from these scenes is of the hard work parents are putting into raising the child's level of activity and responsiveness. The infants smile, look at others, look at their presents, watch the activity around them, play in limited fashion with toys, but need constant prompting from other family members to do so. They fit the profile of 'passive recipients' as described by Burford (1993); most smiled readily, laughed, vocalized and looked in response to others but rarely made the first move. These types of responses are pleasing to adults and mask the fact that the infants are failing to seize the initiative. In fact, all 12 infants show a marked lack of initiation at all the ages observed. While acknowledging that a larger sample of infants and of video examples might show a different picture, one would expect to see infants becoming more active and persistent in seeking adults' attention and guidance in a period of development that is typified by intense curiosity and exploration.

During the 9–12-month period we should see the beginning of gestural requests, pointing, seeking help from adults to demonstrate a toy, waving bye-bye, attempts to name objects and familiar people, and initiating well-known games such as peek-a-boo. Pointing, gestural requests, attempts to name or request names for objects, and seeking adult help to work a toy were not observed on the video examples. A larger sample might yield such observations, but their absence in these examples is interesting, nevertheless, since the infants were observed in contexts that offered good opportunities for exploration and shared activity. Through their passivity the infants are losing valuable opportunities for learning. The 'zone of proximal development' described by Vygotsky (1962) emphasizes the child's contribution to her learning. The adult provides necessary assistance in gaining new knowledge and skills but the partnership is mutual; the child actively seeks guidance in what Rogoff (1990) calls 'guided participation'.

Rett syndrome and autism

A comparative infant home video study of Rett syndrome and autism by Garreau and collaborators (Garreau *et al.* 1996) observed differences in cognitive function and in posture in infants with Rett syndrome in the second year of life. Earlier differentiation between the two groups was not possible however; both Rett and autistic infants displayed difficulties in attention, especially shared attention.

Swettenham *et al.* (1998) found that infants with autism in the second year of life had more shifts of attention between objects than between a person and an object, or between one person and another. The infants with Rett syndrome also rarely shifted attention between a person and an object, but did shift attention between one object and another. Unlike the autistic infants though they readily shifted attention between one person and another, perhaps too readily as has already been suggested. After 9 months infants should develop the capacity to share their attention between a person and an object, most often demonstrated by alternation of gaze (Mosier and Rogoff 1994). Gaze alternation of this nature was not observed in any of the 12 video recordings nor indeed was any attempt made by the infants to engage adults in joint activity.

The picture gained from the video observations is of infants who enjoy being part of the social world. Rett syndrome is commonly misdiagnosed as autism when problems first become apparent, especially during the period of regression when the infant with Rett syndrome becomes difficult and less accessible to human contact. However, the diminished accessibility is temporary. Applying the term 'autism' to girls with Rett syndrome has been challenged for well over a decade. Kerr and Stephenson (1985) called it a misleading and incorrect use of the term since 'autism' implies a loss of interest in personal contact. This was contrary to their observations of the girls' use of eye contact and friendly manner, curtailed by their handicaps rather than motivational limitations. Generally, girls with Rett syndrome show an interest in taking part in social exchanges and forming interpersonal relationships. In contrast, children with autism show little or no interest in social interaction (Volkmar *et al.* 1990, p. 258).

12.3.2 Education and therapy

'Profound learning disabilities' is an all-encompassing categorization of individuals with varying aetiologies who have very severe impairments in cognitive, motor and perceptual development. It is unlikely that development will follow the same course in different aetiological groups; each may have genetic, neurological and biochemical characteristics that produce differences in performance (Hodapp, Burack and Zigler 1990), and therapists and teachers should be aware of the implications of these differences for teaching and therapy programmes. Knowledge and awareness of the cause of a child's profound learning disabilities (and the complex interrelationship of the neurological, psychological and medical aspects of the child's condition) allows practitioners to tailor individual programmes even more effectively to the needs of the individual child. This is not to suggest that the child should be treated merely as a collection of strengths and weaknesses associated with her syndrome. The individual child lies at the heart of any successful therapeutic or educational approach, one that makes best use of the child's strengths rather than focusing on deficits. However, the syndrome will affect the manner and extent to which a child can participate and it is important that teachers and therapists are aware of how this is manifested (Hodapp 1998).

Practitioners also need to be aware of the behaviours that are neurologically driven and are not open to modification. Girls with the Rett disorder have little control over their stereotyped movements, hyperventilation or breath holding and it is important for practitioners to know about this, especially since similar behaviours can also have a psychological origin and can be open to influence (e.g. in other circumstances stereotyped movements can offer therapists a way into an isolated child's world). Nevertheless, music therapy can successfully reduce the level of some Rett behaviours during the session, giving good opportunities for uninterrupted contact and engagement (Eisler, personal communication and Chapter 1). The respite is temporary and the power of the brain soon intervenes to return the behaviours to their full intensity which makes such moments of respite and greater openness to intervention all the more valuable for the girl.

With few exceptions girls with the Rett disorder, despite their rather indiscriminate attention, appear to retain throughout life an easily accessible capacity for an infancy level of communication, despite its disruption during the regression period (Kerr 1995). The style of communication evident in the early months of life of every child offers an effective route for making contact with older people with profound learning disabilities, regardless of the cause of disability (Burford 1988, 1998). During many years of experience both as a movement therapist and researcher, Burford has observed considerable variation in the amount of work and persistence required to activate this basic level of response with people with profound learning disabilities. However, the accessibility of this level of communication in girls with Rett syndrome appears more uniform and reliable for therapists and parents, and can usually be tapped into with relative assurance, though still requiring persistence and sensitivity. This retained capacity for interaction, the girls' greatest strength, should underpin educational and therapeutic strategies to achieve maximum effect. Practitioners can gain many lessons from studying how early communication develops in normal infants. Therapies that follow this basis with people with profound learning disabilities—music therapy and movement therapy—work especially well, offering a sound framework for effective and mutually enjoyable non-verbal interactions.

When searching for ways of helping the children to develop and move forward, the most constructive approach is to seek out what the girls can do, however limited that might seem, and to use this knowledge to gain access to her world. This is not easy to do. A child with poor control of her body needs time before she is able to marshall her body into making a response and runs the risk of being judged unresponsive—the adult moves away because the child has not been able to respond with her movements quickly enough. Some girls communicate likes and dislikes through idiosyncratic movements which seem meaningless to the untrained eye. It can be difficult to recognize when a child is attempting to communicate or to understand the meaning and emotional significance of her actions. However, it is a vital goal since empathic human communication offers essential support for any child's emotional and psychological growth.

12.3.3 Concluding remarks

It seems that the developmental progress that infants with Rett syndrome do make offers a smokescreen that effectively masks their difficulties. However, by 9 months this is becoming an insufficient disguise. This does not mean that by this stage the infant's problems can be easily recognized by parents, but close scrutiny of videos is beginning to uncover early signs of the Rett disorder.

In normal development the carer-infant unit is seen as an intensely dynamic system in which both infant and carer actively participate and influence each other. The child not only responds appropriately, but actively and with curiosity. Even the watching of people and events nearby is an active pursuit in which the infant visually tracks the action and expresses interest and involvement through body movements, alert posture, facial expressions and sounds, or disengages to look away. By contrast, infants with Rett syndrome seem passively interested; they notice and watch events, smile, make spontaneous body movements and sounds, but these lack the variation and independence with responsivity which normally gives an infant's behaviours an attractive vitality.

We can see during the 9–12-month period when great strides should be made that infants with Rett syndrome are already performing poorly in areas that are crucial for development later in infancy, especially a critical period around 18 months. Meltzoff (1990) suggests that there is a 'watershed transformation' in cognition around 18 months in which the infant changes from using representations based on actual experience to being able to hypothesize about the future and make deductions about the past. Thus, the period of regression invariably occurs at a critical developmental stage (Witt Engerström 1992). The loss of skills in communication, hand use and speech deprives the girls of crucial capacities which normally flourish at this stage in infant development, equipping the toddler for wider exploration of her world, greater autonomy and many new experiences which will enhance and encourage yet more learning and progress. Deprived of these possibilities we should view the communicative capacities that girls with Rett syndrome do retain as all the more precious. It is essential that therapists and teachers capitalise on the girls' communicative strengths and their enjoyment of human contact.

References

Aitken, K.J. and Trevarthen, C. (1997). Self-other organisation in human psychological development. *Development and Psychopathology*, **9**, 653–677.

Beebe, B., Jaffe, J., Feldstein, S., Mays, K., and Alson, D. (1985). Inter-personal timing: the application of an adult dialogue model to mother-infant vocal and kinesic interactions. In *Social perception in infants* (ed. T.M. Field and N. Fox), pp. 249–68. Ablex, Norwood, NJ.

Bruner, J. (1983). *Child's talk: learning to use language*. Norton, New York.

Burford, B. (1988). Action cycles: rhythmic actions for engagement with children and young people with profound mental handicap. *European Journal of Special Needs Education*, **3**(4), 189–206.

Burford, B. (1993). Helping with communication through movement. In *Learning disabilities: a handbook of care* (2nd edn) (ed. E. Shanley and T. Starr), pp. 269–89. Churchill Livingstone, Edinburgh.

Burford, B. (1998). Nonverbal paths to communication. In *Hallas' care of people with intellectual disabilities* (9th edn) (ed. W.I. Fraser, D. Sines, and M.P. Kerr), pp. 37–48. Butterworth-Heinemann, London.

Burford, B. and Trevarthen, C. (1997). Evoking communication in Rett syndrome: comparisons with conversations and games in mother-infant interaction. *European Child & Adolescent Psychiatry*, **6**(Suppl. 1), 26–30.

Dawson, G. and Fischer, K.W. (ed.) (1994). *Human behavior and the developing brain*. Guilford, New York.

Donald, M. (1991). *Origins of the modern mind*. Harvard University Press, Cambridge.

Garreau, B., Carmagnat, C., and Sauvage, D. (1996). *Rett syndrome and autism: a comparative study with home movies*. Research Report, Département de Psychopathologie de l'enfant et de Neurophysiologie du Développement, C.H.U. Bretonneau, 37044 Tours Cedex. France.

Halliday, M.A.K. (1975). *Learning how to mean: explorations in the development of language*. Edward Arnold, London.

Hess, W.R. (1954). *Diencephalon: autonomic and extrapyramidal functions*. Grune and Stratton, Orlando, FL.

Hodapp, R.M. (1998). *Development and disabilities. intellectual, sensory and motor impairments*. Cambridge University Press, Cambridge.

Hodapp, R.M., Burack, J.A., and Zigler, E. (1990). New directions in the developmental approach. In *Issues in the developmental approach to mental retardation* (ed. R.M. Hodapp, J.A. Burack, and E. Zigler), pp. 294–312. Cambridge University Press, Cambridge.

Holstege, G., Bandler, R., and Saper, C.B. (ed.) (1997). *The emotional motor system*. Elsevier, Amsterdam.

Jaffe, J., Beebe, B., Feldstein, S., Crown, C., and Jasnow, M. (1999). *Rhythms of dialogue in infancy: coordinated timing and social development*. SRCD Monographs, submitted.

Jeannerod, M. (1994). The representing brain: neural correlates of motor intention and imagery. *Behavioral and Brain Sciences*, **17**, 187–245.

Kerr, A. (1995). Early clinical signs in the Rett disorder. *Neuropediatrics*, **26**, 67–71.

Kerr, A.M. and Stephenson, J.B.P. (1985). Rett's syndrome in the west of Scotland. *British Medical Journal*, **291**, 579–82.

Kerr, A.M. and Stephenson, J.B.P. (1986). A study of the natural history of Rett syndrome in 23 girls. *American Journal of Medical Genetics*, (**Suppl. 1**), 77–83.

Kerr, A.M., Montague, J., and Stephenson, J.B.P. (1987). The hands, and the mind, pre- and post-regression, in Rett syndrome. *Brain Development*, **9**(5), 487–90.

Leonard, H. and Bower, C. (1998). Is the girl with Rett syndrome normal at birth? *Developmental Medicine and Child Neurology*, **40**, 115–21.

Locke, J.L. (1995). The development of the capacity for spoken language. In *The handbook of child language* (ed. P. Fletcher and B. MacWhinney), pp. 278–302. Blackwell, Oxford.

Macleod, H.A., Morse, D., and Burford, B. (1993). Computer support for behavioural event recording and transcription. *Psychology Teaching Review*, **2**(2), 115–9.

Malloch, S.N. (1999). Mothers and infants and communicative musicality. *Musicae Scientiae*, in press.

Meltzoff, A.N. (1990). Towards a developmental cognitive science. The implications of cross-modal matching and imitation for the development of representation and memory in infancy. *Annals of New York Academy of Science*, **608**, 1–31.

Mosier, C.E. and Rogoff, B. (1994). Infants' instrumental use of their mothers to achieve their goals. *Child Development*, **65**(1), 70–9.

Murray, L. and Trevarthen, C. (1985). Emotional regulation of interactions between two-month-olds and their mothers. In *Social perception in infants* (ed. T.M. Field and N.A. Fox), pp. 177–97. Ablex, Norwood, NJ.

O'Rahilly, R. and Müller, F. (1994). *The embryonic human brain: an atlas of developmental stages*. Wiley-Liss, New York.

Panksepp, J. (1998). *Affective neuroscience: the foundations of human and animal emotions*. Oxford University Press, New York.

Panksepp, J. Nelson, E., and Bekkedal, M. (1997). Brain system for the mediation of social separation—distress and social reward. Evolutionary antecedents and neuropeptide intermediaries. In *The integrative neurobiology of affiliation (Annals of the New York Academy of Sciences, Vol. 807)* (ed. C.S. Carter, I.I. Lederhendler, and B. Kirkpatrick), pp. 78–101. The New York Academy of Sciences, New York.

Papousek, H. and Papousek, M. (1987). Intuitive parenting: a dialectic counterpart to the infant's integrative competence. In *Handbook of infant development* (2nd. edition) (ed. J.D. Osofsky), pp. 669–720. Wiley, New York.

Papousek, H. and Bornstein, M.H. (1992). Didactic interactions: intuitive parental support of vocal and verbal development in human infants. In *Nonverbal vocal communication: comparative and developmental aspects* (ed. H. Papousek, U. Jürgens and M. Papousek), pp. 209–29. Cambridge University Press. Cambridge/Editions de la Maison des Sciences de l'Homme, Paris.

Porges, S.W. (1997). Emotion: an evolutionary by-product of the neural regulation of the autonomic nervous system. In *The integrative neurobiology of affiliation (Annals of the New York Academy of Sciences, Vol. 807)* (ed. C.S. Carter, I.I. Lederhendler, and B. Kirkpatrick), pp. 62–78. New York Academy of Sciences, New York.

Reddy, V., Hay, D., Murray, L., and Trevarthen, C. (1997). Communication in infancy: mutual regulation of affect and attention. In *Infant development: recent advances* (ed. G. Bremner, A. Slater, and G. Butterworth), pp. 247–74. Psychology Press, Hove, East Sussex.

Rogoff, B. (1990). *Apprenticeship in thinking: cognitive development in social context*. Oxford University Press, New York.

Schore, A.N. (1994). *Affect regulation and the origin of the self: the neurobiology of emotional development*. Erlbaum, Hillsdale, NJ.

Stern, D.N. (1985). *The interpersonal world of the infant: a view from psychoanalysis and development psychology.* (Second Edition to be published, as Paperback, in 2000, with new Introduction) Basic Books, New York.

Stern, D.N. (1993). The role of feelings for an interpersonal self. In *The perceived self: ecological and interpersonal sources of the self-knowledge* (ed. U. Neisser), pp. 205–15. Cambridge University Press, New York.

Stern, D.N. (1999). Vitality contours: the temporal contour of feelings as a basic unit for constructing the infant's social experience. In *Early social cognition: understanding others in the first months of life* (ed. P. Rochat), pp. 67–90. Erlbaum, Mahwah, NJ.

Stern, D.N., Hofer, L., Haft, W., and Dore, J. (1985). Affect attunement: the sharing of feeling states between mother and infant by means of inter-modal fluency. In *Social perception in infants* (ed. T.M. Field and N. Fox), pp. 249–68. Ablex, Norwood, NJ.

Swettenham, J., Baron-Cohen, S., Charman, T., Cox, A., Baird, G., Drew, A., *et al.* (1998). The frequency and distribution of spontaneous attention shifts between social and nonsocial stimuli in autistic, typically developing, and nonautistic developmentally delayed infants. *Journal of Child Psychology and Psychiatry*, **39**(5), 747–53.

Tager-Flusberg, H. (ed.) (1999). *Neurodevelopmental disorders*. MIT Press, Cambridge, MA.

Teitelbaum, P., Teitelbaum, O., Nye, J., Fryman, J., and Maurer, R.G. (1998). Movement analysis in infancy may be useful for early diagnosis of autism. *Proceedings of National Academy of Science, USA*, **95**(23), 13982–7.

Trevarthen, C. (1979). Communication and cooperation in early infancy. A description of primary intersubjectivity. In *Before speech: the beginnings of human communication* (ed. M. Bullowa), pp. 321–47. Cambridge University Press, London.

Trevarthen, C. (1993*a*). The function of emotions in early infant communication and development. In *New perspectives in early communicative development* (ed. J. Nadel and L. Camaioni), pp. 48–81. Routledge, London.

Trevarthen, C. (1993*b*). The self born in intersubjectivity: an infant communicating. In *The perceived self: ecological and interpersonal sources of self-knowledge* (ed. U. Neisser), pp. 121–73. Cambridge University Press, New York.

Trevarthen, C. (1997). Foetal and neonatal psychology: intrinsic motives and learning behaviour. In *Advances in perinatal medicine* (*Proceedings of the XVth European Congress of Perinatal Medicine*, Glasgow, 10–13 September 1996) (ed. F. Cockburn), pp. 282–91. Parthenon, New York and London.

Trevarthen, C. (1998). The concept and foundations of infant intersubjectivity. In *Intersubjective communication and emotion in early ontogeny* (ed. S. Bråten), pp. 15–46. Cambridge University Press, Cambridge.

Trevarthen, C. (1999*a*). Intersubjectivity. *The MIT encyclopedia of cognitive sciences* (ed. R. Wilson and F. Keil), pp. 413–6. MIT Press, Cambridge, MA.

Trevarthen, C. (1999*b*). Musicality and the intrinsic motive pulse: evidence from human psychobiology and infant communication. *Musicae Scientiae*, in press.

Trevarthen, C. (2000). Intrinsic motives for companionship in understanding: their origin, development and significance for infant mental health. *Infant Mental Health Journal*. (in press).

Trevarthen, C. (2001). The neurobiology of early communication: intersubjective regulations in human brain development. In *Handbook on brain and behavior in human development* (A.F. Kalverboer & A. Gramsbergen, eds.). Dordrecht, The Netherlands: Kluwer Academic Publishers. (submitted).

Trevarthen, C. and Aitken, K.J. (1994). Brain development, infant communication, and empathy disorders: intrinsic factors in child mental health. *Development and Psychopathology*, **6**, 597–633.

Trevarthen, C. and Aitken, K.J. (2000). Intersubjective foundations in human psychological development. *Annual Research Review. The Journal of Child Psychology and Psychiatry and Allied Disciplines*. (in press).

Trevarthen, C. and Hubley, P. (1978). Secondary intersubjectivity: confidence, confiding and acts of meaning in the first year. In *Action, gesture and symbol: the emergence of language* (ed. A. Lock), pp. 183–229. Academic Press, London.

Trevarthen, C., Aitken, K., and Plooij, F.X. (2000). Can age-related brain developments explain behavioural 'regressions' in infancy?. In *Human Development* (special issue) (ed. F.X. Plooij and M. Heimann), in preparation.

Trevarthen, C., Aitken, K.J., Papoudi, C., and Robarts, J.Z. (1998). *Children with autism: diagnosis and interventions to meet their needs* (2nd edn). Jessica Kingsley, London.

Trevarthen, C., Murray, L., and Hubley, P.A. (1981). Psychology of infants. In *Scientific foundations of clinical paediatrics* (2nd edn) (ed. J. Davis and J. Dobbing), pp. 211–74. Heinemann, London.

van de Rijt-Plooij, H.H.C. and Plooij, F.X. (1992). Infantile regressions: disorganisation and the onset of transition periods. *Journal of Reproductive and Infant Psychology*, **10**(2), 129–49.

van Rees, S. and de Leeuw, R. (1993). *The kangaroo method*. (Video) Stichting Lichaamstaal, Scheyvenhofweg 12, 6093, PR Heythuysen, The Netherlands.

Volkmar, F.R., Burack, J., and Cohen, D. (1990). Deviance and developmental approaches to the study of autism. In *Issues in the developmental approach to mental retardation* (ed. R.M. Hodapp, J.A. Burack, and E. Zigler), pp. 246–71. Cambridge University Press, Cambridge.

Vygotsky, L.S. (1962). *Thought and language*. M.I.T. Press, Cambridge, MA.

Wigram, A. and De Backer, J. (1999). *Clinical applications of music therapy in developmental disability, paediatrics and neurology*. Jessica Kingsley, London.

Witt Engerström, I. (1992). Age-related occurrence of signs and symptoms in the Rett syndrome. *Brain and Development*, **14**(Suppl.), S11–20.

Zeifman, D., Delaney, S., and Blass, E. (1996). Sweet taste, looking, and calm in 2- and 4-week-old infants: the eyes have it. *Developmental Psychology*, **32**, 1090–99.

13 Musical responsiveness in the Rett disorder

Björn Merker and Nils L. Wallin

Summary

There are numerous anecdotal indications that music may play a significant role in the lives of Rett patients, but so far no systematic studies of the musical responsiveness of this patient population have been reported. In this chapter we discuss the potential importance of the use of music as a 'window' on the cognitive capacities of Rett patients, as well as the many methodological problems involved in conducting such studies. The developmental perspective is emphasized, since in normal children musical responsiveness is present already in the first year of life, that is, at a time when Rett girls undergo a relatively normal phase of development. Language acquisition, on the other hand, roughly coincides with the onset of Rett regression, a circumstance which may leave language disproportionately affected by the disorder. The study of Rett patients' musical responsiveness therefore may provide important clues to their capacities and sensibilities, and promises to further our understanding and treatment of these severely impaired patients.

13.1 Introduction

Despite numerous informal indications that music plays a significant role in the lives of Rett patients (Chapter 1), there are few reports of research on music in relation to Rett syndrome (Wesecky 1986; Kerr 1987; Hadsell and Coleman 1988; Wigram, 1991; Cass et al. 1993; Wigram and Cass 1995; Wylie 1996; Sigafoos et al. 1996; Burford and Trevarthen 1997; Wigram 1997; Takehisa and Takehisa-Silvestri, n.d.). This chapter accordingly cannot base itself on empirically validated knowledge of Rett patients' relationship to music, but is intended, rather, as a discussion of the potential uses of music as a 'window' on the cognitive capacities of Rett patients, as well as its potential as a means of enhancing their quality of life, provided that evidence concerning Rett patients' responsiveness to music is upheld by future studies. Though our focus here is only on the Rett disorder, some of the approaches, principles and cautions we outline are quite general ones. They may thus prove to be useful also in relation to a number of other developmental and neurodegenerative syndromes such as autism and Alzheimer's dementia.

13.2 The musical challenge in the Rett disorder

Music ranks second only to human language and language-based activities in its potential cognitive complexity. Structurally music is characterized by syntactic structure which, as in the case of language, exhibits hierarchical organization (Salzer 1952; Schenker 1956; Rosner and Meyer 1982; Lerdahl and Jackendoff 1983; Narmour 1990, 1999), but which, unlike language, is not a vehicle for the communication of referential meaning (Staal 1989). This makes music a close to ideal medium by which to explore the cognitive capacities of patient populations lacking language, or exhibiting extreme language impairment, as is the case in the Rett disorder. It is therefore possible that the study of musical responsiveness and preferences on the part of Rett patients could provide a 'window' on their cognitive capacities in the absence of language.

The possibility that Rett patients may show a greater responsiveness to and interest in music than might be predicted from their linguistic abilities as indicators of cognitive function constitutes the musical challenge of the Rett disorder. One reason for believing that musical sensibility and language might be differentially affected in this disorder is that in the normal child, responses to musical stimuli and the capacity to discriminate between them develop quite early and are present in the first year of life (see review by Trehub 1990: Section 13.6). This is considerably before language acquisition and marks the time in infancy when Rett girls undergo a relatively normal phase of development. Language, on the other hand, starts manifesting itself in normal development at about the time when Rett patients start showing overt and conspicuous symptoms, a temporal coincidence likely to leave language disproportionately affected by the disorder.

In exploring this possibility, the motoric automatisms (hand wringing), apraxic and ataxic symptoms of Rett patients (Chapter 1) in combination with their autonomic and respiratory disturbances (Chapter 6) place obstacles in the way of systematic and reliable assessment of their musical sensibilities. It is not their cognitive status as such which is at issue here. Previous experience with response to music in non-Rett children with mental retardation (with or without additional disabilities) tells us that music can be used as a positive reinforcer in learning regimens for these children (Silliman-French *et al.* 1998; Gutowski 1996; Hill *et al.* 1989; Burch *et al.* 1987; McClure *et al.* 1986), that distorted music can function as a negative reinforcer for them (Greene *et al.* 1970), that retarded children not only respond to music (Murphy 1957; Alvin 1959; see also Hanser 1983 and references therein) but show differential responsiveness to different types of music (Sternlicht *et al.* 1967; Staples 1968; Reardon and Bell, 1970) and can express musical preferences when given an opportunity to do so (Cotter and Toombs 1966; Koh and Koh 1966; Dattilo and Mirenda 1987; Hill *et al.* 1989). At issue, rather, is how such questions might be pursued in Rett patients given the many sources of interference with communication, response measures and stable baselines which their motoric and autonomic problems supply. Before turning to this issue, however, some general observations concerning what the study of Rett patients' musical sensibility might teach us concerning these severely disabled individuals, and some general cautions to be observed in pursuing this question.

13.3 Musical background

Music is normally part of the cultural ambience in which every child grows up and acculturates. This means that the musical responsiveness of a given child is shaped by its background of musical exposure, a process we now know has its beginnings even before birth (Busnel and Granier-Deferre 1983; Cooper and Aslin 1989; see review by Lecanuet 1996). Rett girls are no exception in this regard, since they are exposed to the music of their culture in their homes and surroundings and give evidence of having favourite tunes and musical preferences (Hadsell and Coleman 1988). Attention to this fact itself is a first step in approaching the question of their musical responses and preferences. One needs to know, in other words, what types of music are available in the everyday surroundings of a Rett patient, and which types of music were available at different stages of her development. Crucial in this regard is information about music exposure in the premorbid phase of development, and what music preferences may have been formed prior to presentation of overt symptoms. Each stage after this is nevertheless of interest in its own right, since it provides essential information needed to interpret possible evidence for trends or changes of musical taste on the part of Rett patients (see below).

13.4 Musical preferences and antipathies

Musical responsiveness is present whenever music alters a person's state or behaviour, for example, by exerting a calming or activating effect, by becoming the target of focussed attention, or by evoking emotional or motoric reactions. There is no lack of informal indications that many Rett girls display musical responsiveness in such ways. Not only are they musically responsive, but they may exhibit musical preferences in the form of favourite tunes or styles of music. A musical preference or antipathy can be said to exist when a person exercises consistent choice among the set of musical samples to which she is exposed. The choice may be shown explicitly, as when patients control the selection of the music they listen to through requests, multiple choice switches or equivalent arrangements, or it may be exhibited through behavioural reactions indicative of pleasure, interest or aversion when the piece happens to be played or performed for other reasons. Such preferences are of interest from the point of view of cognitive capacities, because the preference by itself implies the operation of discriminative, memory and recognition functions capable of selecting that particular tune from among a set of alternatives. The specificity of preference provides further information: it might range from being focussed on a specific performance of a given tune, over including any version of the tune in question, to embracing the entire genre of which the tune is a member. Do alternate versions of the preferred piece affect the patient's reactions differentially, and if so how?

The existence of a preference need not, however, imply anything specific about the reasons for the preference. It need not signify an aesthetic choice, nor imply a preference for the structural features of the preferred musical item, since there are a number of possible determinants of preferences (and/or aversions) besides the musical qualities of a piece, among which the following two are particularly important:

(a) Acquired familiarity based on differential exposure to a certain kind of music or individual pieces of music (which might take on the character of 'security signal').
(b) Association of certain kinds or pieces of music with significant episodes, persons or experiences (generally of an emotional nature) in the subject's life.

These two sources of preference or antipathy are potential confounding factors in studies attempting to explore the role of structural features of music (parameters such as tempo, rhythmic pattern, melody, periodicity (variance vs redundancy) and timbre) in determining musical preferences.

13.5 Changes in musical preference or taste

Given preferences, one may ask the further question of whether preferences change, and particularly if consistent trends may be said to characterize such changed musical preferences. Do Rett patients show longitudinal change in their musical preferences? Might they develop a preference for a tune to which they were exposed only after the onset of overt symptoms? Questions such as these may provide evidence regarding the cognitive status and learning capacity of Rett patients at different stages of their development. This includes the issue of the extent to which the Rett linguistic deficit is simply one manifestation of a global cognitive deficit, or whether different cognitive capacities are differentially affected in the Rett disorder. A consistent trend in changing musical preference based on listening history implies cumulative cognitive change based on learning mechanisms. The addition of a new favourite tune after regression has set in would mean that discriminative and learning mechanisms needed to support such a change are present and functioning. A change in musical taste from simpler to more complex and demanding musical structures (see below) implies the corresponding discriminative and learning capacity, that is, a capacity to penetrate beneath the surface acoustic flow to the underlying structural content of music. This presupposes, of course, that the changed preference is not a result of associative learning experiences such as those listed in the previous section, but is based on cumulative listening experience leading to a progressively deepening familiarity with the musical materials. If so, it amounts to the acquisition of tacit musical knowledge from experience.

13.6 Comparisons with the developmental progression of musical sensibility in normal children

The receptive musical precocity of the normal human infant is a remarkable developmental fact whose implications have yet to be fully explored. Normal children below 1 year of age show sensitivity to a number of structural features of music which are important in adult musical appreciation such as rhythmic patterns, melodic contour, tempo and phrase structure (see reviews by Trehub 1990; Krumhansl 1990; Fassbender 1996; Dowling 1999; and references in these). The first year of Rett patients' lives generally unfolds without conspicuous symptoms of the coming disorder (Chapter 1), and we may assume that during this stage they share the discriminative musical capacities of normal infants. Rett girls apparently retain a number of these capacities, at least to some extent, even after regression sets in, as evidenced by their ability to discriminate tunes and to favour some over others. What about their access to musical competences which normally develop after the time of onset of overt symptoms of the disorder? Examples of such musical competences are the ability to keep time, upon request, to the beating of a metronome, which develops around 3–4 years of age (Fraisse 1982) and sensitivity to harmonization, that is, melody supported by alternate chord progressions. This develops rather late in normal children, at around 6–7 years of age (Imberty 1969; Zenatti 1969).

Other 'late' aspects of normal childhood musical development which might be explored from this point of view include sensitivity to cadential structure and features of tonality such as the difference between major and minor keys (Imberty 1969), that is, are Rett patients sensitive to an altered cadence in a familiar tune, and are they sensitive to the contrast between major and minor keys (a distinction which actually causes trouble for some normal adults)? Sensitivity to novelty and redundancy might provide further information, that is, how do their reactions to and tolerance of repetition (both within and between pieces) compare to those of normal children? Finally some aspects of musical production should not be overlooked in this regard, despite the severe motoric disturbances of Rett patients. Normal children's production of recognizably musical sequences in the form of ditties, repeated melodic phrases and tunes, by humming, singing or 'vocal play', develops from 2 up to and beyond 5 years of age (Werner 1917; Brehmer 1925; Ostwald 1973; Dowling 1982). It is the ability to keep a stable pitch structure extended in time across a whole tune which takes the longest—some five years or more—to develop (Gardner 1981).

Given these features of normal musical development the question with regard to the Rett disorder becomes the following: which aspects of normally developing musical competence do Rett girls display at different stages after the onset of regression and crucially, do Rett patients possess any aspect of musical competence which normally develops after the time of Rett regression, that is, around 1.5 years of age? We do not at present possess the information needed to answer such questions and before proceeding into ever more hypothetical questions regarding the musical sensibilities of a patient population which so far remains almost unstudied in this respect, it is time to turn to the issue of how the studies needed to address such questions might be carried out, given the severe physical disabilities of Rett patients.

13.7 Nonverbal approaches to the study of musical sensibility in the Rett disorder

In recent decades great advances have been made in our knowledge of infant perceptual and cognitive capacities through the introduction of a number of experimental procedures which utilize orienting movements or other response measures (such as changes in the rhythmicity of sucking movements or heart rate) to circumvent infants' motoric immaturity and lack of language in the assessment of their abilities (Graham amd Clifton 1966; Siqueland and DeLucia 1969; Moore *et al.* 1975; Teller 1979; DeCasper and Sigafoos 1983; Olsho *et al.* 1987; Provasi 1988; see discussions by Fassbender 1996 and Pouthas 1996). Various methods utilizing infants' spontaneous or reinforced orienting movements or autonomic responses to stimulus change or stimulus difference have supplied important information in this regard (see e.g. Melson and McCall 1970 and Trehub *et al.* 1989). An orienting response triggered by a change in a stimulus to which a subject has been habituated by repetition means that the discriminative capacity to detect the change is present, and this in turn means that the subject has the learning capacity to acquire familiarity with specific attributes of the repeating stimulus (Sokolov 1960).

Since they do not require verbal mediation, the methods cited above might seem ideally suited to explore Rett patient responsiveness to music and other stimulus materials. However, great problems are likely to be encountered in this regard because Rett patients are not only language impaired but show severe motoric and autonomic symptoms as well. As already mentioned, their behavioural automatisms, apraxia and ataxia provide multiple sources of interference with testing procedures. Besides the severe physical disability posing general obstacles in this regard, one needs to consider specific factors such as the peculiar tendency of Rett patients to exhibit great and variable response delays in voluntary activities (an aspect of their apraxia, see Chapter 1). Such a tendency is likely to interfere specifically with some applications of nonverbal testing methods based on selective orienting responses. When a Rett patient's overt response to a challenge occurs with a delay of many seconds and even tens of seconds, it becomes difficult to determine the 'reference' of a given orienting movement, movements which normally are assumed to follow the detection of change with short latency (see Sokolov 1960). Response delays in Rett syndrome are a topic of interest in their own right since they imply a disturbance of executive functions in the presence of a relatively intact working memory, but in the context of applying nonverbal testing methods such as preferential looking their role is altogether that of an obstacle.

The same is true of the respiratory and autonomic instability of Rett patients (Chapters 1, 6). This instability has the net effect of interfering with the establishment of proper baseline conditions and with the maintenance of relatively constant state variables as a background for measuring responsiveness. Here recent advances in noninvasive methods of monitoring a number of autonomic variables (Porges 1991; Chapter 6) in combination with routine EEG monitoring may provide a sufficiently rich picture of patient state to allow tests to be applied during epochs of relative stability.

An alternative to testing methods dependent on vulnerable short-latency and 'on-line' responses to stimulus challenge is offered by long-term quantitative assessment of Rett patients' musical preferences and changes in such preferences. This can be done by quantifying listening preferences expressed by Rett patients via deliberate choice among alternate musical selections (see e.g. Koh and Koh 1966; Cotter and Toombs 1966). If such choice is expressed through an apparatus on which Rett patients can select different kinds of music by pressing a 'touch screen' monitor or suitably arranged keys or pads, simple counters or timers attached to each separate pad would provide a longitudinal record of choices through which to assess relative preferences (see Greer and Dorow 1972; Dattilo and Mirenda 1987). Such data would be invaluable aids in addressing the 'musical preference' issues discussed above.

Finally there are indirect routes to gathering information about Rett patients' relationship to music by tapping the knowledge and observations of relatives, therapists, assistants and others in immediate personal contact with the patient. This can be done through interviews, questionnaires, diaries and other records of patient history. At this early stage in the exploration of music as a factor in Rett patients' lives, such indirect methods are essential means of orienting ourselves regarding points at which more demanding and direct studies might fruitfully be applied. In fact, they ought to form the first line of approach for anyone interested in learning more about the important issue of music in the lives of Rett patients. As an aid in gathering such information we present a translation of a questionnaire developed for Swedish Rett Center as a sample in an appendix to this chapter.

Needless to say, should studies along the lines discussed above confirm anecdotal indications of Rett patient responsiveness to and interest in music, this has implications not only for ways of enriching the lives of Rett patients, but potentially for the use of music in therapeutic intervention with these patients as well.

13.8 Conclusions

The symptomatology of Rett patients poses both challenges and obstacles to research on their musical sensibilities. The challenge lies in the possibility that these patients show a greater responsiveness to and interest in music than might be predicted from their linguistic abilities, and that music therefore might provide a 'window' on their cognitive capacities in the absence of language. The obstacles lie in the motoric and autonomic disturbances of these patients, which interfere with the assessment of their musical responsiveness in multiple ways. In this chapter we have tried to discuss how the study of the musical responsiveness of Rett patients nevertheless might provide clues to their capacities and sensibilities, and thus might further our understanding and treatment of these severely impaired patients.

Appendix

Questionnaire for Rett patient parents developed by Märith Bergström-Isacsson, Björn Merker and Ingegerd Witt Engerström for Swedish Rett Center, 1999.

Translated by Björn Merker

1. Is your daughter interested in music? If so, briefly describe the nature of her interest.

2. What kinds of music are available in your daughter's everyday environment?
    (a) music-making or singing in the family
    (b) listening to records/tapes
    (c) radio/television
    (d) does your daughter use a freestyle/headphones?
    (e) other sources of music
    (f) no music
3. What type of music predominates in the sources of music from 2(a)– (e) above to which your daughter is exposed? List the answer, such as pop music, classical music, children's music, after your answers above.
4. Try to estimate the approximate amount of time per day or week which your daughter spends listening to music.
5. Does your daughter receive music therapy, and if so, of what kind?
6. Does your daughter receive other treatments involving music or sound, such as vibroacoustic therapy? If so, what type and how often?
7. Do you remember if you were exposed to song or music or sang yourself in the months before your daughter was born? If so, describe briefly.
8. What kind of music was present in your daughter's environment during infancy and up to the time that she developed noticeable symptoms?
    (a) music-making or singing in the family
    (b) records/tapes
    (c) radio/television
    (d) did you or other family members sing to or with your daughter?
    (e) other sources of music exposure at this time
    (f) no music
9. Does your daughter have any favourite tunes (one or more, which for the sake of simplicity we will refer to as 'favourites' below)?
    If so, please name these with as much additional information as you possess about them, such as whether they are traditional songs, records (and if so which one), etc., to help us identify and analyse these pieces.
10. If she has favourites, does she change preferences, and if so, how often has this happened?
11. If she has favourites, how does she show this?
12. If she has favourites, do you know when she first could have heard them?
13. If she has favourites, do they include any tune she could not have heard until after the time she developed noticeable Rett symptoms? If so, when?
14. Are there any tunes your daughter does not like? If so, describe them, and try to indicate when she first could have heard them.
15. If there are tunes she does not like, how does she show this?
16. Concerning both possible favourites and tunes your daughter might not like, do you know of any special circumstances which might explain her attitude to these tunes? For example, how often was it played or sung, was it associated

with any special situation or person, etc.? If so, briefly describe these circumstanccs.
17. If you use music as 'medicine' for your daughter, what symptoms do you treat?

Acknowledgements

The writing of this chapter was supported by The Institute for Biomusicology and by a research grant from the Bank of Sweden Tercentenary Foundation to Björn Merker.

References

Alvin, J. (1959). The response of severely retarded children to music. *American Journal of Mental Deficiency*, **63**, 988–96.
Brehmer, F. (1925). Melodieauffassung und melodische Begabung des Kindes.
Burch, M.R., Clegg, J.C. and Bailey, J.S. (1987). Automated contingent reinforcement of correct posture. *Research in Developmental Disabilities*, **8**, 15–20.
Burford, B. and Trevarthen, C. (1997). Evoking communication in Rett syndrome: comparisons with conversations and games in mother–infant communication. *European Child and Adolescent Psychiatry*, **6** (**Suppl. 1**), 26–30.
Busnel, M.-C. and Granier-Deferre, C. (1983). And what of fetal audition?. In *The behavior of human infants* (ed. A. Oliveirio and M. Zappella), pp. 126–130. Plenum Press, New York.
Cass, H., Wigram, T., Slonims, V., Weekes, L. and Wisbeach, A. (1993). Therapy issues in Rett syndrome. Paper presented at the Royal Society of Medicine, London.
Cooper, R.P. and Aslin, R.N. (1989). The language environment of the young infant: implications for early perceptual development. *Canadian Journal of Psychology*, **43**, 247–65.
Cotter, V.W. and Toombs, S. (1966). A procedure for determining the music preference of mental retardates. *Journal of Music Therapy*, **3**, 57–64.
Dattilo, J. and Mirenda, P. (1987). An application of a leisure preference assessment protocol for persons with severe handicaps. *Journal of the Association for Persons with Severe Handicaps*, **12**, 306–11.
DeCasper, A.J. and Sigafoos, A.D. (1983). The intra-uterine heartbeat: a potent reinforcer for newborns. *Infant Behavior and Development*, **6**, 19–25.
Dowling, W.J. (1982). Melodic information processing and its development. In *The psychology of music* (1st edn) (ed. D. Deutsch). Academic Press, New York.
Dowling, W.J. (1999). The development of music perception and cognition. In *The psychology of music* (2nd edn) (ed. D. Deutsch). Academic Press, New York.
Fassbender, C. (1996). Infants' auditory sensitivity towards acoustic parameters of speech and music. In *Musical beginnings. origins and development of musical competence* (ed. I. Deliege and J. Sloboda), pp. 56–87. Oxford University Press, Oxford.
Fraisse, P. (1982). Rhythm and tempo. In *The psychology of music* (1st edn) (ed. D. Deutsch), pp. 149–80. Academic Press, New York.
Gardner, H. (1981). The acquisition of song: a developmental approach. *Documentary Report of the Ann Arbor Symposium*, Music Educators National Conference, Reston Virginia.

Graham, F.K. and Clifton, R.K. (1966). Heart rate change as a component of the orienting response. *Psychological Bulletin*, **65**, 305–320.
Greene, R.J., Hoats, D.L. and Hornick, A.J. (1970). Music distortion: a new technique for behavior modification. *Psychological Record*, **20**, 107–9.
Greer, R.D. and Dorow, L.G. (1972). Operant music preference as a dependent measure for music therapists and music educators. Unpublished paper, Teacher's College, Columbia University, New York.
Gutowski, S.J. (1996). Response acquisition for music or beverages in adults with profound mental handicaps. *Journal of Developmental and Physical Disabilities*, **8**, 221–31.
Hadsell, N.A. and Coleman, K.A. (1988). Rett Syndrome: a challenge for music therapists. *Music Therapy Perspectives*, **5**, 52–6.
Hanser, S.B. (1983). Music therapy: a behavioral perspective. *The Behavior Therapist*, **6**, 5–8.
Hill, J., Brantner, J., and Spreat, S. (1989). The effect of contingent music on the in-seat behavior of a blind young woman with profound mental retardation. *Education and Treatment of Children*, **12**, 165–73.
Imberty, M. (1969). *L'acquisition des structures tonale chez l'enfant*. Klincksieck, Paris.
Kerr, A. (1987). The hands and the mind, pre and post-regression in Rett Syndrome. *Brain and Development*, **9**, 487–90.
Koh, S.D. and Koh, T.-H. (1966). Scaling of musical preferences by the mentally retarded. *Science*, **153**, 432–4.
Krumhansl, C.L. (1990). *Cognitive foundations of musical pitch*. Oxford University Press, New York.
Lecanuet, J.-P. (1996). Prenatal auditory experience. In *Musical beginnings. Origins and development of musical competence* (ed. I. Deliege and J. Sloboda), pp. 3–34. Oxford University Press, Oxford.
Lerdahl, F. and Jackendoff, R. (1983). *A generatice grammar of tonal music*. MIT Press, Cambridge, MA.
McClure, J.T., Moss, R.A., McPeters, J.W. and Kirkpatrick, M.A. (1986). Reduction of hand mouthing by a boy with profound mental retardation. *Mental Retardation*, **24**, 219–22.
Melson, W.H. and McCall, R.B. (1970). Attentional responses of five-month old girls to discrepant auditory stimuli. *Child Development*, **41**, 1159–71.
Moore, J.M., Thompson, G., and Thompson, M. (1975). Auditory localization of infants as a function of reinforcement conditions. *Journal of Speech and hearing Disorders*, **40**, 29–34.
Murphy, M.M. (1957). Rhythmical responses of low grade and middle grade mental defectives to music therapy. *Journal of Clinical Psychology*, **13**, 361–4.
Narmour, E. (1990). *The analysis and cognition of basic melodic structures: the implication-realization model*. Chicago University Press, Chicago.
Narmour, E. (1999). Hierarchical expectation and musical style. In *The psychology of music* (2nd edn) (ed. D. Deutsch), pp. 441–72. Academic Press, New York.
Olsho, L.W., Koch, E.G., Halpin, C.F. and Carter, E.A. (1987). An observer-based psychoacoustic procedure for use with young infants. *Developmental Psychology*, **23**, 627–40.
Ostwald, P.F. (1973). Musical behavior in early childhood. *Developmental Medicine and Child Neurology*, **15**, 367–75.
Porges, S.W. (1991). Vagal tone: an autonomic mediator of affect. In *The development of emotion regulation and dysregulation* (ed. J. Garber and K.A. Dodge), pp. 111–28. Cambridge University Press, Cambridge.
Pouthas, V. (1996). The development of the perception of time and temporal regulation of action in infants and children. In *Musical beginnings. Origins and development of musical competence* (ed. I. Deliege and J. Sloboda), pp. 115–41. Oxford University Press, Oxford.
Provasi, J. (1988). Capacités et apprentissages de régulations temporelles chez le nourisson sans l'activité de succion. Unpublished doctoral thesis, Université René Descartes, Paris.

Reardon, D.M. and Bell, G. (1970). Effects of sedative and stimulative music on activity levels of severely retarded boys. *Americal Journal of Mental Deficiency*, **75**, 156–9.

Rosner, B.S. and Meyer, L.B. (1982). Melodic processes and the perception of music. In *The psychology of music* (1st edn) (ed. D. Deutsch). Academic Press, New York.

Salzer, F. (1952). *Structural hearing*, Vol. 1. Charles Boni, New York.

Schenker, H. (1956). *Der freie Satz*. Universal Edition, Vienna.

Sigafoos, J., Laurie, S., and Pennell, D. (1996). Teaching children with Rett syndrome to request preferred objects using aided communication: two preliminary studies. *Augmentative and Alternative Communication*, **12**, 88–96.

Silliman-French, L, French, R., Sherrill, C., and Gench, B. (1998). Auditory feedback and time-on-task of postural alignment of individuals with profound mental retardation. *Adapted Physical Activity Quarterly*, **15**, 51–63.

Siqueland, E.R. and DeLucia, C.A. (1969). Visual reinforcement of non-nutritive sucking in human infants. *Science*, **165**, 1144–6.

Sokolov, E.N. (1960). The neural model of the stimulus and the orienting reflex. *Problems in Psychology*, **4**, 61–72.

Staal, F. (1989). *Rules without meaning. Ritual, mantras and the human sciences*. Peter Lang, New York.

Staples, S.M. (1968). A paired-associate learning task using music as the mediator: an exploratory study. *Journal of Music Therapy*, **5**, 53–57.

Sternlicht, M., Deutsch, M.R., and Siegel, I. (1967). Influence of musical stimulation upon the functioning of institutional retardates. *Psychiatric Quarterly Supplement*, **41**, 323–9.

Takehisa, K. and Takehisa-Silverstri, G. (n.d.). Intermediate results of music therapy in interdisciplinary work with Rett Syndrome in Institut Haus der Barmherzigkeit, Vienna.

Teller, D.Y. (1979). The forced-choice preferential looking procedure: a psychophysical technique for use with human infants. *Infant Behavior and Development*, **2**, 135–53.

Trehub, S.E. (1990). Human infants' perception of auditory patterns. *International Journal of Comparative Psychology*, **4**, 91–110.

Trehub, S.E. (1990). The perception of musical patterns by human infants: the provision of similar patterns by their parents. In *Comparative perception, Vol 1. Basic mechanisms* (ed. M. A. Berkeley and W. C. Stebbins), pp. 429–59. Wiley, New York.

Trehub, S.E., Schneider, B.A., and Endmann, M. (1989). Developmental changes in infants' sensitivity to octave-band noises. *Journal of Experimental Child Psychology*, **29**, 283–93.

Werner, H. (1917). Die melodische Erfindung im frühen Kindalter. Kaiserliche Akademie der Wissenschaften, Vienna, Sitzungsbericht 182.

Wesecky, A. (1986). Music therapy for children with Rett Syndrome. *American Journal of Medical Genetics*, **24**, 253–57.

Wigram, T. (1991). Music therapy for a girl with Rett's Syndrome: balancing structure and freedom. In *Case studies in music therapy* (ed. K. Bruscia), pp. 39–54. Barcelona Publishers, Phoenixville.

Wigram, T. (1997). Vibroacoustic therapy in the treatment of Rett Syndrome. In *Music vibration and health* (ed. T. Wigram and C. Dileo), pp. 149–155. Jeffrey Books, Cherry Hill, NJ.

Wigram, T. and Cass, H. (1995). Music therapy within the assessment process of a therapy clinic for people with Rett syndrome. 1995 BSMT Conference. BSMT Publications, London.

Wylie, M.E. (1996). A case study to promote hand use in children with Rett syndrome. *Music Therapy Perspectives*, **14**, 83–6.

Zanetti, A. (1969). Le developpement génétique de la perception musicale. *Monographies Francaises de Psychologie*, No. 17.

14.1 Behavioural and emotional features of Rett syndrome

Rebecca Mount, Richard Hastings, Tony Charman, Sheena Reilly, and Hilary Cass

14.1.1 Aim of study

To determine which behavioural and emotional features are specific to Rett syndrome.

14.1.2 Background

A number of behavioural and emotional features have been reported in the literature as being associated with Rett syndrome, including hand stereotypies, sleeping difficulties, teeth grinding, screaming and autistic-like behaviours. It is unknown whether these behaviours simply reflect the multiple disabilities found in individuals with severe or profound cognitive impairments with or without Rett syndrome, or constitute a specific profile of behaviours seen only in individuals with Rett syndrome.

14.1.3 Method

Behavioural and emotional problems were assessed in 143 girls with Rett syndrome (age 18 years or younger). They were compared to 84 girls with severe and profound cognitive impairments of mixed aetiologies (age 18 years or younger). Age and level of physical ability were controlled for in the between group analyses. Behavioural and emotional problems were assessed using two parental questionnaires. The Developmental Behaviour Checklist, a well-validated measure of behavioural and emotional disturbance in children with developmental delay (Einfeld and Tonge 1995), was used to assess general behavioural and emotional features. In order to ensure that characteristic Rett behaviours would not go unreported, a checklist of 101 behaviours associated with Rett syndrome was developed called the Rett Syndrome Questionnaire (Mount *et al.* 1998). The 101 items were derived from the existing Rett syndrome literature and clinicians' experience.

14.1.4 Results

The results from the Developmental Behaviour Checklist showed a number of behavioural and emotional features to be significantly more common in girls with Rett syndrome compared to girls with severe and profound cognitive impairments. These features fell into one of two categories: behaviours that are already part of the diagnostic criteria for Rett syndrome (repetitive hand movements and over-breathing) (The Rett Syndrome Diagnostic Criteria Work Group 1988), and behaviours that are currently not included in the diagnostic criteria. The most frequent of these behaviours included repetitive movements such as teeth grinding, facial twitching and mouthing objects, and emotional problems such as laughing for no reason, rapid changes in mood and appearing unhappy.

Analysis of the 101 items from the Rett Syndrome Questionnaire found 46 of the items discriminated between the Rett syndrome and the comparison group of girls with severe and profound cognitive impairments. Factor analyses of the 46 items within the Rett syndrome group suggested an eight factor solution consisting of the following dimensions: general mood, breathing problems, body rocking/lack of facial expression, hand behaviours, night-time behaviours, grimacing, fear/anxiety and walking/standing. These eight groups of behaviour appeared to be common and specific to Rett syndrome and are likely to reflect a specific genetically determined behavioural phenotype of Rett syndrome. The 46-item checklist had good psychometric properties. Test-retest reliability produced intra-class correlations above 0.75 for all sub-scales. Using the Rett syndrome cases, internal consistencies were above 0.6 for all eight sub-scales and 0.9 for the 46 items. Correlations between the Rett Syndrome Questionnaire and the Developmental Behaviour Checklist provide support for concurrent validity. A number of items reported in the literature to be associated with Rett syndrome were found to be not consistently associated with Rett syndrome. These items included self-injury, reduced response to pain, and quality of social contact. These behaviours may therefore reflect disabilities associated with severe and profound cognitive impairments rather than Rett-specific behaviours.

References

Einfeld, S.L., and Tonge, B.J. (1995). The Developmental Behavior Checklist: the development and validation of an instrument to assess behavioral and emotional disturbance in children and adolescents with mental retardation. *Journal of Autism and Developmental Disorders*, 25, 81–104.

Mount, R.H., Hastings, R.P., Reilly, S., and Cass, H. (1998). The Rett Syndrome Questionnaire, Unpublished.

The Rett Syndrome Diagnositic Criteria Work Group (1988). Diagnostic Criteria for Rett Syndrome. *Annals of Neurology*, 23, 425–428.

14.2 Vision in Rett syndrome: studies using evoked potentials and event-related potentials

Daphne L. McCulloch, Ross M. Henderson, Kathryn J. Saunders, and R.M. Walley

Visual interest and apparently good vision is a general feature of women and girls with Rett syndrome. This is remarkable, as severe and profound mental handicap is associated with a very high prevalence of visual impairment particularly from cortical blindness and/or optic nerve atrophy (McCulloch *et al.* 1996). It also appears that vision is useful for cognitive functions, as parents and carers almost invariably report that girls with Rett syndrome respond to familiar faces. Investigations of vision and cognitive visual function may lead in the future to the understanding of the learning processes and to improved communications in Rett syndrome. Behavioural methods for studying vision in Rett syndrome are limited by compliance of the girls and can be difficult to interpret. Ethical and practical considerations make the use of functional MRI, PET and SPECT scanning inappropriate. Encephalographic techniques may have wider applications as visual fixation is generally well maintained and these strategies are relatively tolerant of movement. We have used the visual evoked potential (VEP) to investigate basic functions of the afferent visual system. As basic functions are relatively preserved, another encephalographic technique, the event-related potential (ERP), may be an appropriate tool to investigate basic cognitive visual functions, particularly discrimination and recognition of faces.

14.2.1 The afferent visual pathways

Basic visual function was investigated in 11 girls and young women with Rett syndrome (age range 5–24 years) (Saunders *et al.* 1995). All subjects had a thorough medical and visual history, visual field screening, external and internal ocular examination, refraction and visual evoked potential studies.

We found that all subjects fixated both flash and pattern stimuli for the VEP studies but none produced consistent results for the Acuity Card Test, which requires selective fixation of striped targets (Mohn et al. 1988). None of the subjects were reliable for visual field screening. One subject had a divergent squint, and two had anterior eye disorders (keratoconus and corneal pannus associated with pre-existing ulceration). There were no other serious ocular disorders. Remarkably, none of the optic nerves appeared atrophic. Significant refractive errors were common. Three girls had hyperopia greater than 3 diopters and four others had 3 or more diopters of astigmatism.

In common with some other reports (Verma et al. 1987; Bader et al. 1989; Kalmachey 1990), all of our subjects had reproducible VEPs to flash and pattern, consistent with good function of the central retina and afferent visual pathways. Threshold pattern size, an indicator of visual acuity, ranged from 6 to 24 min of arc (very fine to medium stripes) consistent with visual acuities in the normal to near normal range. Those with higher thresholds tended to be those with the larger refractive errors.

Compared with heterogeneous groups of patients with severe to profound mental handicap, individuals with Rett syndrome appear to have a similar high rate of refractive error but have lower risk of squint and other ocular disorders. However, function of the visual pathway appears to be spared. Correction of refractive error should be considered prior to studies of cognitive visual function as correction provided improved visual attention in some of the individuals in this study.

14.2.2 ERP Studies of Face Discrimination

In normal populations, ERP recordings are characterized by a large positivity (P3) centred over the parietal cortex and associated with infrequently presented stimuli. Recent work has shown that ERPs are often present despite a lack of behavioural response (Nelson and Collins 1991; de Haan and Nelson 1997) and measurable P3s in Rett syndrome have been reported for an auditory paradigm (Bader 1989). Thus, a visual ERP study may be appropriate in Rett syndrome. Rett syndrome is associated with persistent looking at familiar visual stimuli which has been linked to poor cognitive functioning (Von Tetzchner et al. 1996; Fagan 1990). Persistent looking may indicate poor encoding of the stimuli and therefore lack of recognition. An alternative hypothesis is that persistent looking may be linked to difficulties initiating and terminating motor responses (Nelson 1994). The aim of the present study is to assess these underlying neural processes by recording ERPs to two visual paradigms.

Methods: In the first paradigm, face discrimination, a schematic face is presented on 20% of trials and the remainder of trials consist of two different jumbled faces (60% and 20% of trials). The second paradigm is a recognition paradigm where a photograph of a familiar face (mother) is presented with a frequency of 20%. Three other female faces are presented each with a frequency of 20%. The remaining 20% of stimuli are novel faces, female faces seen only once. In both of these ERP paradigms, distinctive ERPs have been shown at 4 years, 8–10 years and in adults with only passive attention.

Eight females with Rett syndrome aged 4–38 years were recruited. An ophthalmologist or optometrist had examined all subjects and five had significant refractive errors. Only one girl wore spectacles, two subjects did not tolerate spectacles and for the other two spectacles had not been recommended. ERPs were recorded while the subjects looked at the stimulus screen and recording was stopped when fixation was lost. In the face discrimination paradigm the stimuli disappeared 500 ms after onset. In the recognition paradigm the stimulus duration was longer (1300 ms). For both paradigms, trials were approximately 2 s apart (random interval of 2200–2350ms).

EEG was recorded from the scalp at 14 sites using tin electrodes secured in an electrode cap. Cooperation and fixation was generally good. Only one subject was uncooperative as she had been agitated prior to testing. Using our standard filtering, an eye movement correction routine (von Driel *et al.* 1989) and rejecting artefacts greater than 300 µV, sufficient artefact-free trials were obtained from three subjects in the discrimination paradigm and four in the recognition paradigm (age range 27–32 years). For all visual stimulation, early peaks are expected at the posterior electrodes. As these were not easily recognized for either paradigm, there is some doubt about the validity of all of the data obtained for the subjects with Rett syndrome.

Face discrimination paradigm: In all three subjects with Rett syndrome the averaged waveforms were too noisy for any definite conclusion.

Face recognition paradigm: Figure 14.2.1 shows the ERP data at the central parietal electrode for four subjects with Rett syndrome and four age matched controls. In addition, grand averaged data for 22 normal adults at the centre of the figure illustrates a distinctive P3, which is recorded to the familiar face only. Reproducible early VEP peaks were present at the occipital midline for all the controls but the parietal ERPs are variable for both groups with only one control subject having a clearly defined P3 to the familiar face. The Rett ERP data have fewer trials in each averaged waveform and higher levels of background noise. Variability among the three repeated faces is a further indication of noisy data. Again, small numbers of subjects and noisy data prevent any conclusions regarding the subjects with Rett syndrome.

Discussion: Most of the subjects with Rett syndrome were cooperative and sufficient data was collected from 50% of them, suggesting that ERP studies are

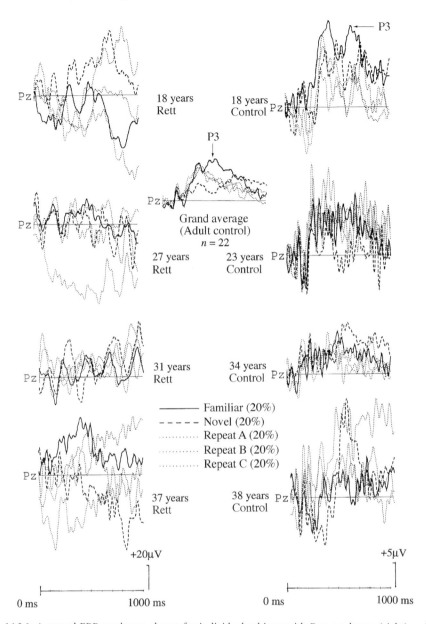

Fig. 14.2.1: Averaged ERP results are shown for individual subjects with Rett syndrome (right) and age matched control subjects (left). The central waveform is the grand average of 22 adult control subjects and clearly demonstrates a P3 for the familiar face only. Earlier peaks are superimposed for the familiar face and three repeated faces. The novel faces (dashed line) produce a negativity (N2) at approximately the same latency as P3. The ERPs for the Rett group have much higher noise levels, although they appear similar as they are displayed with four times less gain (note amplitude scales). ERPs for the Rett group do not demonstrate identifiable components.

feasible in this population. However, the data appears noisy and as the early peaks were not measurable, no conclusions are possible at this point.

14.2.3 Directions of future research

The ERP studies to date have been only partially successful. If the paradigms were modified, modest improvement in the data quality might be achieved. To increase the number of trials recorded, subjects may need to return for a second visit. Also, recent ERP studies have found correlates of familiarity within 1 s in 6-month-old infants (de Hann and Nelson 1997). Therefore, the inter-stimulus interval could be shortened to allow more trials. In addition, greater attention could be given to monitoring fixation, as Jeffreys (1996) has reported that off axis fixation of faces reduces the amplitude of a face-specific ERP peak. Finally, wearing appropriate spectacles or increasing the working distance to reduce accommodative demand may be helpful in improving visibility of the stimuli.

More substantial improvement in ERP studies might be achieved using strategies to improve the signal to noise ratio. We have attempted to reduce noise by subtracting common voltages from local signals (Laplacian derivative, Manahilov *et al.* 1992). For the current data, this did not produce sufficient improvement to allow firm conclusions. Another approach may be to study the frequency spectra of the encephalographic data during visual stimulation. There is some evidence that cortical neurons may fire synchronously within both β and γ bands (20–80 Hz) in response to specific visual tasks (Tallon-Baudry and Bertrand 1999; Shahani *et al.*, in press). This synchronous firing is the basis of the concept of temporal binding, the hypothesis that information about the external world must be temporally bound to specific frequencies for analysis, processing and integration by the nervous system. Studying the frequency spectra in normal controls and in people with Rett syndrome during face recognition may provide insight into these mechanisms of neural processing.

References

Bader, G.G., Engerstöm, I.W., and Hagberg, B. (1989). Neurophysiological findings in Rett syndrome, II: visual and auditory brainstem, middle and late evoked potentials. *Brain Development*, 11, 110–14.

de Haan, M. and Nelson, C.A. (1997). Recognition of mother's, face by six month old infants: a neurobehavioural study. *Child Development*, 68, 187–210.

Fagan, J.F. (1990). The paired-comparison paradigm and infant intelligence. In *Development and neural bases of higher cognitive functions* (ed. A. Diamond), pp. 337–64. New York Academy of Sciences Press, New York.

Jeffreys, D.A. (1996). Evoked potential studies of face and object processing. *Visual Cognition*, 3, 1–18.

Kalmanchey, R. (1990). Evoked potentials in the Rett syndrome. *Brain and Development*, **12**, 73–6.

Manahilov, V., Riemslag, F.C.C. and Spekreijse, H. (1992). The Laplacian analysis of the pattern onset response in man. *Electroencephalography and Clinical Neurophysiology*, **82**, 220–224.

McCulloch, D.L., Sludden, P.A., McKeown, K. and Kerr, A. (1996). Vision care requirements among intellectually disabled adults: a residence based pilot study. *Journal of Intellectual Disability Research*, **40**, 140–50.

Mohn, G., van Hof-van Duin, J., Fetter, W.P.F., de Groot, L., and Hage, M. (1988). Acuity assessment of non-verbal infants and children: clinical experience with the acuity card procedure. *Developmental Medicine and Child Neurology*, **30**, 232–44.

Nelson, C.A. (1994). Neural correlates of recognition memory in the first postnatal year. In *Human behaviour and the developing brain* (ed. G. Dawson and K. Fischer), pp. 269–313, Guildford Press, New York.

Nelson, C.A., Collins, P.F. (1992). Neural and behavioral correlates of visual recognition memory in 4-month old and 8-month-old infants. *Brain and Cognition*, **19**, 105–127.

Saunders, K.J., McCulloch, D.L. and Kerr, A. (1995). Visual function in Rett Syndrome. *Developmental Medicine and Child Neurology*, **37**, 496–504.

Shahani, U., Lang, G., Mansfield, D.C., Halliday, D.M., Weir, A.I., Maas, P., Donaldson, G.B. (in press). Magnetoencephalography and stereopsis: rhythmic cortical activity recorded over the parieto-occipital cortex. *Neuroscience Letters*, submitted.

Tallon-Baudry, C. and Bertrand, O. (1999). Oscillatory gamma activity in humans and its role in object representation. *Trends in Cognitive Sciences*, **3**, 151–61.

Verma, N.P., Nigro, M.A. and Hart, Z.H. (1987). Rett Syndrome—A gray matter disease? Electrophysiological evidence. *Electroencephalography and Clinical Neurophysiology*, **64**, 394–401.

von Driel, G., Woestenberg, J.C. and von Blokland-Vogelesang, A.W. (1989). Frequency domain methods: a solution for the problems of EOG-EEG contamination in ERPs. *Journal of Psychophysiology*, **3**, 29–34.

von Tetzchner, S., Jacobsen, K.H., Smith, L., Skjeldal, O., Heiberg, A., and Fagan, J. (1996). Vision, cognition and developmental characteristics of girls and women with Rett Syndrome. *Developmental Medicine and Child Neurology*, **38**, 212–25.

15 The developmental perspective in the Rett disorder: where next?

Alison M. Kerr and Ingegerd Witt Engerström

Discovery of the gene and growing insight into the pathophysiology of the Rett disorder has answered many important questions. It is now beyond doubt that we are dealing with a prenatal disturbance of growth which profoundly affects cognitive, motor and autonomic functions of the brain and to a lesser extent of the rest of the body, leading to the sequence of events and signs we recognize in the 'Rett syndrome'. Here we consider some implications of these discoveries, what remains to be done, how the new objectives might be achieved and how the knowledge acquired may be directed to produce more effective intervention for people with the disorder and their families.

It is now agreed that mutations on the MECP2 gene (at Xq28) are responsible for the disorder (Amir *et al.* 1999, Wan *et al.* 1999, Cheadle *et al.* 2000). These are mutations with undoubted disease implications, any mutation being currently thought likely to interfere with normal activity of the gene. They have been found in most of the classic cases so far investigated in the UK, and in each new study the number with an identified mutation has increased (Vacca *et al.* 2000). In the rare situations of family recurrence, affected family members show the same mutation. To date the mutation has been unexpressed only in the presence of extreme skewing of inactivation. The early expectations seem likely to be confirmed that although dominant, with high risk for the offspring of a person with disorder the mutation usually occurs '*de novo*' in the germ cells of a normal parent and therefore usually affects only one individual. Such a germ cell mutation could arise in the female or male germ cells.

It is no surprise that there is a wide range in clinical severity in females since the variable pattern of X inactivation will lead to a greater or lesser proportion of the affected X chromosome being active in the various brain tissues. We still know little about the factors which determine patterns of X inactivation although we do know that its timing may differ for the various groups of neurons and that the pattern of X inactivation which is found in the leucocytes and skin, which are readily accessible and therefore commonly tested, may not accurately reflect that in the brain. Mosaicism (possession by one individual of more than one distinct inherited cell lineage) may help to account for survival in an XY male. More difficult to explain is the presence of male as well as female forebears (presumably asymptomatic carriers) in the lineage of people with Rett deriving from small Swedish localities (discussed in Chapters 2 and 5.1).

It is noteworthy that many different mutations are still being found on the gene. This gene is recognized as potentially unstable with an unusually long '3'-prime untranslated region' (this is a long tail after the coding region which is partly conserved and in which some portions are thought to be regulatory). The factors which lead to such instability are only just beginning to be understood. At present we cannot explain why mutations in the gene should affect a particular individual or family however there are clinical clues which should be pursued. The data from Akesson and others suggests that there is an increased probability of recurrence in certain kindreds (Akesson et al. 1992). Several studies have shown a disturbance in pterin metabolism not only in girls with Rett syndrome but also in other family members (Chapters 5.4 and 8). The short fourth digit which occurs in an increased proportion of adults with Rett syndrome has been recorded in other members of their families also (Kerr et al. 1995; Glasson et al. 1998; Leonard et al. 1999). In the British Survey a proportion of families indicate that the girl with Rett disorder may have first or second degree relatives with other neurological disorders. The possibility that a subclinical disturbance might predispose to a Rett mutation should be considered.

The MECP2 gene in its active (transcribed) form MeCP2 is believed to suppress, through the process of methylation, the transcription of a large number of other genes within the nuclei of cells throughout the body, thus terminating their activity at the appropriate times (Nan et al. 1997). In this way the performance of many genes is coordinated. In the presence of an MECP2 mutation, failure to curtail transcription of the secondary genes will be expected to dysregulate their expression and it will be important to identify them and to assess their activities since such interference must be presumed to contribute to the specific profile of disability seen in Rett syndrome. Insight into the consequences of this dysregulation in the Rett disorder will throw new light on problems encountered in other early developmental disorders.

Failure to terminate the transcription of these 'secondary genes' might also be expected to hinder the transcription and performance of genes which should begin production subsequently. On the other hand it seems worth considering that the girl with classic Rett syndrome may make her initial progress during the pre-regression phase of the disease because the mutated MECP2 gene permits early development before the failure to suppress transcription takes full effect.

In addition to loss of function directly related to the genetic failure, the burden of over-produced gene product ('transcriptional noise') may interfere with other cellular activities or exhaust the capacity to recycle the unwanted proteins leading to an energy crisis (Chapter 2). While this might be tolerated by quiescent cells it might be expected to affect most severely those tissues which are most active. It seems likely that the rapid growth and complex functions of the developing brain between 6 and 18 months, when regression usually strikes, might render it particularly sensitive to insult. Such selective vulnerability might be expected also in the respiratory neurons, among the most active in the brain and additionally stressed by the characteristic Rett agitation. Vulnerability to stress might explain anecdotal reports that a severe attack of respiratory or gastrointestinal infection sometimes precedes regression and that in later years an apparently trivial incidental illness may be followed by a 'mini-regression'. Such embarrassment of intracellular function might be expected to remit when the acute stress is relieved, with recovery of function, as is indeed seen after the classical Rett regression unless the individual is very weak or the stress very severe, when sudden death might result. Sudden death and 'near miss' sudden death in Rett syndrome might be investigated for evidence of such exhaustion of the respiratory neurones.

Boys with Rett-like features have been described (Christen and Hanefeld 1995) and also boys with a 'protective' second X of Klinefelter's syndrome (XXY) (Schwartzmann *et al.* 1999). It is now certain that there are (XY) boys with mutations on MECP2 and a Rett-like picture although not the 'classic' syndrome (Schanen and Franke 1998; Meloni *et al.* 2000; Leonard *et al.* 2000). Judging from animal work with mice in which the MECP2 gene has been deleted, such pregnancies with a male embryo are likely to end early in intrauterine life (Tate *et al.* 1996). However some boys may be born with comparable problems to the girls, perhaps more severe, and we still have to learn how to recognize and help such boys and their families. Mosaic inheritance where some cells have a normal X would be expected to facilitate survival.

Rett disorder and the ICF syndrome (immunodeficiency, centromere instability and facial anomalies) are the first two human diseases found to be due to mutations in genes encoding proteins involved in DNA methylation and as such they represent a major advance in understanding the role of methylation in the genome (Hendrich 2000). Their importance will encourage elucidation of the Rett problem and hasten improvements in care.

The anatomical, neuro-physiological and neuro-chemical studies suggest immaturity with lack of brainstem, subcortical and cortical integration and possible deficiency of growth factors (Armstrong 1992; 1995; Chapters 3 and 10.5). The increased receptor densities suggest immaturity or relative unavailability of the major neurotransmitters, monoamines, glutamate and acetylcholine (Chapters 4, 3 and 5.2; Wenk and Hauss-Wegrzyniak 1999; Hohmann and Berger-Sweeney 1998). The early high levels of glutamate receptors, declining later, seem to reflect the early childhood agitation and epilepsy and later seizure remission with a calmer adulthood.

The involvement of MAP2 protein (Chapter 4) with its role in the base plate through which embryonic neurons reach their cortical destinations indicates not only how early the Rett problem is present but also that the essential sensory-motor relationship may be fundamentally disturbed which depends on early interactions between the subplate neurons and thalamic axons (Ghosh 1995).

The disturbances of acetylcholine and glutamate neurotransmission seem likely to contribute to the profound disturbances of cognition, the state of agitation and the lowered threshold for epileptic seizure. Disturbance of the brainstem monoaminergic system and particularly of serotonin (5-HT) helps to explain many of the clinical problems (Chapters 3, 6–8). First of the neurotransmitters to enter the brain, the influence of serotonin is early and widespread but highly selective—an integrative and facilitatory role. Axonal connections are prepared in advance of contact with target neurons but actual contact occurs only during the period of synaptic refinement, just when the Rett regression is seen (Fitzgerald 1991; Dinopoulos 1997). The chief serotoninergic contacts are within the areas most obviously affected by the Rett disorder, frontal, parietal and temporal cortex, the basal ganglia and the dorsal columns of the spinal cord (Fitzgerald 1991, Chapter 3). A better understanding of how all these abnormalities are related will open new possibilities for intervention and the new generation of non-invasive imaging should help the investigation.

While there is deficient growth of the whole brain in Rett there does appear to be a predilection for phylogenetically ancient brain core structures which profoundly influence early development, effectively setting the frame for later sophisticated functions such as speech and fine motor control and providing the integration upon which the mature nervous system depends. In seeking the origins of the disorder suspicion now rests firmly on these directors of early growth.

It is known that the growth, development and maintenance of neurons is highly dependent on normal function and for their continued survival many neurons require growth factors derived from their target (Price *et al.* 1995). It will be no easy task to discover the origin and sequence of the biochemical cascade found in the Rett disorder, however it is only such careful investigation which can lead to really effective intervention. What is found for the Rett situation will prove of value in dealing with other developmental disorders.

Inevitably, so far, the detection of cases has been restricted to people with the readily recognized Rett syndrome and their relatives. We know already that the disorder may be much less severe, although still carrying a high risk of transmission, and it will be important to establish the true prevalence through mutation testing combined with clinical assessment. The final prevalence is likely to be higher than the present UK minimum estimate of 1 in 10,000 females at 14 years (Kerr 1992; Asthana *et al.* 1990).

There are many aspects of the clinical syndrome which must be better understood if we are to offer appropriate help. Investigation of these will also shed light on other disorders which affect the developing brain since similar disease mechanisms are likely to be involved and some of the same therapeutic approaches will apply. The differences between these conditions are likely to prove as instructive as the similarities. Each of the variants carefully described by Hagberg (1995) requires explanation, for which skewed X inactivation can be only one part. Parallels with early autism have been noted (interrupted contact, stereotypy and toe walking) Gillberg 1987. There are features in common with Angelman syndrome (disproportionate involvement of speech and motor coordination) and the early stages of infantile lipofuscinosis (infant regression with hand stereotypy) (Hagberg and Witt Engerström 1990). Respiratory dysrhythmia, regularly seen in Rett syndrome, may also occur in tuberose sclerosis, embryonic tumour and malformation of the brainstem such as Joubert's syndrome (Bolthauser et al. 1987). Cases are known to the British Survey in which there are signs of Rett syndrome with fragile X, Klinefelter's, Down's and mosaic Turner's syndromes. These situations offer valuable insight on normal and deviant regulation of brain development.

Therapeutic intervention in Rett disorder is likely to be most effective very early, but we are not good at detecting the first signs. Because of the normal appearance of the child and her early progress, most cases are missed until many months have passed and the diagnosis is usually reached only after severe disabilities have emerged. Diagnosis under 2 years is unusual. Although measurements of head circumference may show deviation as early as 2 months in some cases (Percy 1992). In the UK many children currently do not have accurate early records of head circumference. This simple but important procedure is an important part of the routine screening of normal babies.

In many cases, early family accounts and videos indicate suspect posture and movement with subtle deviation from expected developmental progress in the early weeks of life in Rett syndrome (Witt Engerström 1987; 1992; Kerr et al. 1987, 1995; Naidu 1997; Leonard and Bower 1998). The studies by Prechtl and colleagues of the spontaneous movements of infants before birth and in the early weeks of life have shown that disturbance of these 'general movements', assessed from video recordings, reliably predicts later motor and possibly cognitive problems (Hadders-Algra 1993; Prechtl 1997; Einspieler et al. 1997). This is relevant to the baby with Rett disorder. Training for health professionals working with babies might include exposure to videos of babies with Rett disorder. Once there is clinical suspicion, genetic testing will be possible and this could be combined with tests for other causes of early developmental delay. Development of a genetic test, equivalent to the Guthrie test, for genetic screening in developmental delay or failure to thrive may become possible in the future.

Too little is known about the regression phenomenon, and although contributory factors have been suggested these have hardly begun to be explored (Table

15.1; Kerr 1995). The clinical impression at the regression stage is of a profoundly stressed child and it seems possible that extreme metabolic demands at this time cause avoidable distress and perhaps even fresh and preventable injury to the developing nervous system. Transiently raised neopterin, lactate, pyruvate and lowered blood glucose have all been recorded in Rett (Chapters 5.4 and 2) but many studies have pooled results across the age range and the need is now to concentrate on specific age bands, including the early regression period. The misconception that the Rett disorder is progressive has impeded progress in diagnosis and research. This arose because physicians have found it difficult to believe that such acute loss of skills could have a developmental basis. The Rett disorder is not alone in producing a period of early infancy regression. This is well known in epileptic syndromes and in autism and we have observed it in Angelman syndrome. The phenomenon of non-dementing regression deserves further study and offers insight into the stages of normal and deviant infant development.

Table 15.1 Suggested factors contributing to the Rett regression (Kerr 1995)

- The child has reached her developmental ceiling
- Programmed cell death prunes early infancy networks
- Myelination reveals the extent of the cortical incompetence
- Cellular immune processes may attack abnormal neurones
- The incompetent cortex fails to control mature subcortical rhythms
- Subcortical movement rhythms interfere with the use of skills
- Seizures and non-epileptic vacant spells interfere with contact
- Non seizure e.e.g. disturbance may interrupt neural pathways
- Dyspraxic breathing leads to hypocarbia, hypoxia, abdominal distension and feeding difficulty
- Agitation exacerbates repetitive movements and distress
- Parental frustration, anxiety or rejection is felt by the child

Reprinted from *Neuropediatrics* 26 (1995) 67–71 with permission from the editor and Hippocrates Verlag, Stuttgart.

We suspect that the autonomic incompetence seen in Rett and associated with low vagal tone and poor sympathetic–parasympathetic balance is one aspect of the brain stem immaturity and that it is responsible for some sudden deaths in the Rett disorder (Chapter 6; Julu *et al.* 1997, 1998; Sekul *et al.* 1994; Chapter 10.1). Such unexpected deaths may represent extreme instances of the very common non-epileptic 'vacant spells' of Rett syndrome and more research is urgently required on their causes and management (Chapter 6; Witt Engerström and Kerr 1998; Cooper *et al.* 1998; Chapters 10.5 and 10.1).

There is increasing recognition among physicians that autonomic incompetence is one of several causes of non-epileptic interruption of consciousness ('pseudo-seizure'). As in Rett the electroencephalogram (e.e.g.) may be abnormal whether epilepsy is present or not, increasing the difficulty of reaching a diagnosis. Careful assessment using extended video, respiratory and e.e.g. monitoring will be required in complex cases in order to provide accurate diagnosis and adequate counselling. The equipment developed by Julu and colleagues will be of value in this (Chapter 6; Julu *et al.* submitted). Correct diagnosis makes economic sense since ill-directed anticonvulsant medication is expensive and increases dependence.

Agitation is a hallmark of the Rett syndrome. The flushed face, widely dilated pupils and excited aspect are part of the charm of the child but also a sign of her disease (Chapter 6; Kerr 2000). Recent research offers some clues to its origins. The affected individual has a poorly integrated brain which is smaller than normal, perhaps insufficiently connected to disperse the impact of stimulation and to modulate response. The increased glutamate receptors reported in young girls suggest increased demand for or turnover of excitatory neurotransmitter and the low vagal tone indicates poor inhibitory regulation. The agitation, rather than an expression of volition, seems to be the product of physiological imbalance. It would appear that in Rett disorder the roots of motivation are effectively disengaged from normal control and themselves determine the mind of the child— 'the tail is wagging the dog'.

That the brainstem is an important player in the problems of mood, respiratory rhythm and intellectual disability in the Rett disorder suggests that closer scrutiny of its role in mental illness will be of value (Kerr and Julu 1999).

Oro-pharyngeal dysfunction, reflux, gaseous distension and constipation are regular problems in Rett syndrome with poor autonomic regulation a chief suspect (Chapters 9, 10.3, and 10.1). They are common also in other severe disabilities including cerebral palsy due to pre- or intra-natal injury and other early developmental disorders in which autonomic status has hardly been explored. A better understanding of the role of autonomic function in all these conditions may open new possibilities in care.

How will the host of new questions be answered? Accurate recording of the clinical problems and course of the disorder remain fundamental to this as to all medical research, and the clinical data must now be matched to the results of continuing genetic research. Neuro-pathological studies have been and will remain of critical importance, possible only when families donate tissues after the death of a person with Rett syndrome.

Animal studies will be essential since only identical animals with a rapid generation time can be thoroughly investigated for the normal role of MECP2 and secondary genes in the brain, the effects of deletion of the gene and the efficacy and risks of intervention. Such studies will help to establish when and how the various neurotransmitters become involved and will indicate potential therapies. Genetic discoveries have direct relevance for patients, and as the full range of mutations on MECP2 becomes known and their consequences understood a genetic test can be developed for the Rett disorder, more comprehensive counselling will be available for families and there will be new possibilities to restore function and support potential for development in the child.

As candidate agents for pharmacological treatment become available, evidence will be required from double blind controlled clinical trials before recommendations can be made for routine use. One of the main obstacles to such trials has been the lack of objective measures. Treatment initiated during regression is apt to be credited with the spontaneous improvement which is usual after this period, and a mistaken expectation of steady degeneration may lead to ill-judged claims of success in treatment when epilepsy remits or new skills appear. Suitable measures may include the increasingly specific and non-invasive brain scanning techniques (Uvebrant et al. 1993) and the monitoring methods described by Julu in Chapter 6. For each medication on trial there must be clear objectives in treatment and measures of success. Comparison must be made between well-matched cases over suitable periods. This calls for collaboration between research centres, the support of families and significant funding.

With its many facets the Rett disorder presents a remarkable opportunity to gain new insights into normal and deviant brain development. Recent advances have led us to the threshold of a revolution in the practice of medicine more profound than the introduction of antibiotics, and for this new age models are required which make accessible to enquiry the intricate patterns of normal brain development and the consequences for later growth of very early defects. The Rett disorder presents us with just such a paradigm.

Acknowledgements

The success of the research into the Rett disorder has been founded on the early commitment of a relatively small number of people among whom we would especially mention Professor Andreas Rett who made the pursuit of understanding and cure for this disorder his life's work, Bengt Hagberg, Hugo Moser and Alan Percy whose enthusiasm has sustained the effort, and Mrs Kathy Hunter whose vigorous and intelligent support of families and of research has encouraged countless people from many disciplines to harness their efforts to this end. Kathy Hunter's phrase 'care today, cure tomorrow' sums up well the spirit which has led the enquiry. We wish to thank the many families, Rett Associations and professional colleagues who have contributed to the Rett studies.

Advice on this chapter is gratefully acknowledged from Brian Hendrich and Angus Clarke. AK receives financial support from the University of Glasgow, the

UK and National Rett Associations and the ESRC. IWE receives funding support from Östersund Hospital Foundation for Medical research and Marcus and Amalia Wallenberg Memorial Fund.

References

Akesson, H.O., Hagberg, B., Wahlstrom, J., and Witt Engerström, I. (1992). Rett Syndrome a search for gene sources. *American Journal of Medical Genetics*, **42**, 104–10.

Amir, R.E., Van Den Veyver, I.B., Wan, M., Tran, C.Q., Franke, U., and Zoghbi, H. (1999). Rett Syndrome is caused by mutations in X-linked MECP2, encoding methyl CpG binding protein 2. *Nature Genetics*, **23**, 185–8.

Armstrong, D.D. (1992). The neuropathology of the Rett syndrome. *Brain and Development*, **14**, 89–98.

Armstrong, D.D. (1995). The neuropathology of Rett Syndrome—overview 1994. *Neuropediatrics*, **26**, 100–4.

Asthana, J.C., Sinha, S., Haslam, J.S., and Kingston, H.M. (1990). Survey of adolescents with severe intellectual handicap. *Archives of Disease in Childhood*, **65**, 1133–36.

Bolthauser, E., Lange, B., and Dumermuth, G. (1987) Differential diagnosis of syndromes with abnormal respiration (tachypnea-apnea). *Brain and Development*, **9**, 462–5.

Cheadle, J.P., Gill, H., Fleming, N., Maynard, J., Kerr, A.M., Leonard, H., Krawczak, M., Cooper, D.N., Lynch, S., Thomas, N., Hughes, H., Hulten, M., Sampson, J.R., and Clarke, A. (2000). Long-read sequence analysis of the MECP2 gene in Rett syndrome patients: correlation of disease severity with mutation type and location. *Molecular Genetics*, 9, 7, 1119–29.

Christen, H.-J. and Hanefeld, F. (1995). Male Rett Variant. *Neuropediatrics*, **26**, 81–82.

Cooper, R.A., Kerr, A.M., and Amos, P.M. (1998). Rett syndrome: critical examination of clinical features, serial e.e.g. and video-monitoring in understanding and management. *European Journal of Paediatric Neurology*, **2**, 127–35.

Dinopoulos, A., Dori, I., and Parnavelas, J.G. (1997). The serotonin innervation of the basal forebrain shows a transient phase during development. *Developmental brain Research*, **99**, 38–52.

Einspieler, C., Prechtl, H.F.R., Ferrari, F., Cioni, G., and Bos, A.F. (1997). The qualitative assessment of general movements in preterm, term and young infants—review of the methodology. *Early Human Development,* **50**, 47–60.

Fitzgerald, M. (1991). The development of descending brain stem control of spinal cord sensory processing. In *The fetal and neonatal brain stem* (ed. M.A. Birke), pp. 127–36. Cambridge University Press, Cambridge. ISBN 0 521 38357 9.

Fiumara, A., Sciotto, A., Barone, R., D'Asero, G., Munda, S., Parano, E., and Pavone, L. (1999). Peripheral lymphocyte subsets and other immune aspects in Rett syndrome. *Pediatric Neurology*, **21**, (3), 619–721.

Ghosh, A. (1995). Subplate neurones and the patterning of thalamocortical connections. In *Development of the cerebral cortex* (ed. G.R. Bock and G. Cardew), pp. 150–72. Wiley, New York. ISBN 0 471 95705 4.

Gillberg, C. (1987). Autistic symptoms in Rett Syndrome: the first two years according to mother reports. *Brain and Development*, **9**, 499–501.

Glasson, E.J., Thomson, M.R., Leonard, S., Rousham, E., Christodoulou, J., Ellaway, C., and Leonard, H. (1998). Diagnosis of Rett Syndrome: can a radiograph help?. *Developmental Medicine and Child Neurology*, **40**, 737–742.

Hadders-Algra, M. (1993). General Movements in early infancy: what do they tell us about the nervous system? *Early Human Development*, **34**, 29–37.

Hagberg, B. (1995). Clinical delineation of the Rett Syndrome Variants. *Neuropediatrics*, **26**, 62.

Hagberg, B. and Witt Engerström, I. (1990). Early stages Rett syndrome and infantile neuronal ceroid lipofuscinosis—a difficult differential diagnosis. *Brain and Development*, **12**, 20–2.

Hendrich, B. (2000). Human genetics: methylation moves into medicine. *Current Biology*, in press.

Hohmann, C.F. and Berger-Sweeney, J. (1998). Cholinergic regulation of cortical development and plasticity. *Perspectives on Developmental Neurobiology*, **5**, 401–25.

Julu, P.O.O., Kerr, A.M., Hansen, S., Apartopoulos, S.F. and Jamal, G.A. (1997). Functional evidence of brain stem immaturity in Rett Syndrome. *European Child and Adolescent Psychiatry*, **6**, 47–54.

Julu, P.O.O., Kerr, A.M., Hansen, S., Apartopoulos, F., and Jamal, G. (1998). Cardio-respiratory instability in Rett Syndrome suggests medullary serotononergic dysfunction. In: Witt Engerström I., Kerr, A.M. meeting report. Workshop on Autonomic Function in Rett Syndrome. Swedish Rett Centre, Froson, Sweden, May 1998. *Brain and Development*, **20**, 323–6.

Julu, P.O.O., Kerr, A.M., Hansen, S., Apartopoulos, F., Witt Engerström, I., and Engerstrom, L. Characterisation of the breathing and autonomic abnormality in Rett Syndrome, in preparation.

Kerr, A.M. (1992). Rett Syndrome British longitudinal study (1982–1990) and 1990 survey. (ed. J.J. Roosendaal), pp. 143–5. *Mental Retardation and Medical Care*, 21–24 April 1991. Uitgeverij Kerckbosch. Zeist ISBN 9067201219.

Kerr, A.M. (1995). Early clinical signs in the Rett disorder. *Neuropediatrics*, **26**, 67–71.

Kerr, A.M. (2000). Behaviour in the Rett disorder. In *Developmental disability and behaviour* (ed. C. Gillberg and G. O'Brien). McKeith Press, Lavenham. ISBN 1 898683 18 2.

Kerr, A.M. and Julu, P.O.O. (1999). Recent insights into hyperventilation from the study of Rett Syndrome. *Archives of Disease in Childhood*, **80**, 384–387.

Kerr, A.M., Armstrong, D.D., Prescott, R.J., Doyle, D., and Kearney, D.L. (1997). Analysis of deaths in the British Rett Survey. *European Child and Adolescent Psychiatry*, **6**, 71–4.

Kerr, A.M., Mitchell, J.M., and Robertson, P. (1995). Short fourth toes in Rett Syndrome: a biological indicator. *Neuropediatrics*, **26**, 72–4.

Kerr, A.M., Montague, J., and Stephenson, J.B.P. (1987). The hands, and the mind, pre- and post-regression in Rett syndrome. *Brain and Development*, **9**, 487–490.

Leonard, H. and Bower, C. (1998). Is the girl with Rett Syndrome normal at birth? *Developmental Medicine and Child Neurology*, **40**, 115–21.

Leonard, H., Thomson, M.M., Lasson, E., Fyfe, S., Leonard, S., Ellaway, C., Christodoulou, J. and Bower, C. (1999). Metacarpophaloangeal pattern profile and bone age in Rett Syndrome: further radiological clues to the diagnosis. *American Journal of Medical Genetics*, **83**, 88–95.

Leonard, H., Silberstein, J., Falck, R., Howink-Monville, J., Ellaway, C., Raffaele, L.S., Witt Engerström, I. and Schanen, C. (accepted 2000). Rett syndrome in males. *Journal of Child Neurology*.

Meloni, I., Bruttini, M., Longo, I., Mari, F., Rizzolio, F., D'Adamo, P., Denvriendt, K., Fryns, J-P., Toniolo, D. and Renieri, A. (2000). A mutation in the Rett Syndrome gene, MECP2, causes X-linked Mental retardation and progressive spasticity in males. *American Journal of Human Genetics*, **67**, 982–5.

Naidu, S. (1997). Rett Syndrome: a disorder affecting early brain growth. *Annals of Neurology*, **42**, 3–10.

Nan, X., Campoy, F.J., and Bird, A. (1997) MeCP2 is a transcriptional repressor with abundant binding sites in genomic chromatin. *Cell*, **88**(4), 471–81.

Percy, A.K. (1992). Neurochemistry of the Rett Syndrome. *Brain and Development*, **14**, S57–62.

Philippart, M. (1990). The Rett syndrome in males. *Brain and Development*, **12**, 33–36.

Prechtl, H.F.R. (1997). State of the art of a new functional assessment of the young nervous system. An early predictor of cerebral palsy. *Early Human Development*, **50**, 1–11.

Price, D.J., Beau Lotto, R., Warren, N., Magowan, G., and Clausen, J. (1995). The roles of growth factors and neural activity in the development of the neocortex. In *Development of the cerebral cortex* (ed. G.R. Bock and G. Cardew), pp. 231–50. Wiley, New York. ISBN 0 471 95705 4.

Regional cerebral blood flow: SPECT as a tool for localisation of brain dysfunction. In *Rett syndrome—clinical and biological aspects* (ed. B. Hagberg), pp. 80–5. Clinics in Developmental Medicine, Vol. 127. MacKeith, London.

Schanen, C. and Franke, U. (1998). A severely affected male born into a Rett Syndrome kindred supports X-linked inheritance and allows extension of the exclusion map. *American Journal of Human Genetics*, **63**, 267–69.

Schwartzman, J.S., Zatz, M., Vasquez, L.D.R., Gomez, R.R., Koiffmann, C.P., Fridman, C. and Otto, P.G. (1999). Rett Syndrome in A boy with 47,XXY karyotype. *American Journal of Human Genetics*, **64**, 1781–5.

Sekul, E.A., Moak, J.P., Schultz, R.J., Glaze, D.G., Dunn, J.K., and Percy, A.K. (1994). Electrocardiographic findings in Rett Syndrome: an explanation of sudden death. *Journal of Pediatrics*, **125**, 80–2.

Tate, P., Skarnes, W., and Bird, A. (1996). The methyl-CpG binding protein MeCP2 is essential for embryonic development in the mouse. *Nature Genetics*, **12**, (2), 205–8.

Uvebrant, P., Bjure, J., Sixt, R., Witt Engerström, I., and Hagberg, B. (1993).

Vacca, M., Filippini, F., Budillon, A., Rossi, V., Mercadante, G., Manzati, E., Gualandi, F., Bigoni, S., Trabbanelli, C., Pini, G., Calzolari, E., Ferlinin, A., Meloni, I., Hayek, G., Zappella, M., Renieri, A., D'Urso, M., D'Esposito, M., MacDonald, F., Kerr, A.M., Dhanjal, S. and Hulten, M. (accepted 2000). Mutation analysis of the MECP2 gene in British and Italian Rett sysdrome families. *Journal of Molecular Medicine*.

Wan, M., Lee, S.S.J.L., Zhang, X., Houwink-Manville, I., Song., H.-R., Amir, R.E., Budden, S., Naidu, S., Pereira, J.L.P., Lo, I.F.M., Zoghbi, H.Y., Schanen, N.C., and Francke, U. (1999). Rett Syndrome and beyond: recurrent spontaneous and familial MECP2 mutations at CpG hotspots. *American Journal of Human Genetics*, **65**, 1520–9.

Wenk, G.L. and Hauss-Wegrzyniak, B. (1999). Altered cholinergic function in the basal forebrain of girls with Rett syndrome. *Neuropediatrics*, **30**, (3), 125–9.

Witt Engerström, I. (1987). Rett Syndrome: a retrospective pilot study of potential early predictive symptomatology. *Brain and Development*, **9**, 481–6.

Witt Engerström, I. (1992). Rett Syndrome: the late infantile regression period — a retrospective analysis of 91 cases. *Acta Paediatrica Scandinavica*, **81**, 167–72.

Witt Engerström, I. and Kerr, A.M. (1998). Workshop on Autonomic Function in Rett Syndrome. Swedish Rett Centre, Froson, Sweden, May 1998. *Brain and Development*, **5**, 323–6.

Abbreviations and Glossary

% sREM	percentage of stage REM sleep
% SWS	percentage of stage SWS
3H-LSD	3H-lysergic acid diethylamide 3-methoxy-4-hydroxyphenylethylene glycol
5-HIAA	5-hydroxyindolacetic acid
5-HT	5-hydroxytryptamine, serotonin
5-HT 1A receptors	serotonin 1A receptor
5-HTP	5-hydroxytryptophan
6-OH-DA	a selective catecholamine neurotoxin
ACh	acetylcholine
AChE	acetylcholine esterase
AChRs	acetylcholine receptors
AMPA	adenosine monophosphate acid
AMPA	alpha-amino-3-hydroxy-5-methyl-4-isoxazole propionic acid
ANS	autonomic nervous system
AR-EPDF	autosomal recessive early onset parkinsonism with diurnal fluctuation
AVP	arginine vasopressin
BDNF	brain-derived nerve growth factor
BH4, BA4	tetrahydrobiopterin
BMPs	bone morphogenetic proteins
BNM	nucleus basalis of Meynert
CA	catecholamine, catecholaminergic
CAM	cell adhesion molecule
CC	corpus callosum
c-fos	cellular-feline osteosarcoma virus
CGRP	calcitonin gene related peptide
ChAT	choline acetyltransferase
Cho	choline
CIT	coordinated interpersonal timing
CMCT	central motor conduction time

CNS	central nervous system
CNTF	ciliary neurotrophic factor
CO2	carbon dioxide
COX	cyclooxygenase
CpG	a dinucleotide of 5methylcytosine followed by guanosine
CREB	cyclic adenosine monophosphate response element binding
CSB	cardiac sensitivity to baroreflex
CSF	cerebrospinal fluid
CT	computed tomography
cVRG	caudal ventral respiratory group of neurons
CVT	cardiac vagal tone
Cx	cortex
Cx I, VI	cerebral cortex layer I and VI
Cx IV	cerebral cortex layer IV
DA	dopamine
DA D2	dopamine D2 receptor
Dab1	disabled 1 (gene)
DBH	dopamine beta hydroxylase
DBH-IR	dopamine-ß-hydroxylase immunoreactivity
DCX	doublecortin double cortex syndrome/lissencephaly gene
dJP	dystonic type of juvenile parkinsonism
DMD	duchenne muscular dystropy
DOPA	3,4-dihydroxyphenylacetic
DOPAC	3,4-dihydroxyphenylacetic acid
DQ	developmental quotient
DRG	dorsal respiratory group of neurones
DS	Down's syndrome
DSPS	delayed sleep stage syndrome
EAA	excitatory amino acids
ECG	electrocardiogram
EEG, e.e.g.	electroencephalogram
EGF-family	epidermal growth factors and transforming growth factor-alpha
EGFs	epidermal growth factors
EIA	early infantile autism
EM	electron microscopy
ENK	enkephalin
ENS	enteric nervous system
ERP	event related potential
FGF 1-9	fibroblast growth factor family
FGF	fibroblast growth factor fluctuation

FMR1	Fragile X mental retardation 1
fMRI	functional magnetic resonance imaging
FMS	friendliness-muricide-self-mutilation
fPET	functional positron emission tomography
GABA	Gamma-amino-butyric acid
GABAb	gamma aminobutyric acid b
GAD	glutamic acid decarboxylase
GAP	growth-associated protein
GAP-43	growth associated protein-43
GCH-I	GTP-cyclohydrolase I
GDNF	glia derived neurotrophic factor
Genotype	the genetic constitution of an individual
GER	Gastro-esophageal reflux
GFAP	glial fibrillary acidic protein
GI canal	gastrointestinal canal
GI tract	gastrointestinal tract
GLUD2	glutamate dehydrogenase 2
GluRs	glutamate receptors
GM	grey matter
GMs	gross movements
GRIP	glutamate receptor interacting protein
GTP	cyclohydrolase I (GCH-I) deficiency
HF	high frequency
HPD	hereditary progressive dystonia with marked diurnal fluctuation
HRV	heart rate variability
HVA	homovanillic acid
IC	insular cortex
ICE	interleukin-1-beta-converting enzyme
IEGs	immediate-early genes
IGF I and II	peptides in the insulin family
IGF	insulin-like growth factor
IL 1-15	Interleukins
IL-1	interleukin-1
IMF	intrinsic motive formation
IP	Incontinentia pigmenti
IQ	intelligence quotient
IR	immunoreactivity
LC	locus coeruleus
LIS1	lissencephaly 1
LSD	lysergic acid diethylamide
l-threo-DOPS	l-threo 3,4-dihydroxyphenylserine

LVS	linear vagal scale
MA	monoamine, monoaminergic
MAO	monoamineoxidase
MAP	microtubule-associated protein
MAP-2	microtubule-associated protein 2
MASH	mammalian achaete-scute homologous
MECP2	gene for methyl-CpG-binding protein 2 (also *MECP2*)
MeCP2	methyl-CpG-binding protein 2
MEP	motor evoked potentials
MHPG	3-methoxy-4-hydroxyphenylethylene glycol
MLR	midbrain locomotor region
MOA	monoamine oxidase
MPTP	1-methyl-4-phenyl-1,2,3,6-tetrahydropyridine
MRI	magnetic resonance imaging
MRSI	magnetic resonance spectroscopic imaging
MZ	monozygotic
NA	noradrenaline
NAA	*N*-acetyl-aspartate
NCAM	neural cell adhesion molecule
NGF	nerve growth factor
NMDA	*N*-methyl-*D*-aspartate
nNOS	neuronal nitric oxide synthase
NO	nitric oxide
NPY	neuro-peptide Y
NREM	non-rapid eye movement
NRPo	nucleus reticularis pontis oralis
NS	nigrostriatal
NSE	neuron specific enolase
NSF	*n*-ethylmaleimide-sensitive fusion protein
NT 3-5	neurotrophin 3-5
NT	neurotrophin
NTS	nucleus of the tractus solitarius
OCT	ornithine carbamoyl transferase
ORNT1	ornithine transporter gene
p38 ®C	synaptophysin
p75 NGFR	low affinity (p75) NGF receptor
PAFAH,	platelet activating factor acetylhydrolase
PAG	periaqueductal grey matter
PARP	poly (adenosine diphosphate ribose) polymerase
pCO2	partial pressure of carbon dioxide
PET	positron emission tomography
PGO	ponto-geniculo-occipital area

PII	phasic inhibition index
phenotype	the clinical characteristics associated with a genotype
PKA	protein kinase A (cAMP dependent)
PKC	protein kinase C (calcium dependent)
PLC	Phospholipase C
PNMT	phenyl-*N*-methyltransferase
PNMT-IR	phenyl-*N*-methyltransferase immunoreactivity
PNS	peripheral nervous system
PPN	pedunculo-pontine nuclei
PS	paradoxical sleep
PSD	postsynaptic density
PSG	polysomnography
PSVNM	presympathetic vasomotor nerves
QTc	corrected QT intervals
REM	rapid eye movement (stage during sleep)
REMs	rapid eye movements
RD	Rett disorder
RS	Rett Syndrome
RSA	respiratory sinus arrlythmia
RTT	Rett syndrome designation in McKusick Catalogue: 312750
SAR	slowly adapting pulmonary stretch receptors
SCG	superior cervical ganglion
SCN	suprachiasmatic nuclei
SERT	serotonin transporter
SFG	superior frontal gyrus
SHH	sonic hedgehog gene
SMA	supplementary motor area
SN	substantia nigra
SNAPs	soluble NSF attachment proteins
SNc	substantia nigra, pars compacta
SNr	substantia nigra, pars reticulata
SOM	somatostatin
SP	substance P
SPECT	single photon emission CT imaging
sREM	rapid eye movement sleep stage
S-W	sleep-wake cycle
SWR	sleep-wake rhythm
SWS	slow wave sleep
syndrome	a group of consistently associated signs assumed to result from the same disorder
TGFs	transforming growth factors
TGF-ß	a transforming growth factor

TH	tyrosine hydroxylase
TH-IR	TH-like immunoreactive
TMS	transcranial magnetic stimulation (electromagnetic stimulation)
TMs	twitch movements
TNF	tumour necrosis factor
TPA	tissue plasminogen activator
TPR	total peripheral resistance
TRH	thyroxine releasing hormone
Trk	tyrosine kinase
tRNA	transcription ribonucleic acid
TSC2	tuberous sclerosis 2
UGI	upper gastrointestinal tract
UPD	uniparental disomy
VAChT	vesicular transporter of ACh
VEP	visually evoked potential
VIP	vasoactive intestinal peptide
VLM	rostral ventrolateral medulla
VTA	ventral tegmental area
WM	white matter
XDML	X-linked dominant male-lethal
XLIS	X-linked lissencephaly
Xp	X chromosome, short arm
Xq	X chromosome, long arm

Index

abdomen, distension with air 13, 351
N-acetyl-aspartate (NAA) 87, 107
acetylcholine (ACh) 229–30, 233, 347–8
  see also cholinergic system
acetylcholinesterase (AChE) 229, 277
achondroplasia 30
Acuity Card Test 340
adenosine monophosphate acid (AMPA) receptors 97–8
adrenal medulla 133
adrenergic neurons, medulla 235
adrenergic receptors, heart 138
aetiology of Rett syndrome 220
age, corpus callosum morphology and 278
agitation 13, 18
  pathogenesis 169–70, 351
Aicardi syndrome 29
amygdala 141
ancestors, common, Rett cases 5, 37
Angelman syndrome 269, 353, 354
angiotensin-II 141
ankle clonus 10
anticonvulsant drugs 13
aphasia, post-stroke 288
apneustic breathing
  brainstem serotonin receptors and 70
  clinical intervention 177
  in RS 14, 152, 157
apnoea
  central 157, 159, 177
  during swallowing 255–6
  reflex 154
apoptosis 66
arachidonic acid 177
aspiration, food 256
ataxia, truncal 11
atonia
  in NREM 192, 213, 218
  sREM 190, 191, 212–13
atropine 163
attachment relationships 312
attention, difficulties in 314–20
atypical Rett syndrome, see variants, Rett syndrome
auditory evoked potentials 16, 289
Auerbach's (myenteric) plexus 142, 232
autism (including early infantile autism, EIA)
  CSF NGF levels 129
  monoaminergic involvement 192, 194–5, 198, 215
  sleep-wake cycle 192, 194, 195, 212
  vs animal lesion studies 196
  vs RS 58, 210, 304, 313, 320, 353, 354
'autistic' behaviour, in pre-regression RS 5, 210
autonomic dysfunction (in Rett syndrome) 131–81, 354–5
  clinical features 13–14, 131–2, 218, 244–5
  clinical intervention 176–7
  during inadequate ventilation 172–6
  feeding/swallowing difficulties and 257–61
  neurophysiological studies 31–2, 61–2
  role of insular cortex 107
  serotonin receptor binding studies 70–7
  skeletal and ECG abnormalities and 265–7
  sudden death and 249–53, 351, 354
autonomic function, brainstem
  baseline, in RS 164–7
  clinical evaluation 155–67
    appraisal of methods 178
    assessing musical responsiveness 332–4
    cardiovascular function monitoring 162–7
    measurement of breathing rhythms 155–62
    patient and carer preparation 155
  during breath holding in RS 171–2
  during hyperventilation in RS 168–70
autonomic ganglia 230, 231
autonomic nervous system (ANS) 227–48
  central 234–6
    development 134, 135–9
    functional organization 140–55
    see also brainstem
  gender specific development 243–4
  general organization 228–30
  historical aspects 132–4
  neurotrophic factors 236–8
  peripheral
    development 234
    higher centres innervating 234–6
    pre- and postganglionic neurons 230–3
  plasticity 238–40
  reciprocal sympathetic/parasympathetic innervation 133–4, 233–4
  see also parasympathetic nervous system; sympathetic nervous system
autoradiography, receptor 71, 74–6, 98

autosomal recessive early onset parkinsonism with diurnal fluctuation (AR-EPDF) 193–4, 195, 197, 198
axonal changes 66–7, 87–8

Babinski response 10
baroreceptors 144
  cardiac sensitivity, *see* cardiac sensitivity to baroreflex
  in cardiorespiratory integration 149
  development 139
  interaction with other afferent inputs 153, 154
  regulation of cardiac vagal tone 147, 148
basal ganglia
  disorders, early onset dopa-responsive 193–4, 197
  neuronal degeneration 66–7
  in RS 206, 209
  substance P 77–9
basal nucleus of Meynert, *see* nucleus basalis of Meynert
bcl-2 protein 129
BDNF, *see* brain-derived neurotrophic factor
behavioural features of Rett syndrome 60–1, 339–41
benzodiazepine binding sites 98
biopterin 31, 125–6, 206–7
Biot's breathing 160, 162
bladder, autonomic control 133
blood pressure (BP)
  beat-to-beat 162
  maintenance 149
  mean arterial (MAP)
    in brainstem storm 174
    during breath holding 171–2
    during hyperventilation 168–9, 170
    during inadequate ventilation 172, 173
    during Valsalva's manoeuvre 160, 161
    in RS 164, 165
  monitoring 162
body movements
  during sleep in RS 213–14
  see also movement disorder; twitch movements
body weight 15, 59
bone growth 265–6
Bötzinger complex 146, 152
bradycardia
  rebound, during Valsalva's manoeuvre 160, 161
  reflex 155
brain
  development 134
    gender specific 243–4
    genetic and environmental factors 183–203
    infant motives and 302–3
  growth deficiency 6, 352
  immaturity in RS 67–8, 176, 351
  size 59–60, 62–3, 86–7
  volume 59, 63–4, 87
  weight 60, 62, 86
  see also brainstem; cerebral cortex; *other specific areas*

brain-derived neurotrophic factor (BDNF) 101, 127–8, 236
  CSF levels 129
  gene 129
  receptor 127, 237
brainstem
  autonomic function, *see* autonomic function, brainstem
  epilepsy 175–6, 177
  intrauterine development 134, 135–9
    heart as means of studying 137–9
    neural projections from 137
  monoamine (MA) deficiency 207
  parasympathetic centres 141–4
  role in RS 351
  serotonin receptor binding studies 70–7, 96, 176
  shutdown 172–3, 177
  storm 173–5, 177
  substance P 77–9
  sympathetic centres 140–1
  see also autonomic dysfunction; medulla
breath holding 13, 14, 156
  autonomic tone during 171–2
  recordings of chest movements 157, 158
  regular 157, 158
breathing
  atypical 161–2
  deep 159, 160
  depth, in RS 156
  during swallowing 255–6
  dysrhythmia of RS 7, 31, 132, 349
    assessing musical responsiveness and 329
    clinical characteristics 13–14, 156–62
    clinical intervention 176–7
    clinical measurement 155–6
    monoamine hypothesis and 95–6
    pathogenesis 152–3, 218
  feeble 157, 159
    abnormal brainstem function during 172–6
    clinical intervention 177
  forceful 158–9, 160
  movements
    monitoring 155–6
    normal, in RS 156
  periodic rhythms 160–1, 162
  rapid shallow 157, 159
  shallow 157, 159
  unclassifiable rhythms 161–2
  see also respiration; ventilation, pulmonary
Broca's motor speech areas (44 and 45) 277, 279
  during hand/arm movements 285–7
  morphological studies 279–80
  in RS 286, 291–5
bruxism (tooth grinding) 10, 12, 289, 340
buspirone 177

calbindin 65, 98, 187
calcium binding proteins 187, 281
calorie requirements 15
calretinin 187
candidate genes, in Xq28 41–2

carbachol 215
carbon dioxide, partial pressure (pCO$_2$) 31, 149
  in brainstem storm 173, 174, 175
  transcutaneous monitoring 156
cardiac arrest
  abnormal brainstem function causing 175
  reflex-induced 153, 154
  risk in RS 177
cardiac output, integrated control 144–5, 149
cardiac sensitivity to baroreflex (CSB) 163–4
  during breath holding 171–2
  during inadequate ventilation in RS 172, 174, 175
  in RS 165–7
cardiac vagal tone (CVT) 14, 151
  baseline, in RS 166, 167, 176
  during breath holding 171–2
  during hyperventilation 168–9, 170
  during inadequate ventilation 172, 173, 174, 175
  during Valsalva's manoeuvre 161
  generation of baseline 147–8
  integrated control 149
  interactions between afferent inputs regulating 153–5
  intrauterine recordings 138–9
  monitoring 163, 178
cardiorespiratory integration
  common autonomic pathways 149–51
  in RS 167–76
cardiorespiratory motor neurons 145–8
cardiorespiratory neurons (medullary) 144–5
  sensory inputs 144–5
  serotonin receptors in RS 71, 72
cardiovagal motor (cardiac parasympathetic) neurons 142, 147–8
caregivers (including parents, mothers)
  assessing musical responsiveness 334–6
  attachment relationships 312
  communication with infant 309–11, 312
  evaluation of brainstem function and 155
  face recognition in RS 345–7
  role in infant development 303, 305, 307
catecholaminergic (CA) neurons
  in immature brains 188–9
  trophic/morphogenetic functions in early development 228, 240–3
caudate nucleus 63, 67, 209
central motor conduction time (CMCT) 271–2
cerebral blood flow, distribution 61, 176
cerebral cortex (including neocortex)
  development 136, 137, 304
    role of monoaminergic neurons 241–3
  in RS 68, 85–106, 303–7
  functional lateralization, see hemispheric lateralization
  general changes in RS 85–90, 209
  molecular pathology in RS 92–4
  monoaminergic function in RS 209
  monoaminergic innervation 184–9
  neurotransmitters in RS 94–9
  pathogenesis of RS 99–101

  selective involvement in RS 90–2
cerebral palsy 19, 355
cerebrospinal fluid (CSF), increased proportion 91
chemoreceptors
  central 144
  interactions with other afferent inputs 153, 154
  peripheral (arterial) 144, 149, 153
  regulation of cardiac vagal tone 148
Cheyne–Stokes breathing 161, 162
choline (Cho) 89, 107
choline acetyltransferase (ChAT) 229
  animal lesion studies 100
  MeCP2 deficiency and 100–1
  NGF actions 128
  in RS 31, 96–7, 209
  in speech areas 277
cholinergic system 229–30
  animal experiments 100
  intrauterine development 138
  regulation of sleep 190, 212–13
  in RS 96–7, 209, 215
  in RS pathogenesis 216, 219
chromatin, neuronal 89
cingulate cortex, monoaminergic innervation 186, 187
cingulate gyrus 141
circadian clock 121, 211
  in RS 121–2, 211–12
classification of Rett syndrome 2–3
clinical features of Rett syndrome 210–11
  post-regression 8–18
  pre-regression 5–6, 210
  range in severity 19–20
  regression period 6–8
  related to autonomic dysfunction 13–14, 131–2, 218, 244–5
clinical trials 352
coeliac ganglion 231, 232
cognitive approach, infant development 308
cognitive function
  pathophysiology of defective, in RS 218–19
  in RS 17–18
  see also mental retardation/disability
communication 277–301
  facilitation in RS 305
  motives for learning by 308–14
  normal development 309–11, 312–13
  preverbal, in RS 287, 304
  in RS 284–5, 287–9, 304–5, 314–23
    future research needs 296–7
    preserved potential 289
    therapeutic interventions and 295–6, 321–2
  see also speech
computed tomography (CT), brain size studies 86–7
computer, use of 18
conditioned learning 17–18
confocal microscopy 290–1
consanguinity 37
constipation 15, 245, 355
Coordinated Interpersonal Timing (CIT) 311

'co-regulation', between infant and caregiver 307
corpus callosum (CC)
    gender differences 244, 281–2, 283–4
    heterogeneity of development 282–3
    morphological studies 281–4
cortical plate 136, 137
cranial nerve nuclei 141–2
critical period
    language development 296
    regression period and 322
cyclooxygenase 2 (COX-2) 65, 94
cytoarchitectonic studies 89
cytogenetic studies 38–9
cytoskeletal proteins 93–4, 209–10

DA, see dopamine
death
    rates in RS 19
    sudden, see sudden death
defence response 141
delayed sleep stage syndrome (DSPS) 193, 195
dementia, lack of, in RS 58
dendritic arborization
    in cholinergic-lesioned mice 100
    in Down's syndrome 64–5, 92
    molecular studies 93–4
    pathogenesis of impaired development 99–101
    reduced, in RS 63–4, 87, 90
    regional cortical changes in RS 91–2
    speech areas 280–1
development, see brain, development; infant development
Developmental Behavior Checklist 339–41
diagnosis of Rett syndrome 352–4
diagnostic criteria for Rett syndrome 2
digits, shortened fourth 9, 32, 265, 350
3,4-dihydroxyphenylacetic acid (DOPAC) 95
distractibility 318
diving reflex 145, 155
DNA
    methylation 42–4, 351
    triplet repeat expansions 33, 112–14
dopamine (DA), in RS brain 94–5, 208
dopamine β hydroxylase (DBH) 188, 189, 229
dopamine (DA) neurons 183–4
    animal experiments 196, 197–9
    clinical correlates of early dysfunction 194–5
    hypofunction in RS 208–9, 213, 214, 215
        pathophysiological role 216, 217–18
    in mature and immature brains 184, 185–8
    in neuropsychological disorders of infancy/childhood 192, 193–4, 197–8
    trophic/morphogenetic functions in early development 228, 240–3
dopamine (DA) receptors
    D_2 subtype 191, 197, 198, 208–9
    D_4 subtype 197
    supersensitivity 207, 214
dopa-responsive early onset disorders 193–4, 197
dorsal respiratory group (DRG) 146
dorsal vagus nucleus 142

Down's syndrome (trisomy 21, DS) 353
    5HT system dysfunction 192, 194, 195
    cytoskeletal proteins 93–4
    dendritic arborization 64–5, 92
Duchenne muscular dystrophy (DMD) 30
dysautonomia, see autonomic dysfunction
dysmorphism in Rett syndrome, lack of 59
dyspraxia 11–12
dystonia
    postural
        pathophysiology 217–18
        in RS 12, 211, 217–18
    in Segawa's disease 194, 195
    in RS 2, 3, 10
dystonic type juvenile parkinsonism (dJP) 193–4, 195, 198

eating, see feeding
Edinger—Westphal nucleus 142
education, in RS 320–2
EEG, see electroencephalography
electrocardiographic (ECG) abnormalities 32, 249–53
    autonomic dysfunction and 265–7
electroencephalography (EEG)
    in autonomic function monitoring 164
    in RS 31–2, 61, 131–2, 176, 269–73
        during regression 7, 269, 271
        face discrimination study 345
        post-regression stage 13, 270, 271
        pre-regression 6, 269
electromagnetic stimulation, see transcranial magnetic stimulation
embryonic brain stem tumours 19, 353
emotional features of Rett syndrome 17–18, 339–41
emotional motor system 306–7
encephalitis, acute 269
β-endorphin 31, 177
endothelin 233
enkephalin (ENK) 230
enteric nervous system (ENS) 142, 232–3
    dysfunction in RS 261–2
entorhinal cortex 66
epilepsy 12–13, 132, 211
    before regression 19, 34
    brainstem 175–6, 177
    EEG recordings 268
    and mental handicap, limited to females 30
    see also seizures
epileptic seizures, see seizures
ergotropic activities 306, 313
event-related potentials (ERP) 343, 344–7
eye hand coordination 7
eye-pointing 12, 289

face
    appearance in RS 9
    discrimination in RS 344–7
    recognition in RS 345–7
facial nerve, autonomic motor nuclei 142, 143
facial twitching 340

familial Rett syndrome, possible 4–5, 32–4, 350
family, *see* relatives
fatty acids, essential 177
feeding
    ability in RS 6, 12
    difficulties in RS 15, 255–6, 257–61, 288–9
feet
    cold and moist 13, 244–5
    growth 9, 59, 266
females
    carriers, sex-linked disorders 28–9
    restriction of RS to 27
Finapres BP monitor 162
'foreign accent syndrome' 289
formes fruste of Rett syndrome 20, 34
fractures 9
fragile site in Xp22 38
fragile X syndrome 108, 112, 353
    gene (*FMR1*) 99
frontal cortex
    molecular pathology 65, 94
    monoaminergic innervation 185–6, 199, 218
    neurotransmitter systems 97
    selective involvement in RS 90–2
    substance P 77–9
frontal lobe
    reduced dendritic arborization 63, 64
    reduced volume 63
    GABAergic neurons
    cardiac vagal tone and 147
    in cardiorespiratory integration 150, 151
    in respiratory rhythm generation 152

gait abnormality 211
games, person-person 312
γ-aminobutyric acid (GABA) receptors 42, 98
gangliosides 31
gastric secretions, autonomic control 143
gastrin-releasing peptide receptor 42
gastrointestinal tract (gut)
    autonomic control 143–4, 233–4
    autonomic innervation 134, 142, 232–3
    disturbances in RS 351
    upper, dysmotility in RS 257–61
gastro-oesophageal reflux (GER) 15, 261
gastrostomy feeding 256
gender differences
    brain development 243–4
    corpus callosum 244, 281–2, 283–4
    speech areas 244, 280
genes
    additional (secondary) mutation 111–14
    candidate, in Xq28 41–2
    MeCP2-regulated 99, 350
genetics of RS 27–55, 111–15
    inheritance 27–38
    investigations 38–47
genetic testing for Rett syndrome 353
glial-cell-line-derived neurotrophic factor (GDNF)
        127, 128, 129
glial fibrillary acidic protein (GFAP) 66, 89

gliosis 66, 67, 89
glossopharyngeal nerve 142, 143, 144–5
glutamate 347–8
    cortical changes 97–8
    CSF levels 97, 128
    receptors 97–8, 348
glutamate dehydrogenase-2 (GLUD2) 42, 98
glycine receptor α2 subunit 42
Goltz syndrome 29
G-protein coupled receptors 237
    sympathetic tone and 140–1
grey matter (GM), cortical
    age-dependent changes 89–90
    neuronal changes 89
    reduced volume 63, 87, 91
gross movements (GMs), during sleep in RS
        213–14
growth associated protein-43 (GAP-43) 240
growth disorder in Rett syndrome 3, 9, 59
growth factors, neuronal 236, 237–8, 348
GTP-cyclohydrolase I (GCH-I) deficiency 193, 197
gut, *see* gastrointestinal tract

handedness
    corpus callosum structure and 281–2
    delayed development, in autism 194–5, 196
    normal development 280
    in RS 12, 211, 288
        asymmetry of speech areas and 291–2, 295
    speech dominance and 277–8, 279
hand movements
    abnormal, in RS 5, 7, 211, 313
    normal development 311
    in pre-regression RS 314
    speech processing and 285–7
    stereotyped 10, 12, 211
        asymmetry 288
        pathophysiology 217
        vs severe cognitive impairment 340
hands
    function in RS 61, 199, 210–11
    growth in RS 59, 265–6
head circumference
    growth deceleration 6, 59, 86, 211
        pathophysiology 218
    motor handicap and 59
    routine recording 353
hearing
    normal development 310–11
    in RS 16
heart
    autonomic control 133, 134, 142
    autonomic function in utero 137–9
heart rate (HR)
    baseline, in RS 166, 167
    during breath holding 171–2
    during hyperventilation 168–9, 170
    during inadequate ventilation 172, 173, 174
    during Valsalva's manoeuvre 160, 161
    integrated control 149
    intrauterine responses 138–9

heart rate (HR)—*continued*
 monitoring 162
 variability 14, 178, 249–53, 265
height
 brain weight for 60
 deceleration in growth 59
 final 9, 32
hemispheric lateralization
 normal development 284
 in RS 288, 295–6
 speech, *see* speech, dominance
 see also handedness
hereditary progressive dystonia/dopa-responsive dystonia (HPD/DRD), *see* Segawa's disease
hippocampus, neuronal changes 66, 92
histone deacetylase 44, 238
holocytochrome c-type synthetase 42
homovanillic acid (HVA) 31, 208
5-HT, *see* serotonin
Hunter, Mrs Kathy 1
6-hydroxydopamine (6-OH-DA) 242–3
5-hydroxyindoleacetic acid (5-HIAA)
 CSF in RS 70, 208
 gender differences 244
 in Rett brain 69–70, 208
5-hydroxytryptamine (5-HT), *see* serotonin
5-hydroxytryptophan (5HTP) 192, 194, 212
hyperammonaemia 35, 206
hypercapnia, in brainstem storm 173–4
hyperornithinaemia—hyperammonaemia—homocitrullinuria (HHH) syndrome 42
hypertonia 2, 3, 9
hyperventilation (over-breathing) 13, 14, 156
 autonomic tone during 168–70
 brainstem shutdown after 172–3
 EEG abnormalities during 270
 recordings of chest movements 158, 160
 specificity for RS 340
 sudden death risk 177
hypothalamus
 autonomic modulation 141
 circadian clock 121, 211
 regulation of cardiac vagal tone 147–8
hypotonia, in RS 2, 3, 9
hypoxia, in brainstem storm 173–4
hypsarrhythmia 13, 34, 270

immune activation 125
immunoblotting studies 93–4, 97
immunochemical methods 93–4, 229
immunodeficiency, centromere instability and facial anomalies (ICF) syndrome 351
immunofluorescence, indirect 290
incidence of Rett syndrome 3–4
incontinentia pigmenti 29
infant development
 motives for learning by communicating 308–14
 normal 309–14
 in pre-regression period 5, 6, 210, 304, 314–20
 psychobiological factors 303–7
 role of caregiver responses 305, 307, 308–9

 subtle deviations, in RS 30, 314–20, 353
 transitions/difficult periods 313
 video recordings in early RS 314–19
infantile degenerative disorders 19
infants
 early intelligence 303–26
 motives, brain development and 306–7
inferior mesenteric ganglion 231, 232
inferior olivary complex, serotonin receptor studies 72–3
inferior salivatory nucleus 142
inheritance 27–38, 111–15
 metabolic studies 35–6
 other models 36–8
 RS phenotype and 30–2
 RS variants 34
 sex-linked 27–30
initiation, lack of 319
injury, autonomic plasticity after 239–40
inspiration, protracted 157, 158
insular cortex (IC)
 autonomic modulation 141
 magnetic resonance spectroscopy 107
 neuroimaging study 91, 107–10
insulin-like growth factor-1 (IGF-1) 127
 CSF levels 128, 129
insulin-like growth factor-2 (IGF-2) 127, 129
integrative inhibition
 concept 150–1
 defective, in RS 167, 172
intellectual function, in RS 17–18, 61, 210
intelligence, early infant 303–26
International Rett Syndrome Association 1
interneurons, reduced numbers 65
intrinsic motive formation (IMF) 304, 305
iris
 autonomic control 133, 134, 142, 233
 development of innervation 139
 joint contractures 11

Joubert's syndrome 349
juvenile parkinsonism (JP) 197
 dystonic type (dJP) 193–4, 195, 198
 kainate (KA) receptors 98

'kangarooing' 307
Klinefelter syndrome 39, 353
 incontinentia pigmenti with 29
 RS with 4, 20, 27, 351
Kölliker-fuse nucleus 146
kynurenine 208

lacrimatory nucleus 142
lactic acidosis 35, 36
lamotrigine 13
language
 cortical representation 277–84
 critical period for development 296
 lateralization, *see* speech, dominance
laughter 18
lead poisoning 269

learning
  conditioned 17–18
  disability, see mental retardation/disability
levodopa (L-Dopa) 194, 195, 212
light reflex, pupillary 142
limbic nuclei 141
limbic regions, insular cortex and 108–9
Linear Vagal Scale (LVS) 163
  in RS 166, 167
linkage studies, genetic 40–1
lipofuscin
  quantitative analysis 291
  in Rett brain 66, 67, 89
lipofuscinosis, infantile 19, 353
literary talent, outstanding 278
locomotion
  animal experiments 196–7
  development 191
  disorder in RS 10–11, 210
    pathophysiology 215–17
locus coeruleus (LC) 184, 188
  animal experiments 196, 218
  control of sleep 190
  development 241
  hypofunction in RS 215
  substance P 78
looking, persistent 344
lung inflation 153, 154
lung receptors, regulation of cardiac vagal tone 148
3H-lysergic acid diethylamide (LSD) binding
    studies 70–1, 72, 75–6, 96, 176

M6b 42
magnetic resonance imaging (MRI)
  brain volumetric studies 59, 63, 87
  corpus callosum morphology 281–2, 283
  functional, speech processing 279, 283, 286
  left-right cortical asymmetry 277–8
  regional cortical changes 91
magnetic resonance spectroscopy (MRS)
  cerebral cortex 87
  insular cortex 107
  RS girls with seizures 89
magnetocardiography, fetal studies 138–9
males with Rett syndrome 4, 20, 27, 32, 351
MAP-2, see microtubulin-associated protein 2
mean arterial pressure (MAP), see blood pressure
    (BP), mean arterial
mechanoreceptors, heart 144
MECP2 gene 42, 44, 58, 237–8
  future research needs 46–7, 355–6
  instability 350
  knockout mice 351
  protein product, see methyl-CpG-binding protein 2
  X inactivation 46
MECP2 mutations 44–5, 349–50
  additional mutation hypothesis 111–14
  metabolic abnormalities and 36
  monoamine hypothesis and 220
  in pathogenesis of RS 45–6, 99–101, 350
  phenotypic variations 4

medulla
  cardiorespiratory neurons, see cardiorespiratory
    neurons
  sympathetic centres 140–1
  ventrolateral, see ventrolateral medulla
MedullaLab system 155–6
Meissner's (submucosal) plexus 142, 232
melanin
  in brainstem neurons 206
  in substantia nigra 62–3, 66, 67, 208, 209
melatonin 121–2
  circadian rhythm in RS 122
  in pathophysiology of scoliosis in RS 218
  therapy in RS 122, 212
memory 18
menarche 9, 62
Menkes disease 29
menstruation 9
mental age 17
mentalis muscle, twitch movements (TMs) 214
mental retardation/disability
  behavioural and emotional problems, vs RS
    339–41
  in RS 17, 131, 210, 320–1
  visual problems, vs RS 344
metabolic interference, X-linked locus 36–7
metabolic studies 35–6
metatarsal (and metacarpal), shortened fourth 9,
    32, 263–4, 350
3-methoxy-4-hydroxyphenylethylglycol (MHPG)
    208
1-methyl-4-phenyl-1,2,3,6-tetrahydropyridine
    (MPTP) 217
methylation, DNA 42–4, 351
methyl-CpG-binding protein 2 (MeCP2) 42–5
  function 44, 99, 350–1
  gene, see MECP2 gene
  genes regulated by 99, 350–1
Meynert nucleus, see nucleus basalis of Meynert
microdysgenesis, Rett brain 67
microtubulin-associated protein 2 (MAP-2)
  changes in RS 65, 68, 93, 94, 209–10
  in pathogenesis of RS 99–100, 218, 219, 352
microtubulin-associated protein 5 (MAP-5) 94, 99
midbrain
  locomotor region (MLR) 191
  monoamine (MA) deficiency 207
  reduced volume 63
'mirror neurons' system 283
'mirror' reactions, in early development 300, 301
miscarriages 33
mitochondria, abnormalities 35–6
mitochondrial inheritance 36
molecular genetics 40–1
molecular pathology, RS cortex 92–4
monoamine hypothesis of Rett syndrome 95,
    205–25
monoaminergic (MA) neurons 183–203, 228,
    302–3
  animal studies 196–9
  in central autonomic nervous system 229, 235–6

monoaminergic (MA) neurons—*continued*
  clinical correlates of early disturbances 194–5
  clinical and neurophysiological correlates of maturity 190–1
  in mature and immature brains 184–9
  in neuropsychological disorders of infancy/childhood 192–4
  pathophysiology of RS and 215–20, 352
  in RS 206–15
  trophic/morphogenetic functions in early development 228, 240–3
mood 17–18, 131
mosaicism 32–3, 111, 350
mothers, *see* caregivers
motives
  infant, brain development and 306–7
  for learning by communicating 310–14
motor coordination
  normal development 310, 311, 313
  in regression period 7
motor cortex
  involvement in RS 91–2, 287
  neuronal proteins 65
  reduced dendritic arborization 63, 64
  speech areas 280
  speech processing in RS and 285–6
motor evoked potentials (MEPs) 275
motor speech areas, *see* Broca's motor speech areas
mouthing objects 340
movement disorder 11–12, 131, 210
  involuntary 7, 12
  pathophysiology 217
  speech processing in RS and 281–3
  voluntary 11–12
movement therapy 321
MRI, *see* magnetic resonance imaging
muscle tone, disorder of 9–10
musical responsiveness 18, 289, 327–38
  challenge of 329–30
  changes in preference/taste 330–1
  facilitating communication 305
  musical exposure and 329
  nonverbal approaches to study 332–4
  preferences and antipathies 329–30
  questionnaire for parents 334–6
  vs normal children 331–2
musicians, brain asymmetry 278–283
music therapy, in RS 321
mutation rate, for RS 30
myenteric plexus 142, 232

N-acetyl-aspartate (NAA) 87, 107
Na/K-ATPase 97
naloxone 69, 177
naltrexone 31
neocortex, *see* cerebral cortex
neopterin 125–6, 198, 206–7
nerve growth factor (NGF) 101, 127–8, 236, 237
  cortical levels in RS 97
  CSF levels
    in other disorders 128, 129

  in RS 31, 128, 129
  hereditary deficiency 237
  low affinity receptor (p75) 97, 237
neural crest 234
neurodegenerative disorders, neurotrophic factors 128
neurodevelopmental disorder, RS as 127
neuroendocrinology 62
neurofilaments 65, 94, 281
neuroimaging studies 86–7, 89–90
  functional, speech processing 279–80, 283, 284–5
  insular cortex 91, 107–10
  see also magnetic resonance imaging
neurological disorders, in families of RS girls 126, 346
neuronal proteins 65, 92–4
neurons
  aberrant migration/maturation 67–8, 99–100
  degenerative changes 66–7
  dendritic arborization, *see* dendritic arborization
  increased packing density 63, 66, 89, 209
  numbers in Rett brain 66
  reduced size
    in RS brain 63, 66, 89, 209
    in speech areas in RS 292, 293, 295
neuropathology of Rett syndrome 30–1, 57–84, 88–9
  anatomic features 62–8
  chemical features 31, 68–79
  unanswered questions 66–8
neuropeptides (peptides)
  cortical 98
  medullary, modulating sympathetic tone 140–1
  preganglionic neurons 230
neuropeptide Y (NPY) 65, 98
neurophysiological studies 31–2, 61–2, 211–15
neuropsychological testing 61
NeuroScope monitoring system 14, 138–9, 162–3
neurotensin 230
  receptors 98
neurotransmitters
  in RS brain 68–79, 351–2
  in RS neocortex 94–9
neurotrophic factors 127–9, 236–8, 352
  in clinical disorders 128
  in RS 128–9
neurotrophin-3 (NT-3) 101, 127, 237
neurotrophin-4/5 (NT-4/5) 127, 237
neurotrophins 101, 127, 236–7
newborn infants 304–5, 312–13
NGF, *see* nerve growth factor
nicotinic cholinergic receptors 97
nigrostriatal-dopamine (NS-DA) neurons 186–7, 214
  development 190, 191
  early lesions 193–4, 198, 214
  hypofunction in RS 199, 217–18
nitric oxide (NO) 230, 233
NMDA (*N*-methyl-D-aspartate) receptors 97–8, 276
non-rapid eye movement sleep (NREM)
  development 190
  see also REM-NREM cycle

noradrenaline (NA, norepinephrine)
  neurotransmitter function 229–30, 233
  in RS brain 95, 122, 208
noradrenaline (NA, norepinephrine) neurons 183–4
  animal experiments 196, 218
  in dystonia and scoliosis of RS 217–18
  hypofunction in RS 215–17, 218
  in mature and immature brains 184, 185, 188–9
  in sleep-wake cycle 189, 190, 191, 213
  trophic/morphogenetic functions in early development 228, 240–3
normotonia (mild hypertonia) 2, 3, 9, 10
nucleus ambiguus 142, 146, 147, 149
  interactions between afferent inputs 153, 154
nucleus basalis of Meynert 66, 196–7
  neurochemical changes 69
  in RS pathogenesis 219, 220
nucleus raphe dorsalis 66
nucleus reticularis pontis oralis (NRPo) 215–17
nucleus of solitary tract (NTS) 145, 235
  in cardiorespiratory integration 149
  integrative function in RS 165
  interactions between afferent inputs 153, 154
  measuring integrative function 163–4
  regulation of cardiac vagal tone 147–8
  serotonin receptor studies 71, 72, 73
  substance P 77–8
  viscerotopic organization of sensory input 145
nutrition 15

object permanence 17
objects
  mouthing 340
  playing with 312, 316–17
obsessive compulsive disorders 192, 195, 197
occipital cortex
  involvement in RS 91, 92, 219
  molecular pathology 94
occipito-frontal circumference, see head circumference
occurrence of Rett syndrome 3–5
ocular disorders 344
oculocardiac reflex 145, 148
oculomotor nerve 142
oesophageal dysmotility 259–60
opioid antagonists 177
μ-opioid receptors 98
opioids 69
organotopic arrangement, autonomic representations 140, 141
organ weights 60
orienting responses, for assessing musical responsiveness 332–3
ornithine carbomyl transferase (OCT) deficiency 29, 35
oropharyngeal dysfunction 255–6, 257–61, 355
orotic acid, urinary excretion 35, 36
osteopenia 266
osteoporosis 9
over-breathing, see hyperventilation

oxygen, partial pressure (pO_2) 31, 149
  in brainstem storm 173, 174
  transcutaneous monitoring 156
p38-IR, see synaptophysin immunoreactivity

pacemaker neurons, medullary 140, 144
pain, responses to 16
paradoxical sleep (PS)
  'off-cells' 212
  'on-cells' 212, 213
parasympathetic nerves 133
parasympathetic nervous system 229–30
  brainstem centres 141–4
  cardiorespiratory integration 144
  historical aspects 132–4
  pre- and postganglionic neurons 230–3
  reciprocal sympathetic innervation 133–4, 233–4
paravertebral ganglia 230, 231–2
parents, see caregivers
parkin gene 193
parkinsonism
  autosomal recessive early onset, with diurnal fluctuation (AR-EPDF) 193–4, 195, 197, 198
  juvenile, see juvenile parkinsonism
parvalbumin 187
passiveness, infants with RS 5, 315
pathogenesis of Rett syndrome 45–6, 99–101
  monoamine hypothesis 215–20
  neurotrophic factors 127–9
pedunculopontine nuclei (PPN) 196–7, 215–17, 220
peptides, see neuropeptides
periambigual area 146
periaqueductal grey (PAG) 141, 142
PET, see positron emission tomography
pharyngeal motility problems 255
phasic inhibition index (PII) 214–15
phenyl(ethanolamine)-N-methyltransferase (PNMT) 188, 229
pineal gland, development 139
planum temporale, left—right asymmetry 277–8
plasticity, autonomic nervous system 238–40
play
  in post-regression period 17
  in pre-regression period 6, 316–17, 318
plethysmograph 155–6
polysomnography (PSG)
  in early onset neuropsychological disorders 192–3
  in foetal period 190
  in RS 206, 211, 212–15
pons
  autonomic motor nuclei 142
  lower ventrolateral 152
  parabrachial nuclei 141, 146
ponto-geniculo-occipital (PGO) spikes 212
positron emission tomography (PET) 208
  speech processing 278–9, 283, 284, 289
postganglionic neurons 230–3
post-regression period 2, 8–18
postural augmentation 191

postural control, normal development 311
postural disorders
    pathophysiology 217–18
    in RS 10–11
    see also dystonia, postural
pre-Bötzinger complex 146, 151
prefrontal cortex
    involvement in RS 91–2
    speech processing 274
preganglionic neurons 230–3
    innervation by higher centres 234–6
premutations, unstable 32, 33
pre-regression period 2, 5–6, 210
    infant video recordings 314–20
    intellectual function 304
presympathetic neurons
    rostral VLM 144, 146
    in RS 165
presympathetic vasomotor neurons (PSVMN) 140, 150
prevalence of Rett syndrome 3–4, 348–9
prevertebral ganglia 232
protoconversations 310–11
protolanguage 304, 312
pseudo-seizures 355
    see also vacant spells, non-epileptic
pterin metabolism 125–6
    in family of RS girls 126, 350
    inherited disorders 198
    in RS 125–6, 206–7
pulmonary slowly adapting stretch receptors (SAR) 144, 153, 154
pupillary light reflex 142
pupilloconstrictor reflex 142
putamen
    cholinergic system 96
    dopamine (DA) system 208–9
    role in speech processing 289
    serotonin metabolites 208
pyramidal neurons
    in catecholamine-depleted rat brain 242, 243
    left/right asymmetry in RS 65, 292, 293, 294
    reduced dendritic arborization 63, 91–2
pyruvic acid 35

QT interval 32
    corrected (QTc) 249–53, 265
    Rab GDP-dissociation inhibitor I 42

raphe nuclei 188
    development 241
    hypofunction in RS 215
    serotonin receptor studies 72, 73–4, 96
rapid eye movement sleep (sREM) 212–13
    development 190–1
    in RS 213, 219
    see also REM—NREM cycle
recurrent laryngeal nerve 153, 154
refractive errors 344, 345
regression period 2, 61, 354
    clinical features 6–8

developmental effects 304–5, 322
pathogenesis 351, 354
vs transitions of normal infancy 313
relatives
    neurological disorders 126, 350
    pterin metabolism abnormalities 126, 350
REM—NREM cycle 189, 212
    development 190, 191
    in RS 213
respiration
    integrated control 144–5
    observations in RS 156–62
    rhythm generation 151–3
    see also breathing; ventilation, pulmonary
respiratory neurons 144, 146
    functional interactions with autonomic neurons 153–5
    rhythm generation 151–3
    vulnerability to stress 351
respiratory rate, in RS 156
respiratory sinus arrhythmia (RSA) 149
reticular formation 73, 78
Rett, Andreas 1, 206, 207
Rett Syndrome Checklist 340
Rett syndrome (RS, RTT), defined 131
rhythmic movement, facilitating communication 305
rickets, vitamin D-resistant, hypophosphataemic 29
RS, RTT, see Rett syndrome

salivary glands, autonomic control 134, 142, 143
scoliosis 11, 211
    pathophysiology 217–18
screaming 7, 218
Secondary Intersubjectivity 312
secretomotor nerves 133
Segawa's disease (hereditary progressive dystonia/dopa-responsive dystonia, HPD/DRD) 193, 197, 198
    L-dopa therapy 195
    postural dystonia 194, 217
seizures 12–13
    MRS studies 89
    RS variant with early 19, 34
    see also epilepsy
sensory faculties 16
sensory speech areas
    morphological study in RS 290, 292–5
    see also Wernicke's sensory speech area
serotonin (5HT)
    brain content, gender differences 244
    CSF in RS 70
    functions 76
    in respiratory rhythm generation 152
    in Rett brain 69–70, 95–6, 122, 208
serotonin (5HT) neurons 183–4
    animal experiments 196–7
    in central autonomic nervous system 235–6
    clinical correlates of early dysfunction 194–5
    gender differences 244

hypofunction in RS 76–7, 215–17, 219, 351–2
in mature and immature brains 184–5, 189
in neuropsychological disorders of
infancy/childhood 192, 193
in sleep-wake cycle 189, 190, 213
trophic/morphogenetic functions in early
development 228, 240–3
serotonin (5HT) receptors
binding studies in RS 70–7, 96, 176
type 4 (5-HT$_4$) 165
sex differences, see gender differences
sex-linked inheritance 27–30
sexual characteristics, secondary 9, 62
shallow breathing 157, 159
rapid 157, 159
Sin3 44, 238
single photon emission computerized tomography
(SPECT) 18, 176, 208
sino-atrial node (SA node) 163
skeletal abnormalities in RS 263–5
sleep disturbances 7, 15, 61, 131–2
melatonin therapy 121–2, 212
monoamine hypothesis and 95
neurophysiological studies 211–15
sleep-wake (S-W) cycle 121
development 190–1, 197
development of handedness and 196
in infantile autism 192, 194, 195, 212
role of monoaminergic neurons 189
in RS 121–2, 211–12
slowly adapting pulmonary stretch receptors (SAR)
144, 153, 154
slow wave sleep (SWS)
development 190–1
in RS 213
in Tourette's syndrome 193
smiling, in infancy 310, 317
social interactions
infants 309
in RS 17, 319, 320
somatosensory cortex
involvement in RS 16, 219
monoaminergic innervation 184, 185
somatostatin (SOM) 230
somatotopic organization, autonomic
representations 141
SPECT (single photon emission computerized
tomography) 18, 176, 208
speech
ability in RS 6, 16–17, 131, 288
development in RS 304–5
dominance
factors influencing 277–8
functional neuroimaging 278–9, 287
morphological studies 280–4
factors affecting, in RS 288–290
normal development 310–11, 312
processing
functional imaging 278–9, 283, 285–6
future prospects 296–7
in RS 284–7

speech areas 277–8
cytoarchitecture 279–80, 290–1
in RS 292, 293
dendritic architecture 280–1
gender differences 244, 280
morphological studies
in normal subjects 279–84
in RS 65, 290–96
neurochemistry 281
in RS 284–5
spinal cord
monoaminergic function 215
peripheral autonomic nervous system 230–1
substance P 77–8
squint 16, 345
stages, Rett syndrome 2
stature, short 9, 32
stereotyped movements 7
stroke, aphasic 289
subiculum 63, 66
submucosal plexus 142, 232
subplate, aberrant development 93, 99–100
subretrofascial nucleus 235
substance P (subP) 230
deficiency in RS 77–9, 98, 252, 259–60
functions 78
substantia nigra (SN)
animal experiments 197–8
development 241
dopamine neurons 187
dysfunction in RS 217–18, 220
hypopigmentation 62–3, 66, 67, 94, 208, 209
serotonin receptor binding studies 76
sudden death 19, 351
autonomic dysfunction and 249–53, 354–5
clinical intervention 176–7
role of insular cortex 107
sudden infant death syndrome 252
superior cervical ganglion (SCG) 238–40
superior mesenteric ganglion 231, 232
superior salivatory nucleus 142
supplementary motor area (SMA) 186, 187, 217
suprachiasmatic nucleus (SCN) 121, 211
supraoptic area 244
suprarenal glands 133, 134
swallowing problems 255–6, 257–8, 259–61
sweating, autonomic control 133, 233
SYBL1 gene 112
sympathectomy, surgical 245, 266
sympathetic chain 230
sympathetic nerves 133
sympathetic nervous system 229–30
activity, non-invasive monitoring 162–3
historical aspects 132–4
medullary centres 140–1
over-activity in RS 132, 245, 265–6
plasticity 238–40
pre- and postganglionic neurons 230–3
reciprocal parasympathetic innervation 133–4,
233–4
supra-medullary centres modulating 141

sympathetic tone
  baseline, maintenance 140
  central modulation 140–1
synaptic organization
  in developing brain 189
  pathogenesis of RS and 100, 218–19
  in RS 63–4, 90
  in speech areas in RS 65, 293–5
synaptophysin immunoreactivity (p38-IR)
  quantitative analysis 291
  in RS brain 67
  in speech areas in RS 65, 293–5
tachypnoea, recordings 158–9, 160

Talairach grid 108, 109–10
tear production 142, 143
temporal binding 347
temporal cortex
  molecular pathology 94
  reduced dendritic arborization 63, 64
  selective involvement in RS 90–2
tendon reflexes, deep 10
testosterone 244
tetrahydrobiopterin (BH$_4$) 125–6
  in RS 208
  in Segawa's disease 193, 197
therapy
  breathing dysrhythmia of RS 176–7
  RS 320–2, 353, 356
theta (θ) rhythm 13, 270
l-threo 3,4-dihydroxyphenylserine (l-threo-DOPS) 212, 214, 215
tics 195, 198
toileting 15
tongue movements 12
tooth grinding 10, 12, 340
total peripheral resistance (TPR) 149
Tourette's syndrome 192–3, 195, 197, 198
toys, playing with 316–17, 318
transcranial magnetic stimulation (TMS) 32, 275–7
  speech processing 286–7, 297
transcription
  derepression in RS 45, 350
  non-specific increase ('transcriptional noise') 44, 45, 351
  repression by MeCP2 44, 99
tremor 12
trigeminal nerve 153, 154, 155
triplet repeat expansions 33, 112–14
trisomy 21, see Down's syndrome
Trk (tyrosine kinase) receptors 127
trophotropic activities 307, 313
tryptophan hydroxylase 184
tuberose sclerosis 19, 34, 353
Turner's syndrome 39, 243, 353
twins, monozygotic (MZ)
  with RS 4–5, 19, 33–4
  X inactivation 28
twitching, facial 340
twitch movements (TMs)
  developmental changes 190, 191
  in early onset neuropsychological disorders 192–3
  in RS 213–14
tyrosine hydroxylase (TH) 184, 229
  in early-onset dopa-responsive disorders 193, 197
  in immature brains 188–9, 191
tyrosine kinase (Trk) receptors 127, 237

ulnar variance, negative 265
uniparental disomy (UPD), X chromosome 39, 40
upper motor neuron pathways 10
urea cycle defects 35
urinary retention/urination problems 13, 245

vacant spells, non-epileptic 14, 132, 270
  autonomic dysfunction and 354–5
  in pre-regression RS 315
vagal tone, see cardiac vagal tone
vagus nerve
  control of gut function 143–4
  motor nuclei 142
  sensory inputs to cardiorespiratory neurons 144–5
valproate, sodium 13, 35
Valsalva's manoeuvre 14, 159–60, 161
  brainstem shutdown after 172
variants, Rett syndrome 2–3, 19–20, 34
  with early seizures 19, 34
vas deferens, development of innervation 139
vasoactive intestinal peptide (VIP) 266
vasomotor nerves 132–3
vasomotor tone
  autonomic control 233
  baseline, in RS 164–5
  in cardiorespiratory integration 149, 153
  hand and foot growth in RS and 266
ventilation, pulmonary 31, 153
  excessive, in RS 158–9, 160–1
  inadequate, in RS 157, 158
    abnormal brainstem function during 172–6
  see also breathing; respiration
ventral respiratory group 152
  caudal (cVRG) 146, 152
  rostral (rVRG) 146
ventral tegmental area (VTA) 218
ventrolateral medulla (VLM)
  activation during hyperventilation 170
  cardiorespiratory motor neurons 146–7
  caudal 146, 147, 235
  intermedial 235
  rostral 146, 235
    cardiorespiratory neurons 144
    integrative function 149–51
    sympathetic centres 140–1
vesamicol 96
vesicular transporter of acetylcholine (VAChT) 96–7, 101, 229
Video Logger 315
video recordings
  infants later diagnosed with RS 314–20

monitoring of brainstem function in RS 155–6, 178
RS vs autism 320
vigabatrin 13
viscerotopic organization, sensory input to nucleus of solitary tract 145
vision
    methods of study 343
    normal development 309–10
    in RS 16, 219, 343–8
visual acuity 61, 345
visual cortex, monoaminergic innervation 184, 185, 186
visual evoked potentials (VEP) 16, 343–4
visual pathways, afferent 343–4
vocalizations
    normal infants 310–11, 312
    in RS 7, 218
    see also speech
volume receptors 144

walking 6, 7, 11
Wernicke's sensory speech area (22) 277, 297
    hand/arm movements and 285–7
    morphological studies 280, 281
    in RS 290, 292–5
Western blotting (immunoblotting) 93–4, 97
white matter (WM), cortical
    age-dependent changes 89–90
    MAP-2 immunostaining 93
    reduced volume 87, 91
X chromosome
    candidate genes in Xq28 41–2
    deletion of distal Xp 38
    'excluded' loci 40–1
    presumptive RTT gene 112–14
    translocations 38–9
    uniparental disomy (UPD) 39, 40

X chromosome inactivation 39–40
    MECP2 gene 46
    patterns 28–9, 349–50
    skewed 32, 33, 39–40
X-linked dominant disorders 27–9
X-linked dominant, male-lethal (XDML) inheritance 29–30, 32–3, 37–8, 40, 111
X-linked locus, metabolic interference 36–7
X-linked recessive disorders 27
XqYq recombination, postulated 112–14